Clinical Trials

Regulative Legal Controls on Bio-Logical Warfare

Clinical Trials
Regulative Legal Controls on Bio-Logical Warfare

Editor-in-Chief
Prof. (Dr.) Shefali Raizada

Editor
Ms. Ekta Gupta

Technical Support
Dr. Rupinder Kaur

Student's Editorial Board
Mr. Akshdeep Gupta
Ms. Vanshika Jha
Mr. Pratyush Shounikya
Ms. Vaani Vishal
Ms. Ananya Kukreti

BLOOMSBURY
NEW DELHI • LONDON • OXFORD • NEW YORK • SYDNEY

BLOOMSBURY INDIA
Bloomsbury Publishing India Pvt. Ltd
Second Floor, LSC Building No. 4, DDA Complex, Pocket C – 6 & 7,
Vasant Kunj, New Delhi, 110070

BLOOMSBURY, BLOOMSBURY PRIME and the Diana logo
are trademarks of Bloomsbury Publishing Plc

First published in India 2021
This edition published 2021

ISBN: 978-93-54353-14-7
2 4 6 8 1 0 9 7 5 3 1

Printed and bound in India by Replika Press Pvt. Ltd.

To find out more about our authors and books visit www.bloomsbury.com
and sign up for our newsletters

Foreword

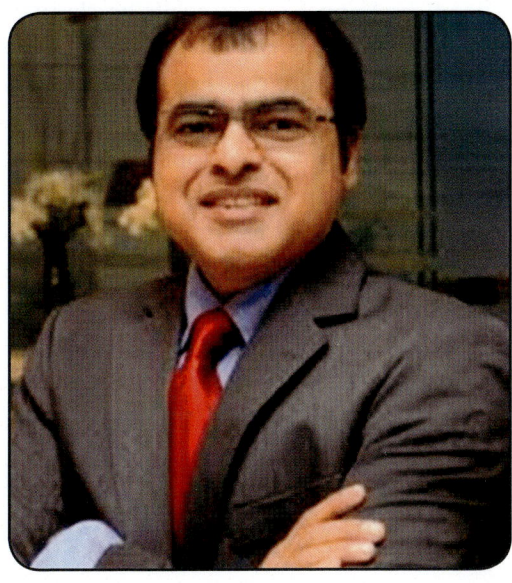

If India has to become a developed country, we need to focus and invest in research and development. According to my study in the area of innovation, the most significant innovations have come from the university led consortiums. I am so happy that Amity University has taken the lead and come out with timely book on Clinical trials.

If India has to become a super-power, it has to become a healthcare super-power, and for that, clinical research is critical.

Clinical trials are research studies conducted on people aimed at evaluating a medical, surgical, or behavioural intervention. Clinical trials are the most crucial way researchers determine if a new treatment, such as a new drug, diet or medical device (for example, a pacemaker), is safe and effective in humans. Other clinical trials test ways to detect illness early, sometimes before there are symptoms. Still, others are examining ways to prevent a health problem. A clinical trial can also investigate how to improve the lives of people with a life-threatening illness or a chronic health problem. Clinical studies sometimes examine the role of caregivers or support groups.

The term biological warfare is not that different from clinical trials if connected and compared. Generally it conjures up images of medieval warriors throwing dead cattle on the city walls or clandestine government agents releasing mysterious microbes into hostile territory. Of course, biological warfare involves such activities, but the vast majority of biological warfare is much more common. Since life revolved around 3.8 billion years ago on Earth, organisms have developed continuously new ways to kill each other. Any organism that uses toxins - from bacteria to snakes- is engaged in the form of biological warfare. People who participate in biological warfare do so using these toxin-producing organisms and there is much more to this topic than these few lines and definitions, which I am sure that this book will fulfil all these societal questions and give answer to suffice each one of them. I am sure academia and researchers will benefit immensely from this timely book.

Prof. Rajendra Pratap Gupta
Policymaker and Former Advisor to
Union Minister of Health & Family Welfare
Government of India

Blessings from

Hon'ble Founder President,
RBEF and President,
Amity Law Schools, AUUP

FOUNDER PRESIDENT

Dr. Ashok K. Chauhan

Founder President, Ritnand Balved Education Foundation (RBEF)
(The Foundation of Amity Institutions and the Sponsoring Body
of Amity Universities) & President, Amity Law School,
NOIDA, Amity University, UP

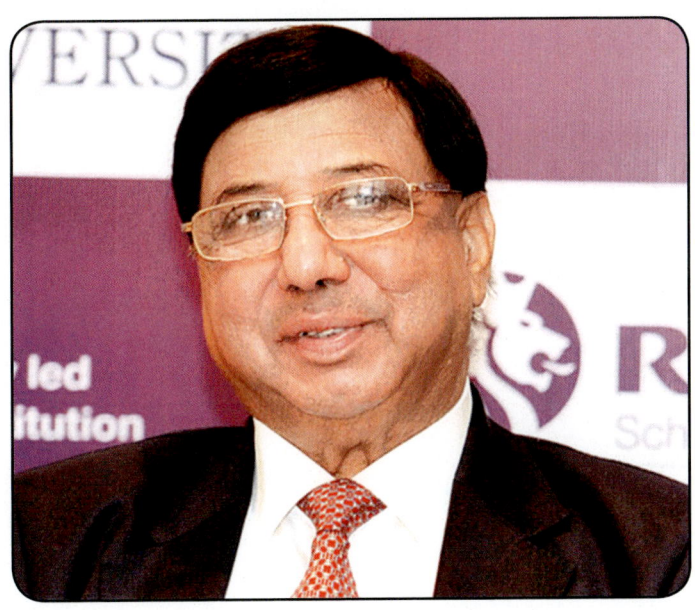

Best Wishes from
Hon'ble Chancellor, AUUP

CHANCELLOR

Dr. Atul Chauhan

Chancellor, Amity University, NOIDA, AUUP
President, Ritnand Balved Education Foundation (RBEF) and CEO,
AKC Group of Companies

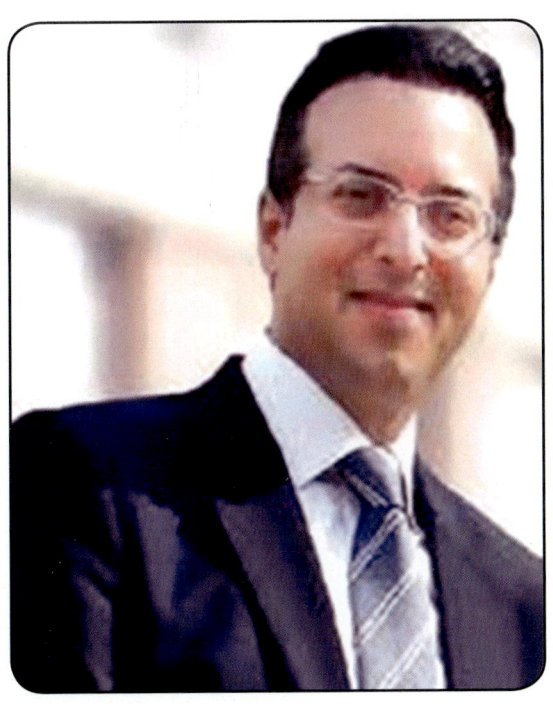

___

Motivation and Inspiration from
Hon'ble Vice-Chancellor, AUUP

VICE CHANCELLOR

Prof. (Dr.) Balvinder Shukla
Vice Chancellor, Amity University, Uttar Pradesh

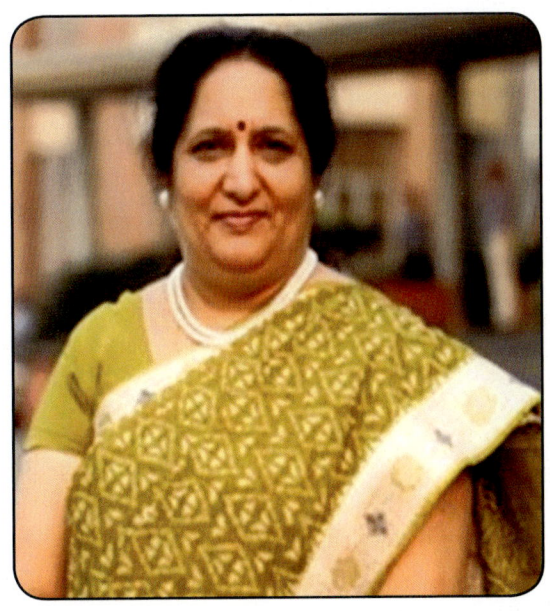

Message from
Chairman, Amity Law Schools,
Advisor to the Founder President

CHAIRMAN

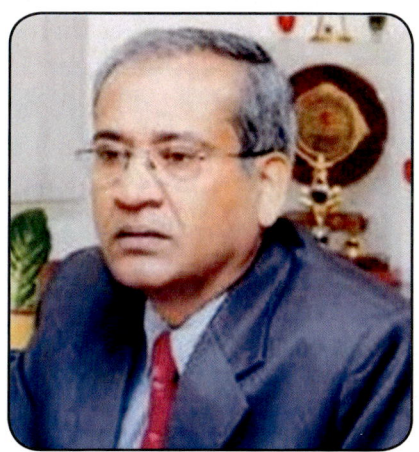

Pandemics have always been a significantly capricious in the events of history; it has set the world in a revolutionary cycle into deciding the way the human live their lives. Clinical trials embark and regulation into the controlling and the usage of the biological warfare. The concept of biological warfare is an amalgamation of nuclear, chemical and radiological warfare which all together fall under the purview of biological warfare. There have has been various initiatives that have seen to be meted out in order to curb and contain the usage if biological warfare amongst different states and neighboring nations.

In the light of COVID-19 pandemics, our dependence on the usage and adaptability towards clinical trials has increased in a massive scale. The concept of clinical trials is currently globally active, clinical trials functions as fundamental in nature, acting as a research tool for the adaptability of bringing in effort in order to develop and with the creation of new products, through the process of gaining data that is to be required by the regulators.

Clinical trial at the current stance have created a surrounding of dependability upon them in order for the creation of vaccines or the cure that is to be required at the global arena, Moreover, it would not be wrong to say that the pandemic has accelerated the rate towards the adoption of new methods and technology through the process of clinical trials to curtail the spread of the COVID-19.

All the disciplines of study have been using the concept of clinical trials as their disposal for an effective outcome. At the global arena, we are witnessing the collaboration of various nations into coming together and lending help to one another, during such difficult times of the pandemic. The study of clinical trials has seen to portray advances and their effect on discipline of studies have yielded exponential results in terms of efficiency and precision.

This book "Clinical Trials: Regulative Legal Controls on Bio-Logical Warfare" is aimed to provide wide and unrestricted dissemination of knowledge of law and the understanding of the concept of clinical trials and the advancing of regulations that are required to abided with it. The book is devoted to the discussion of the usage of clinical trials, the concept of biological warfare, the guidelines and the regulations that are propounded in order to abide to the regulations, the complexities of the issues and the practice of law, as the issues of law and clinical trials are pervasive and complex in nature. The book focuses to delve into the study of these issues in detail and strives to suggest probable solutions and way-forwards for the same.

I believe that the confluence of law and clinical trials would bring a positive change in the way humans evolve with respect to making the world a better place to live in. This book is a rich collection of scholarly articles and research papers on the latest developments in these areas. With articles and information from leaders in the business and legal communities, the book is an essential resource for members of the bench, the bar, and academia. I feel proud of the immense contributions made by the students and the faculty members under the guidance of Jt. Head Prof. (Dr.) Shefali Raizada to bring out this book. I wish them all the success in their endeavor.

Prof. (Dr.) D.K. Bandyopadhyay
Chairman, Amity Law Schools
& Advisor to the Founder President

Preface

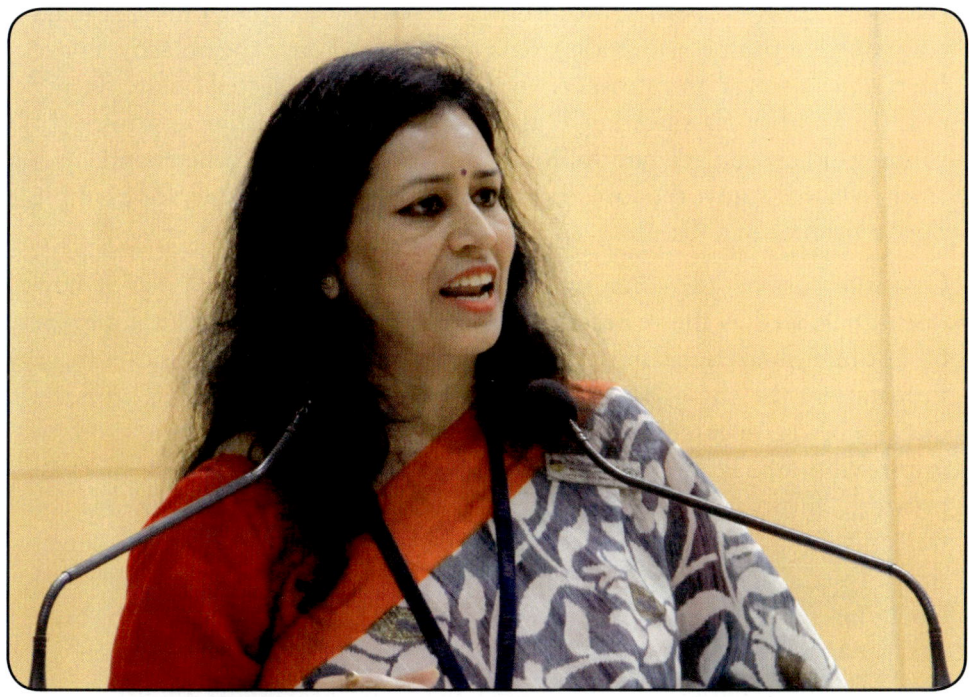

"Learning is not attained by chance it must be sought for with ardor and attended to with diligence."

—Abigail Adams
(Former first lady, United States)

It is well known that humans crave for development but this development must go hand-in-hand with our environment and with the well being of people we live with. Since the end of the last World War, there have been a number of treaties dealing with restrictions, reductions and elimination of the so-called weapons of mass destruction and their transportation systems (commonly known as delivery). Some of the treaties are bilateral, others multilateral or, in rare cases, universal.

Clinical trail research can be defined as research in which a researcher deals directly with human subjects or materials of human origin. It contains the mechanisms of human disease, therapeutic interventions, the development of new technologies, epidemiological and behavioral studies, and results and research on health services. The types of clinical research can be classified as retrospective/prospective, referring to the time of data collection. In prospective studies, data are collected once the objectives have been set. However, in retrospective studies, data is collected before setting targets. Another classification is that of cohort/cross-sectional studies. In cohort studies, subjects are followed over time. On the other hand, in a cross-sectional study, the subjects are examined at a given time, for example the occurrence of a disease.

Over the past decade, there have been threats of the emergence of new diseases, as well as the re-emergence of old diseases and the development of antimicrobial resistance and its spread to new geographical areas. Preparation for these drugs requires comprehensive knowledge of the disease, better research and training facilities, diagnostic facilities and an improved public health system. This review of biological warfare agents will provide information on biological warfare agents, their means of transmission and distribution, and the tracking systems available to detect them. In addition, current information on the availability of available and emerging technologies against biological warfare agents has also been discussed. The risk associated with the use of these drugs in war or bioterrorism scenarios can be mitigated by the availability of improved detection technologies.

The purpose of this book is to bring out the harmony of these two topics and unite them under the umbrella of legal studies and scholar ideas. India's biotechnology industry is growing rapidly thanks to its extensive and advanced dual-use pharmaceutical industry. The security and standardization of institutions and facilities dealing with biological material remains a challenge. India has ratified the Biological and Toxic Weapons Convention (BTWC) and has promised to fulfill its obligations. There is no clear, circumstantial or other evidence that directly points to an offensive biological warfare program. India has a defensive biological warfare (BW) and has done research to combat various diseases. Even with such capabilities and given the current global pandemic, this issue seems to be of the highest priority with no remedy available. Therefore, people should be concerned with regulations which, in turn, can provide protection against such disasters in the future. It is one of the most important aspects of community well-being, as it affects human health and the environment, and is documented as a serious need for the economy.

With this objective the book- "Clinical Trials: Regulative Legal Controls on Bio-Logical Warfare" is presented. The aim of the book is to provide a platform where issues are addressed in the area of warfare and its affect mainly on day today life. Authors of all articles have given new elucidations and tried to give new meanings of the concept, where it may be either the best or worst. Problems faced due to these advance topics, a new face to this question has been given. Bio-warfare aims to save one-self from destruction and clinical trials are a new way towards development, but the questions remains at what cost we achieve development in today's time. This book also aims at giving a review about this young and still heterogeneous and dynamic research field, certainly inclusive of the legal field. As the editor – in-chief of this book, I believe that it is important to establish some ground rules and some legal sanction in the way we see these in future. This issue of the book is a compilation of a rich collection of scholarly articles and research papers focused on latest developments in these areas. I have confidence that this book will provide great contributions to academic literature and will provide an essential resource for the members of the legal fraternity.

I am extremely grateful to our Founder President Sir Dr. Ashok K. Chauhan for all blessings and motivation and to give the opportunity to work with Amity. There is always an inspiration in his vision to do something extraordinary and certainly for research and publications as well. I also convey thanks to Hon'ble Chancellor, AUUP, Dr. Atul Chauhan and Hon'ble Vice Chancellor Prof. (Dr.) Balvinder Shukla AUUP for good wishes and inspirations. I am extremely thankful to our Chairman Amity Law Schools Prof Dr. D.K. Bandyopadhyay for his continuous guidance and support. Research papers received for this book with varied themes and expressions from academicians, scholars, researchers, students, practitioners etc., deserve a lot of appreciation and applause.

I congratulate the editor of this book Ms. Ekta Gupta, Assistance Professor for this commendable work. My heartfelt wishes and thanks to them for dedication and determination to achieve this task. I congratulate and acknowledge the contribution of faculty technical coordinator Dr. Rupinder Kaur, Asst. Professor and my worthy student committee for editing and other technical works their hard work and enthusiasm for completion of the work is praiseworthy. I am thankful to Prof. Rajendra P. Gupta, Member – Central Advisory Board, Ministry of Labour & Employment, Govt. of India, for his contribution in the form of foreword. Last but not least, I am thankful to the publisher Bloomsbury India for publishing this book and for cooperation throughout the time.

Best wishes to all and sundry.

Prof. (Dr.) Shefali Raizada
Editor-in-Chief
Addl. Director/Joint Head
Amity Law School, NOIDA, AUUP

Message from the Editor

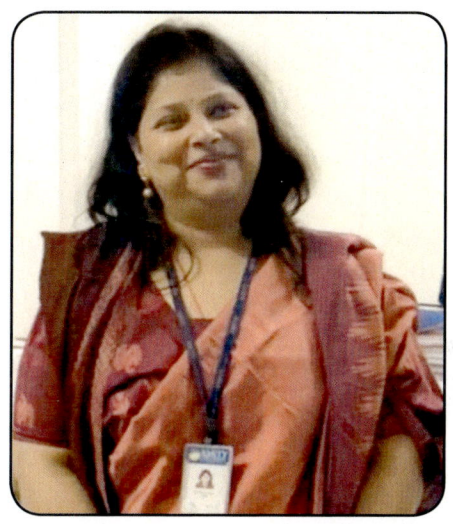

The concept of the pandemic has always been quite mercurial in nature. It not only states the advantages towards the diction of health and purity but rather also in relation to concept of the modern rationality in the due course but it has approved and administered in idea of the creation of demarcation line, wicket gate and quarantines, the current state of pandemic which has affected the world community alike. The track record that has been seen especially in the field of medical sciences remains unassailable from the field of clinical trials to the production of manufacturing a cure for such pandemic related viruses. Ever since the declaration of COVID-19 as a Pandemic, the WTO has seen to be conducting various sessions and press conferences relating to the concept of clinical trials and creation of an cure for all nations, keeping in mind the sole objective of disseminating knowledge pertaining to clinical trials among maximum countries and the public at large. The COVID-19 has leaded an advent of speculations into the involvements of nations to the preparedness during the spread of any such virus at such an global level and the mode to tackle the situation at such an mass level.

The concept of biological warfare is an amalgamation of nuclear, chemical and radiological warfare which all together fall under the purview of biological warfare. There have has been various initiatives that have seen to be meted out in order to curb and contain the usage if biological warfare amongst different states and neighboring nations. Clinical trial at the current stance have created a surrounding of dependability upon them in order for the creation of vaccines or the cure that is to be required at the global arena, Moreover, it would not be wrong to say that the pandemic has accelerated the rate towards the adoption of new methods and technology through the process of clinical trials to curtail the spread of the COVID-19. At the global arena, we are witnessing the collaboration of various nations into coming together and lending help to one another, during such difficult times of the pandemic. The study of clinical trials has seen to portray advances and their effect on discipline of studies have yielded exponential results in terms of efficiency and precision.

This book "Clinical Trials: Regulative Legal Controls on Bio-Logical Warfare" is aimed to provide wide and unrestricted dissemination of knowledge of law and the understanding of the concept of clinical trials and the advancing of regulations that are required to abided with it. The book is devoted to the discussion of the usage of clinical trials, the concept of biological warfare, the guidelines and the regulations that are propounded in order to abide to the regulations, the complexities of the issues, the practice of law as the issues of law and clinical trials are pervasive and complex in nature. The book focuses to delve into the study of these issues in detail and strives to suggest probable solutions and way-forwards for the same. I am blessed to have a wonderful family who has always been there, my special friends and at last 'Almighty' without their existence and blessing I am nothing and not able to achieve anything. I want to show my gratitude with special thanks to Ms. Jyoti Mehrotra. Thanks to Hon'ble Founder sir for the blessings, Hon'ble Chancellor sir for the wishes, Hon'ble Vice-chancellor ma'am for her words of motivation, and Hon'ble Chairman Sir for his constant guidance. I also want to thank our Addl. Director Prof. (Dr.) Shefali Raizada ma'am for giving us this opportunity. I want to extend my special thanks to Dr. Rupinder Kaur for giving her constant support. I want to thank my colleagues for contributing to, institutional staff for immeasurable help. Also, without my Student Editorial Team Mr. Pratyush Shounikya,

Ms. Vaani Vishal & Ms. Ananya Kukreti especially Mr. Akshdeep Gupta and Ms. Vanshika Jha, they have given their day and night of hard work to this project, this piece of creation would not have been possible. This book is an attempt to bring creative minds together and to create something which will really give some valuable contribution to the society and if in any way I am not able to justify this aim then I sincerely apologize.

Ms. Ekta Gupta
Assistant Professor - II
Amity Law School, NOIDA, AUUP

Contents

Women Empowerment in COVID Period— The Real Trial of Human Rights

Prof. (Dr.) Shefali Raizada* and Ms. Apoorva Roy**

नारीराष्ट्रस्यअक्शिअस्ति
(Meaning thereby, woman is the eye of the nation)

Hence, women need empowerment and an upgraded status than what the society is providing to them right now. Women comprised almost equal population in the whole world and India is no different with this respect as well. The question therefore lies as to why there is need for uplifting the women and the most plausible answer is, despite uttering:

नारीअस्यसमाजस्यकुशलवास्तुकाराअस्ति
i.e. Woman is the perfect architect of the society.

We are yet to give the women the status that they deserve. India is a complex country. We have a social structure and strong and strengthen system of social fabric that binds the unit of our society i.e. our family. Yet, within the family itself there are numerous impediments towards the women. We had traditions of considering the newly-wed bride to be equated with "Goddess Laxmi" i.e. Fortune-bearer and yet the same bride sometimes are getting subjected to domestic cruelty. The instant subject presently is plaguing the society including hygiene awareness and sanitation for women. Apart from this spreading of awareness about the movements like me-too and other campaigns which brought the plight of women out in the open.

In certitude it can be said that, constant public awareness and some prompt action taken by the law enforcement authorities off-late have provided

* Addl. Director, Amity Law School, NOIDA, AUUP.
** Assistant Professor, Amity Law School, NOIDA, AUUP.

these issues a prominent platform to talk about in our society. Although issues with respect to domestic violence, cruelty against women in generally still are matter of social-taboo like before, however, at the advancement of various social media arena, the reporting of these issues are being taken up more frequently and at the same time the said are being addressed in no time. Undoubtedly, there are more to be done, but any positive step towards ending these atrocities can surly be welcomed.

The post-modern feminist jurisprudence, quintessentially, seeks to understand the gender spectrum; which is not so narrow anymore.

The idea of a training program and educating the set target group in Assam had been a remarkable way forward with respect to gender awareness among public. At the same instance, horrors of discrimination that spew around that term also need to be acknowledged and understood to mitigate the inequity and promote substantive equality. Assam and other north-eastern states have been in fact successful in deliberating the issues regarding women empowerment and gender equality after repeated attempts from the side of the governmental authorities and we can see the result already, where majority of the Indian states are still dealing with issues regarding female feticides or women infanticides, the north-eastern states and their societies are actually doing well in their commitments to protect all sorts of specific rights to be given to women member of the society and in bringing a much awaited equality in the social life among male and female.

Through these training programs, it will be possible for the government to understand the issue be dealt with by the females in the society various coordinates relating to other aspects of identity issues.

These training projects are not just limited to the relation of gender with society, or how gender and law are related. It attempts to traverse into the questions pertaining to State Policy. In the words of the Minister of Women and Child Development of Assam: *"It is a matter of deliberation and research whether State-Policy should be gender-neutral or gender-specific, and by a logical extrapolation-identity-neutral or identity specific. Historical, contemporary, and transnational analyses of how gender and sexual formations arise in different contexts such as colonialism, nationalism, and globalization can be mentioned as important points of discussion."*

This idea will navigate through various cross-sections of gender, society and law. Every minute component of this endeavor will have gendered implications. Therefore, it becomes imperative to understand the chemistry of this term and the sociology of the context in which it is used in common parlance. A befitting tribute to current social conditions and an informative handbook on the gender spectrum and the laws relating to such marginalized communities.

Interdisciplinary studies are a standard for today's education scenario and it is sure that training/learning and research about this interesting field area of gender will substantiate the objective of this project. In today's times, law is not only limited to conventional areas. And this academic simulation is a great step in achieving the great goal of overall complete academic excellence with multiple outcomes.

The present training project will be able to initiate eliminating violence against women; to yield the importance of Human Rights and dignity of women/girls; to pursue the sustainability in development processes; to end to the discrimination in workplace and family; to encourage girls to get education; to prepare women to participate in governance to end violence against women.

LEGISLATIVE APPROACH ON PROTECTION OF WOMEN

Following are some of the provisions from different legislations dealing with the issue of providing legal protection to women and thereby empowering them:

> Section 498A of the Indian Penal Code (IPC) may be taken as an instance here to be a pioneering provision against the cruelty towards women committed by in-laws.

> Section 497 of the IPC, talks about the offence of adultery, is also another provision falling in the same category.

Along with these, issues like Medical termination of Pregnancy, Eve teasing, Projection of a derogatory image of women in cinematograph films and advertisement, Female feticide, Prostitution (whether forced or not), bride burning, Legal position of Eunuchs, Rights of a second wife in case of a polygamy are some of the burning issues on women rights and mostly for all of them the legislators have intended to make specific laws and hence, the protection part at least legally is possible.

The issues regarding Honor killing, Sexual harassment of women in workplaces are also some of the topics which got major attentions from the legislators and as a result we have got some of the Acts and provisions dealing with all of them.

Judiciary also has contributed with their part in cases like the infamous Vishakha and Others vs. State of Rajasthan case which talks about the issue of sexual harassment in workplace.

ISSUES RELATING TO GENDER INEQUALITY

Gender Justice: The phrase gender justice had been coined in the late 20th century academicians and social activists to ensure firstly an acknowledgement of the fact that, gender roles are responsibilities are still pre-ordinated in most of the societies and hence, it is creating a problem for the growth of an equal and commensurate status for both the genders. At the same time, it could gather the attention of the policy-makers towards the women-centric issues to be addressed properly hopefully in near future.

Consent of a Mental Retarder for Abortion Necessary: In *Suchitha Srivastava and anr v. Chandigarh Administration* we can find the much needed observant role of the Supreme Court in dealing with such an important issue which has the potential to change the entire course of medico-legal field.

Gender Inequality: The issue of gender equality and addressing the same in our society shows, how much work still needs to be done to make the world safe for both the genders.

Domestic Violence in Marriage: Any type of violence against any human being is condemnable and legally susceptible. However, when it is subjected to only one gender that too within the walls of their home and the aggravator is their husband or other members of their in-laws, it reaches a new level and therefore, requires special attention from the law-makers and the enforceable agencies.

CHANGING FACETS OF SEXUAL OFFENCES

Prostitution in India: Although prostitution is being condemned by both law and the society as such, however, the same could not stop the atrocities being committed against the women who are being victimized of their socio-economic status which are compelling them to take this path despite possibly hating the same.

Trafficking in Women: Related to the above-mentioned, trafficking of women has plagued our society. Sometimes, the reason is directly associated with the purpose of forcing them to get into the business of prostitution while in others, forced marriages or domestic helps are the veils in front of the trafficking which are being purported to the end result of prostitution only.

Rape: Whether Textual or Psychological: Textual or documentary ways of violating women is a common form now-a-days. Wherein, the sexual violence is being either documented by the perpetrators or the violence in fact is being committed in the way of using social media platforms.

Legal Position of Rape: Rape is a heinous crime in our world and the civilized country have enacted their own legal provision for such kind of crime. The status of women has improved because of the enactment of laws. In a developing country like India, women are still struggling for their dignified status in the society. Many provisions talk about the protection of women rights but still the position of the women need to strengthen more in a patriarchy society.

PROVISIONS ENSURING RIGHTS OF INDIAN WOMEN

Law must exist, in order to improve the socio-economic status of women, by giving them a wide platform so that they can utilize their potential for personality growth and also for the betterment and contribution of positivity towards the growth of their country. The present scenario shows that development of our country is also dependent upon the socio-economic status of the women. Therefore, the provisions enhancing the value of present could be as following:

1. Constitutional provisions
2. Other provisions in Law.

In our society, awareness regarding the provisions of constitution and other ancillary laws are comparatively less and hence, it is pertinent for the authorities to understand the situation and act accordingly so that, normal people can understand the consequences of these crimes which have already been sanctioned by the parliament.

CONSTITUTIONAL PROVISIONS TO ENSURE THE DIGNITY OF WOMEN

"Make sure that constitution of India safeguards the social and legal rights of women."

—*Dr. B.R. Ambedkar*

Hence, we should have provisions that will ensure both the dignity of women and at the same time self-respect to the women.

Article 14 deals with ensuring, "The equality before the law or the equal protection of the laws within the territory of India," Therefore, "Article 14 provides that equal legal protection to women against any women based crime, paving the way for other various laws or acts to provide protection and also enforcement of the legal rights of women in the country."[1]

Article 15 states, "no one should create any sort of discrimination only on the grounds of religion, race, caste, sex or place of birth or any of them within the territory of India. During the time of Independence, women were facing discrimination in the country which was abolished after the introduction of the Article 15. Article 15(3) of the constitution provides that the "state has the authority to make any special provision for women and children."[2]

Article 16 deals with the "equal employment opportunity to every citizen of India".

"Any kind of discrimination related to the employment opportunity based upon the grounds of religion, race, caste, sex, descent, and place of birth, residence or any of them should be renounced". In the words of the Honorable Delhi High Court: "In the present time where women are participating in different sectors equally and holding responsible positions different private stakes or government institutions like Chandakochhar or Indira Nooyi, Sonia Gandhi, Sushma Swaraj and this never ending list goes on."[3]

Article 39 of the Constitution of India also, "secures the benefit of the directive principles of state policy to the women being the **guiding principles** by framing of laws by the government at different state level".

---

[1] B.R. Ambedkar, Constituent Assembly Debate.
[2] Supra note 1.
[3] Naz Foundation vs. Union of India.

While Article 39(a) certify to directs the state "to apply policies focusing upon both the genders men and women to have an equal right of adequate means of livelihood and it also ensures equal pay for equal work for both men and women."

Article 42 states, "A duty on every employer by ensuring just and humane conditions of work and including *maternity relief*."

Article 243 on the other hand deals with "the reservation of seats in gram panchayat for women."

"Opportunity to ensure representation of women in the village area also hence, have been provided here".

Some of the offences which are acknowledged as crime against females can be classified as follows:

Adultery against women in India is a major crime affecting married women. Adultery can be defined in other words as: *"having voluntary sex with someone other than the spouse."* Section 497 of the Indian Penal Code, 1860, deals with the offence of adultery as *"sexual intercourse with a married woman without the consent of her husband when such intercourse is not committed for rape."*

Adultery can be legally defined with various meaning in different countries.

Section 497 Indian Penal Code states, "The offender shall be punished with imprisonment for a term of *five years, or with fine, or with both*". In the country like India, the wife shall not be punishable as a partner in crime.

Child marriage is also a serious offence against the children harming the future of child on one hand and also damaging social values on the other hand. Moreover, the reports of the doctors also showed that, "child marriage being a serious cause for the poor health condition of female child in India. Child marriage restricts the social development resulting in reduction of educational and employment opportunities in the global market making a burden to practice this unwritten custom in our country."

Female feticide means illegally identifying and killing of female fetus before they take birth, making it the most brutal way of killing women. The tradition related to killing of female girl child is practiced in our society since ancient times.

Burning of human flesh and sometimes even damaging bones and eyes of the victim due to throwing acid at them has also become a new phenomenon in the list.

According to Swati Maliwal, the President of the National Commission of Women:

> "Few victims are forced to leave their education or occupation due to the results of acid throwing. It is quite sad that despite of so many cases of acid attacks on women, we do not have a dedicated and specific law to deal with such cases. The National Commission for Women (NCW) is asked for a well-defined law to deal with such casualties. The NCW has introduced a draft of the Prevention of Offences (by Acids) Act, 2008, which is with now with the Union Ministry of Women and Child Development for the purpose of vetting and final recommendations. Once the Union Ministry of Women and Child Development approved the Bill, it will be sent to the law ministry to be tabled in Parliament. After the approval in Parliament it will become applicable as law."

The scope of fraudulent marriages has increased in the recent past at the instance of the parents of a girl being extremely lusty for NRI grooms who would be able to provide a decent lifestyle to the girl. To the extent, they do not even care to check the back-ground of the prospective groom before the fixing of the marriage. Many a time, we have seen that, after the marriage the evil side of the man prevails over the groom and he uses the marriage as an opportunity to exploit the girl.

An observation with respect to the crime relating to molestation and rape had been made by eminent jurist on criminal law Prof. K.D. Gaur:

> "Rape is another very heinous crime against women in our society and this crime is increasing day by day like anything. Reporting of rape and abduction cases has become very common in print and electronic media which is indeed a very sad affair for all of us. Increasing rape cases are enough to prove that our moral values are still very low and we still to learn how to respect their dignity."

He also added that, "The manifestation of dowry is other social evil, dragging the women since medieval age in India. There are many different legal provisions in the country to combat with this problem though the media reports show that how dowry and domestic violence cases are so prominent. The payment of dowry was prohibited in the year 1961 by civil law of India. Moreover, the Indian Penal Code, 1860 also incorporated with Sections 304B and 498A, allowing the victim to file such complaint and also in seeking restoration of her rights in the serious instances related to harassment by the family of her husband. The crucial reason behind the increase of domestic violence is 'Dowry'.

In India, thousands of dowry deaths along with mental trauma cases are reported and registered every year and also in such cases 'incidents' like burning, suicides, physical and mental torture of women is very common by husband and his family. Due to the increasing number of cases related to the dowry deaths, one more legislative provision was drafted as Protection of Women from Domestic Violence Act 2005, which was introduced in order to reduce domestic violence cases and to protect women's rights."

With having so many different interests over the women issues, there is no doubt that, women empowerment would not be very easy. Nevertheless, 21st century being a called a century of new hope and emancipation are showing rays of positivity towards a better tomorrow for the women.

History of Bio-warfare:
Reviewing it at Global Arena

Ms. Ekta Gupta* and Ms. Puja Pallavi**

The threat of bioterrorism is real and significant; it is neither in the realm of science fiction nor confined to our nation. Infectious diseases has taken gargantuan number of lives, roughly estimated to be over 500 million, during the past century. A huge number of these deaths were caused due to the intentional release of toxins and pathogens. A considerable amount of causality was witnessed during World War II against China, by the Japanese, as a war strategy. To mitigate such events, biological weapons were outlawed by 2 international treaties which took place in 1925 & 1972 respectively. However, both were proved nugatory in stopping the countries from carrying on research for offensive weapons and to stop the production of biological weapons at a large scale.

With advancement in science and technology, we are becoming more and more acquainted with the biology of disease causing agents like toxins, viruses and bacteria. Hence it would be a colossal mistake to neglect the issue of modified pathogens resulting in potential devastating adversity via use of biological warfare. Chemical and conventional weapons have now become somewhat less efficacious than the bio warfare agents and production of such weapons has been further simplified by the progress made in biochemistry and biotechnology in the past century. A widespread of bio weapons has been observed due to the technical knowhow, broad availability and ease of production of bio agents; making it alluring to developing countries. This alleviated threat of terrorism is the reason why there exists a need for better understanding of the historical development and use of bio agents as well as a thorough evaluation of various micro-organisms as biological weapons & assess risk attached to them. In this

*Assistant Professor-II, Amity Law School, NOIDA, AUUP.
**Graduate, Amity Law School, NOIDA AUUP & LLM from Cambridge, U.K.

research paper we will be going through the concept of biological warfare, its utilization, stages of development and the endeavors to curb its proliferation throughout history.

EARLY USE OF BIOLOGICAL WARFARE

Infectious disease was recognized as a potential weapon back in 600 BC.[1] Use of animal carcasses, cadavers and contagion had pernicious effect and enfeebled the enemy.[2] A common strategy which has been used since centuries, including multiple European wars, American civil war and even till recently is to pollute the water sources of enemy and compromising their strength.

It was the middle ages when military leaders understood that they can weaponize the victims of an infectious disease to their advantage. In 1346, an epidemic of plague was experienced by the attacking Tarter force during the seizure of a Genoese-controlled, well-fortified, seaport called Caffa, now known as Feodosia in Ukraine.[3] Soon the Tarter utilized their misfortune and used it for their advantage by placing the dead bodies of their lamented soldiers inside the city and with that commencing an epidemic in the form of plague which later resulted in the retreat of Genoese forces. In the 14th century, the pandemic soon travelled through North Africa, Europe and the Near East and become known as the Black Death. The origin still remains uncertain with suggestions of it being originated from the Far East, China, central Asia, India, and Mongolia. It is still referred as one of the most devastating public health disaster in recorded history.

A notary born in Piacenza north of Genoa, Gabriel de Mussie, described the saga of Caffa in the year 1348 or 1349.[4] Two main points that were claimed by him in his description of the incident were; First that the diseased cadavers were intentionally placed into the besieged city and secondly that the plague reached Mediterranean seaports via the escaped

---

[1] Edward M. Etizen Jr. & Ernest T. Takafuji, *Historical overview of biological warfare*, MED ASP415, 418 (1997).

[2] Andrew G. Robertson & Laura JR, *from asps to allegations*, 160 MIL MED 369, 160 (1995).

[3] Mark Wheelis, *Biological warfare at the 1346 siege of Caffa*, 8 EMG DIS 971, 973 (2002).

[4] V.J. Derbes, *De Mussis and the great plague of 1348*, 196 JAMA 59, 60 (1966).

Italians from Caffa.[5] In fact, it has been contended that the second plague pandemic was caused due to the ship which sailed through Venice, Constantinople, Genoa and other Mediterranean seaports, and carried plague infected refugees (and allegedly rats) with them. However, it may be oversimplification to surmise, given the complex epidemiology and ecology of plague, that a single bio attack could have caused the Caffa epidemic and the 14th century pandemic in Europe. Nonetheless, Caffa incident is a robust reminder that appalling ramifications may be witnessed when disease are used as a weapon.

Simultaneous to the plague pandemic that took place in 14th century, resulting in death of around 25 million, there is an indication that poisons and diseases were commonly used during the war. For example, in 1422, the ranks of the enemy were catapulted by dead bodies of soldiers. During the war between Swedish forces and Russian troops in Reval in the year 1710, a similar strategy was noticed that used the cadavers of the plague victim. The historical recordings mention use of bio agents multiple times during the past 2000 years in form of filth, human and animal cadavers, disease, etc. Few examples of chemical and biological warfare used in past are mentioned below:

600 BC During the siege of Krissa, a purgative herb hellebore was used by solon.

1155   Water wells were poisoned by Emperor Barbarossa in Tortona, Italy by putting human bodies inside.

1346   Siege of Caffa took place. Tartar forces used infected bodies of plague victim by planting it inside city walls.

1495   A Spanish mix wine with the blood of a patient having leprosy was sold in Naples, Italy to their French foes.

1675   It was agreed by French and German forces to not use "poisonous bullets".

1710   Swedish cities had plague victims human bodies catapult by the Russian troops.

1763   Native Americans were distributed blankets by the British from smallpox patients.

---

[5] John Norris, *East or west? The geographic origin of the Black Death*, 51 Bull Hist Med 1, 17 (1977).

1797   To enhance the spread of malaria, plains of Mantua, Italy was flooded by Napoleon.

1863   During the US Civil War, clothing were sold by the confederates which originally belonged to smallpox and yellow fever patients.

WW I   Anthrax and Glanders were used by French and German.

WW II   Several countries developed by experimenting bio weapons; Anthrax, plague and other diseases were used by Japan.

1980-88 During the Persian Gulf War, tabun, mustard gas and sarin were used by Iraq against Iran and ethnic groups inside Iraq.

1995   Sarin gas was used by Aum Shinrikyo in the Tokyo Subway System.

HISTORY OF BIOLOGICAL WARFARE IN THE LAST CENTURY

19th century witnessed a more sophisticated use of bio warfare. The production and isolation of stocks of certain specific pathogens were made possible by the development of modern microbiology and the conception of Koch's postulates.[6]

World War I

There exits material evidence which evinces the existence of a more progressive form of bio warfare program during WWI in Germany. There was also word that Germany had attempted to ship, to the USA and other countries, cattle and horses inoculated with bacteria which produces disease, such as *Pseudomonas pseudomallei* (glanders) and *Bacillus anthracis* (anthrax).[7] Also, an export which was to be made to Russia of Romanian sheep witnessed the infection by same agent. This was followed by allegations on Germany trying to spread plague in St. Petersburg in Russia and Cholera in Italy.[8] These allegations were refuted by Germany including the accusation that they have dropped biological bombs over British positions.

---

[6] *Supra* note 2.

[7] Jones M.H., *Wickham Steed and German biological warfare research*, 7 INT & NATSEC 379, 392 (1992).

[8] *Id.*

No concrete evidence was found against Germany to prove that they employed the bacteriological arm of warfare but involvement of chemical warfare was indicated by some documents when Temporary Mixed Commission, a subcommittee of League of Nations, in 1924, looked into the matter.[9] After the incidents of horror of WWI created by chemical warfare were witnesses, to limit such usage of chemical and bio weapons, International diplomatic efforts were made. In furtherance of that, Geneva Protocol of 1925 was signed by 108 countries which included the present UN's 5 Permanent members of Security Council. But the Protocol lacked on multiple fronts. For example, it failed to differentiate between virus and bacteria and no address of compliance or verification in the agreement was made, which rendered the document less meaningful and 'toothless'.[10] Countries like Canada, Great Britain, the Netherlands, Japan, Belgium, The Soviet Union etc. started developing bio weapons soon after the ratification of Geneva Protocol 1925 whereas The United States of America did not ratify the agreement all together till 1975.[11]

World War II

The usage of biological warfare saw an amplification during World War II. Multiple charges and countercharges were bought in against countries involved. Research of bio weapon was conducted by Japan from 1932 till the end of WWII. Shiro Ishii (1932–42) & Kitano Misaji (1942–45) led the research and the center of the bio-warfare program of Japanese were later known as 'Unit 731' which was located in the town of Pigfan, Manchuria.[12] The scale of this program was massive and included more than 3000 scientists, 150 buildings and 5 satellite camps. They showed interest in *Yersiniapestis, B. anthracis, Shigella* spp, *Neisseria meningitides* and *Vibrio cholera*.[13] These research experiments resulted in death of more than 10,000 prisoners, who were used as lab rats, out of which almost 3000 were prisoners of war. Apart from this, Japan was also alleged to develop a plague which reportedly resulted in 10,000 casualties amongst

---

[9] 1 SIPRI, the Rise of CB Weapons, 125–140 (1971).

[10] US ACD Agency, *Arms Control and Disarmament Agreements,* WASHINGTON DC: US ARMS 18, 24 (1996).

[11] *Id.*

[12] *Supra* at 1.

[13] Sheldon H. Harris, Factories of Death, 201 (2d ed. 2002).

other bio attacks. Later in the history, Japanese officials called these experimental programs as "most regrettable from the view point of humanity".[14]

In Dec. 1949, trial of 12 Japanese prisoners of war took place by Soviet military tribunal in Khabarovsk. They were alleged to have prepared and used biological weapons. The former head of Unit 731's section 1st, 3rd and 4th, Major General Kawashima, testified that on average 600 prisoners were killed every year at Unit 731. This, in turn, met with an accusation by Japanese government on the Soviet Union that they were experimenting on bio weapons as well and referred to the recovered organism of *V. cholera, B. anthracis* and *Shigella* from Russian spies.

Whereas, no charges were bought against Germany regarding their research and experimentation on organisms like malaria, *Rickettsia prowazekii* and hepatitis A virus which led to death of prisoners.[15] It was alleged that Hitler had prohibited the use of such bio weapons due to his own pernicious experience during WWI with chemical agents. However, this did not stop Germans, they began their research on bio weapons after receiving help from German high ranking officers.[16] Despite all these efforts, allegedly, their offensive bio weapon programs never materialized as they lagged behind. On the other hand, it was noticed that Germans started accusing their allies of using bio weapons. One of the German Nazi politicians named Joseph Goebbels accused British of importing the yellow fever from West Africa to India[17] which was largely believed as British were indeed experimenting on at least one bio warfare weapon on Gruinard Island near the coast of Scotland.[18]

In 1942, the United States, under the direction the War Reserve Service, started an offensive bio warfare program.[19] Initially *Brucellasuis* and *B. anthracis* were organism of interest and roughly five thousand bombs

---

[14] *Id.*

[15] *Supra* at 1.

[16] Sheldon H. Harris, *Japanese biological warfare research on humans,* 666 ANN SCI 21, 45 (1992).

[17] *Supra* at 1.

[18] Stewart R&Manchee R., *The decontamination of Bacillus anthracis on Gruinard Island,* 24 CHEM BR 690, 691 (1988).

[19] *Supra* at 1.

filled with spores of *Bacillusanthracis* were produced by them but it was observed that the facility lacked adequate safety measures, leaving them vulnerable to their own experiments.

Bio-warfare Programs after WWII

Soon the WWII ended, the newspapers were covered with articles about intentional outbreak of diseases by foreign agents.[20] At the time of the Korean War, countries like North Korea, Soviet Union and China publicly accused United States of using offensive bio weapons against North Korea.[21] In the later years, the United States did admit that it had the technological advancement and means to produce such bio-warfare weapons but denied using the same against North Korea during the War. However, the credibility of the United States was bought into questioning when it publicly acknowledged its own offensive bio-warfare program, didn't ratify the Geneva Protocol, 1925 and was conjectured to be in an alliance with Unit 731 scientist.[22]

In fact, an expansion of the United Nations Biological warfare program was observed during the Korean War (1950–53) with the establishment of a new facility in Arkansas. To add to this, a new defense program which had an objective of developing antisera, therapeutic agents and vaccines among other countermeasures was launched in the year 1953 to safeguard their army personnel from any possible bio attack. Soon by the end of 60s, the United Nations military had its hands on a bio arsenal, which could induce famine, and included numerous pathogens of fungal plants, toxins and bio pathogens.[23]

Multiple other countries like France, Canada, Soviet Union and Britain were also keeping up with the bio weapons and continued researching on them. In the year 1951, the Microbiological Research Department of the UK, originally established in 1947, was expanded.[24] They continued the

---

[20] James A. Poupard & Linda Miller, *History of biological warfare*, 666 ANN SCI 9, 13 (1992).

[21] *Id.*

[22] *Id.*

[23] *Supra at 1.*

[24] GBCarter, *Biological warfare and biological defense in the UK,* 137 RUSI JOURNAL 67, 69 (1992).

research to develop bio agents and made pilot warfare plans. Several bio-warfare agent trials were also conducted by Britain to refine their weapons in Scottish waters, Bahamas and the Isles of Lewis. However in the late 1950s, the British government decided to further pursue the defensive research of biological agents and abandoned the offensive research in 1957 following it by destroying stockpiles.[25] Whereas, the Soviet Union, during the same time, decided to accelerate its work on both defensive as well as offensive bio-warfare R&D.[26] Although the Soviet Union stayed firm on its statement to not be in possession of any chemical or biological weapons, there were reports in the 1960s & 70s of their offensive research.

Few other allegations of post WWII:

- An allegation was made by China against USA for causing the 1961 epidemic of cholera in Hong Kong.
- An accusation against the "imperialistic aggressors" were made for using bio weapons in the Middle East, by Egypt in 1969, for causing Cholera epidemic in Iran in the year 1966 among other things.
- *Pravda,* a Soviet newspaper in the year 1964 made an assertion that bio agents were used against the peasants in Bolivia and Colombia by the Columbian troops & United States Military Commission.
- A statement was made against Britain that they have used bio weapons against Oman in 1957 by the Eastern European press.
- Allegation was made by China that United States was behind the Hong Kong cholera epidemic that took place in 1961.

Biological Weapons Convention, 1972

By this time, it was quite evident that Geneva Protocol, 1925 had failed to achieve its objecting of controlling the speedy growth of bioweapons. It was July of the year 1969 when a proposal was submitted to the United Nations by Britain which outlined the necessity to proscribe the development of bioweapons, its production and stockpiling.[27] Unlike the Geneva Protocol, this proposal was comparatively more detailed and also proffer measures required for inspection & control of biological weapons

---

[25] *Id.*

[26] *Supra at 1.*

[27] 4 SIPRI, CB Disarmament Negotiations, 193–221 (1971).

as well as laid down procedures which needs to be followed in case of violation. Soon after the submission of this proposal by the Great Britain, under the lead of the Soviet Union, the Warsaw pact nations also submitted to the United Nations a similar proposal. But unlike the Britain proposal, this one lacked the provisions for inspection.

Subsequently in the year 1972, Biological Weapons Convention, also known as BWC, was developed. As suggested in the proposal, the treaty interdicts development of bioweapons, its production and stockpiling of toxins or pathogens in "quantities that have no justification for protective, prophylactic, or other peaceful purposes"[28]. This convention also disallowed the exchange or transfer of bio warfare expertise or technologies between countries. It further went ahead and stated that within 9 months of the ratification of the treaty by a country, there must be compulsory destruction of production equipment, stockpiles and delivery system by them. The Treaty went into effect in March of 1975 after its ratification in the month of April, 1972 with 103 nations cosigning it.

However, even BMC lacked to provide an adamantine guideline for the adherence to the treaty or the control & inspection of disarmament. To add to this, it saw an absence of guidelines on cases of violation and enforcement, the "defensive research" definition[29] as well as to qualify as benevolent research the quantity of pathogens were uncertain.[30] The United Nations Security Council was to be informed in case of any alleged violation of the Biological Weapons Convention which upon such report may initiate an inspection on the violation of BMC of the accused party as well as provide with ways to correct it. However, this provision is undermined by the veto right of the permanent members of the Security Council.

After the year of BMC

The ineffectiveness of the convention was well observed when signatories to the agreement reached in 1972 indulged in activities which were strictly prohibited by the treaty.[31] Even though the exact identity and

---

[28] *Supra at 28.*

[29] 5 SIPRI, Technical Aspects of Early warning and Verification, 89–118 (1971).

[30] 3 SIPRI, *CBW and the Law of War,* 217–279 (1973).

[31] *Supra at 1.*

number of the nation which participated in the disobedience by further pursuing offensive bio research is a classified data, it is no rocket science to gather that such numbers have grown multiple fold in the last three decade 3 minutes ago. To add to this, we have witnessed terrorist attacks which aren't state sponsored as well as several assassination attempts and attacks.

In the 1970s, the bioweapons were started to be get used for covert assassinations. An assassination which was later known as 'umbrella killing' took place in London where one Gaorgi Markov, a Bulgarian exile, was killed in 1978. The nick name was given as the weapon used to kill, which made Markov severely ill and caused his death 3 days later after it was discharged into subcutaneous tissue of his leg, was disguised as an umbrella.[32] Similar assassination attempt was made on the life of Vladimir Kostov, another exiled Bulgarian, in Paris just 10 days before the death of Markov. While traveling via metro, at the time of his exit, he felt a sharp pain in his back and saw a man running away with an umbrella. He got examined by French doctors, two weeks later when he learned of Markov's death and a similar pellet was removed from his body which encompassed toxin ricin. In the later years, it was revealed that Soviet Union supplied the technology to the communist secret services of Bulgaria for the assassination.[33]

In addition to these military related and state sponsored biological warfare programs, cases has been taken notice of civilian and private groups who have attempted to develop, use and distribute such chemical and biological weapons. In September of 1984, one such incident was reported where salad bars in restaurants were intentionally contaminated by Rajneeshee cult in Oregan.[34] *Salmonella typhimurium* was discerned as the causative organism and 751 total cases were reported of severe enteritis. After the incident, suspension was drawn towards Rajneeshees but no conclusive evidence about the origin of the epidemic was found by the Centers for Disease Control (CDC) and the Oregon Health Department. However, a member of the cult, later in the year 1985, confirmed that it was an intentional biological attack by the cult.[35]

---

[32] US AMRI for Infectious Diseases, *MMBC Handbook* 34 (4d ed. 2001).
[33] *Id.*
[34] LC Caudle, *The biological warfare threat*, MEDICB451, 459 (1997).
[35] *Id.*

Unfortunately, it isn't abstruse to descry the intentional use of bioweapons. A large quantity of a toxin named botulinum was found, which apparently never has been used[36], in the possession of Red Army Faction's safe house in Paris, France in mid 1990s. The resurfacing of the biological terrorism was then seen on March 18, 1995 where sarin gas was dispersed by the Aum Shinrikyo in Tokyo subway system. Evidence showing a primitive bioweapons program was unearthed when the investigation of the Tokyo subway incident took place. Allegedly, 3 unsuccessful attempts were made by the cult using botulinum and anthrax toxin before the subway incident. Moreover, in 1992, the cult tried to get their hands on the Ebola virus in Zaire. However, not all the information was disclosed to the public and Japanese police and intelligence could only find out a small portion of the entire bioweapons program. Till this date, nobody knows the full extent of the program by the Aum Shinrikyo.

Suggestion and Conclusion

Bioweapons are preferred as it's hard to detect the origin and have a delayed effects. These factors further helps in causing confusion, panic, paralyzing uncertainty and fear among its victims. Carrying an objective to blindside a nation, disrupt its economic and social activities, impairment of military responses, enfeeble the economy, cause recession, and the breakdown of government authority, these attacks can bring any nation to its knees.

Considering the technological advancements and available resources, in the contemporary world, the threat of biological warfare is no blague. Although not yet certain, the Covid 19, which the whole world is battling with at the moment, has been alleged to be one of such bio-warfare. As of today, India along with 61 other nations have showed concern and asked for a detailed enquiry for the origin of the virus. Allegations have been made back and forth between China and the United States for intentionally releasing the virus. In addition, many countries are demanding compensation from China (ground zero for the virus) if it is proved to be a malicious act of the Chinese government to crash the economy of all its competitors.

Politics aside, the present scenario has made us wonder the reforms that needs to be made to the healthcare facility and calls for a uniform law to

---

[36] *Id.*

deal with such pandemic. As bio-warfare is no longer something of a blue moon, it's in our best interest if the medical community as well as general public familiarize themselves with control measures and epidemiology to increase the chances of a calm response. Furthermore, hospitals must be equipped to handle such pandemic or any biological warfare scenario and further investment needs to be made to recognize such potential threat in timely manner.

To tackle biological warfare, primary prevention is to devise a robust global norm that condemns the development of such bio weapons. Prompt treatment and an early detection can be identified as secondary prevention in the case of biological warfare and the medical community has a vital role in this. They must take part in surveillance and instant disease reporting if any primary indication of bio-warfare is suspected. Furthermore, improved effective response plans, diagnostic capabilities and therapeutic agents along with continued research on improvement of disease surveillance will further vitalize the secondary prevention measures further. Finally the tertiary prevention measure is to limit the disability that follows the disease. Unfortunately, at present, we have an imperfect prevention measures to deal with such circumstances and Covid 19 is a perfect example to display that. We must, if not perfect, then at least improve the preventive measure. While the BMC does assist bio-warfare affected nation, it is in the best interest to be self-reliant and be ready for any such circumstances.

Code of Conduct in Clinical Trials and its Historical Perspective and Contemporary Importance

Mr. Saju Jakob*

*ABSTRACT: **Ever since the dawn of 2020**, mankind has only one chant "break the chain" of corona virus infection. In the beginning of the year 2020, many countries were literally shocked at the spread out of covid-19 virus and its impact on their citizen. As on today, 21ˢᵗ of June 2020, the corona infections in India rose to 4.25 lakhs. Globally infection rate is nearing to 9 million. Every day, name of one or another country finds its new place in the front page of all newspapers across the globe with a report of its new ranking in the rate of covid infected patients. The said virus has not only attacked the health of the people but declared emergency on the entire activities of mankind at large. The whole world is at war against the virus of covid 19 pandemic and tall leaders of various countries fell prey to the attack of such virus. Everyone's freedom is largely affected or limited to the minimum requirements of life. Each new dawn begins with the one and same question, "if there is any drug already invented against this viral attack or any vaccination available?" Naturally, the horizon of a human being's interest is expanded to the new areas of wisdom and quite naturally, the term, clinical trial has become a common man's term in their daily vocabulary in today's world of distress and panic due to the covid-19 viruses. Sole objective of clinical trials is to figure out if a new medicine is effective in human body to protect from deceases and to enhance the knowledge of it's working in human biology for the protection of health and thereby of the mankind. Where the extent of medical science has reached its new heights,*

---

* The author [LL.B (IND), LL.M. (GER), MBA (USA)], is the Advocate practising in the Supreme Court of India. He is the Member of Law Society, London; Member of Bar Council, Cologne, Germany; Life Member of Supreme Court Bar Association; Solicitor of U.K. and Germany, and the Senior Counsel in the law firm Lily Thomas and Saju Jakob. His expertise lies in constitutional law, criminal law and international contracts.

clinical trials have become the prime research tool to check the effectiveness of new drugs. Clinical trial is the experiments conducted on several humans at once to test the reaction of that drug on human bodies within different variables. Whereas its importance cannot be challenged, the process poses a serious threat on the fundamental rights of those humans on whom the drug is tested, known as 'trial subjects', as well as those infected people on whom the new drug is inflicted for the first time, who are known as 'post trial subjects'. Whereas, every person on account of being a human, holds the freedom to impose himself into any situation of his choice, the way of exercising the right to choice holds the constitutional questions of the choice or consent being free and informed. Several questions arise in the mind on this aspect. Whether a trial subject volunteering to undergo the clinical trial due to abject poverty can be considered to have given free consent?

If the procedure of legal/ medical recourse is not known by the trial subject, can his consent be considered as an informed consent? Whether the right to freedom and right to life of an individual can be put under scrutiny for the benefit of the public at large? Whether the consent of a legal heir of the 'trial subject' or 'post trial subject' can be considered as the consent of 'the subject'? When the countries relax the rules of clinical trials, in the light of emergency due to the pandemic, do the need to give up all the constitutional right of individuals or they need to strike a balance at the heart of democratic values? Many more questions with regard to the ethical regulations have arisen in the minds of various jurists and authorities. The need to bring in the morality of democratic ethics was felt way back, which has been discussed later in the research paper. The current research paper aims to find out not only the constitutional aspect of clinical trials, but also the modus operandi of conducting clinical trials in general and resultant injury and deaths, if any. The research paper examines the global code of conduct existing across the globe, and also its historical perspective.

Keywords: Clinical trials, Historical Perspective, Indian Perspective, ICCPR, World Medical Association.

CHAPTERIZATION: The Part I of the paper deals with the introduction to the constitutional aspect of clinical trials. Part II deals with the historical perspective of clinical trials which includes Prussian code, Helsinki declaration, Nuremberg code, ICCPR guidelines, CIOMS guidelines and u.n charter. Part III deals with the global perspective of clinical trials. Part IV deals with Indian perspective and Part V deals with conclusion of the research paper.

INTRODUCTION

The history of clinical trials and ethical regulations can be traced way back to 1747, when first controlled clinical trial was done by James kind to find that citrus fruit could be used to prevent and cure scurvy.[1] The first recorded clinical trial, though not of medicine, was done by king Nebuchadnezzar in babylon,[2] when he ordered his people to eat only meat and wine as their diet. The order of the kind was objected to by some royal blood who preferred a vegetarian diet. For the first ten days, these royal bloods were allowed to eat legumes and water, however after ten days the vegetarian appeared to be healthier than the meat eaters and hence the king allowed them to continue on their diet. Whereas during that era, people were bound by the order of the king and had no alternative but to abide by king's order, today, we are protected by constitutional and enshrined right there under. Our every action is guided by constitutional framework and protected by constitutional right and Indian constitution provides for quality of life as fundamental rights. Informed consent forms the ethical and constitutional backbone of clinical trials and the consequences of a party being subjected to a clinical trial must be known to the patient. The consent of the patient must be gleaned from the person by informing him of varied implications which could arise from the entire process of human experimentation. The term informed consent first was used in Helsinki declaration, 1964[3] which also provided for the subject to withdraw his consent to participate without reprisal. Informed consent was defined as *"informed consent is a decision to participate in research, taken by a competent individual who has received the necessary information; who has adequately understood the information; and who, after considering the information, has arrived at a decision without having been subjected to coercion, undue influence, inducement or intimidation."*

The two tests which governed the standard of informed consent in medical filed are the prudent patient test and reasonable doctor test are

---

[1] Katkade, Sanders and Zou, *"real world data: an opportunity to supplement existing evidence for the use of long-established medicines in health care decision making"*, Journal *of multidisciplinary healthcare*, dove press, 2018.

[2] Anonymous, *"The history of clinical trials is fascinating,"* Boston clinical trials: bridging the gap between compound and cure, 2014.

[3] Principle 25 of Helsinki declaration (1964).

two,[4] while in former the doctor discloses only the material information which a patient considers material, the later standards, originated from American case laws,[5] connotes disclosure of all[6] details which another doctor would disclose in the same instance. In these standards, a consideration is kept about the health and effect of the information on the patient, however in clinical trial these standards cannot be adopted. It must be much more than the information sought by the subject, as the patient may not be aware of intricate details and effects for the drug is still on trial stage and the reasonable doctor test cannot be the guiding standard as the subject would be rendered to guinea pigs with no bodily autonomy, if the decision of how much information to be disclosed is left over on the physician. Hence in clinical trials, informed consent signifies a complete disclosure of it, from the method used, to the effect and the aftermaths of the clinical trial.

Another aspect which needs contemplation is body autonomy of an individual which has been recognized by the apex court[7] and it is one's right to decide with respect to one's body that is the idea that people should be able to rule themselves rather than be ruled by others,[8] hence the concept of informed concept relies on one's exercise of his right to bodily autonomy. The un charter mandates the need for consent and lays emphasis on human dignity and informed consent and with the outbreak of covid-19, the importance of informed consent with the need for a vaccine during health emergencies cannot be emphasized. Hydroxychloroquine has been in the news for being a potential drug to treat corona virus infected patients and related side-effects. The instance of use of hydroxychloroquine, with no conclusive proof of its benefit and without testing its effect on a corona-virus infected patient, renders the covid-19 patient as research subject, without consent let alone informed

---

[4] International ethical guidelines for biomedical research involving human subjects (2002).

[5] *Canterbury v Spence* (464 f.2d. 772, 782 d.c. Cir. 1972.

[6] *Salgo v Leland Standfordjr. University board of trustees*, 154 cal. App. 2d 560 (1957).

[7] *Nalsa v union of India and puttaswamy (i) v union of India,* writ petition (civil) No. 400 of 2012.

[8] Harigovind, P.C., "*Informed consent in clinical trials and the role of institutional ethics committees: A sociol-legal analysis*", *Christ university law journal*, 3, 1 (2014), 1–16, ISSN 2278–4322.

consent. In this emergency health crisis, the question which needs to be answered is whether the most important and ethical aspect of clinical trials can be surpassed and patients can be reduced as a research subject. Though the theory of utilitarianism may justify subjecting people to pain for the benefit of the larger populace, however in this run for a lifesaving drug, an individual autonomy being protected by constitution cannot be forced to take a back seat. This research paper traces the history of clinical trial and the concept of informed consent. Paper analyses various international guidelines and framework which may or may not be binding yet are ethically to be observed while carrying out a clinical trial. The researcher seeks to analyse the constitutional aspect of clinical trial in light of the various new guidelines issued by the government of India.

HISTORICAL PERSPECTIVE

19th century marked desideratum of human trials, specifically in the field of bacteriology, venereology, immunology and virology to study the effect and consequences of drugs along with the evaluation of its dosage. During this time human experimentations were carried on hospitalised patients without their consent giving rise to the facets of medical ethics and human rights. In 1767, john hunter, a Scottish surgeon, renowned for advocating research and experimentation and propagator of scientific methods in medicine,[9] performed a human experiment, where he injected pus from one patient who was suffering from gonorrhoea into penis of another man who was perfectly normal. But later on it was discovered that the man developed both the disease simultaneously gonorrhoea and syphilis at the same time. This paved the way for surgeons to believe that gonorrhea and syphilis had the same source of origin.[10] later, Philippe Ricord, the French physician conducted almost 2500 experiments on humans in the form of inoculations between 1831–1837. Although with these experimentations, he was able to find out the difference between syphilis and gonorrhea as well as finely trace the three stages.

---

[9] Kelly a Kapp and Glean e. Talboy, "*John hunter, the father of scientific surgery*", American college of surgeon, 2017.

[10] Ameeta e. Singh and Barbara Romanowski, "*Syphilis: review with emphasis on clinical, epidemiologic, and some biologic features*" clinical microbiology reviews, American society for microbiology (1999).

Of syphilis,[11] but he believed that it was absolutely wrong to inoculate healthy people with diseases whose consequences were unpredictable.

Prussian Code and Neisser Case (1901)

In 1892 by Albert Neisser, head of Nematology, at the University of Breslau in Prussia found gonococcus bacterium, which was bacteria causing sexually transmitted genitourinary infection gonorrhea.[12] He developed a study for syphilis prevention which was achieved through human experimentation. His study was categorised into two categories based on the age of the subject. The first group consist of female subjects between the age of adolescence and maturity i.e. 10–24 years of age these subjects were injected with serum from the infected patients which lead to them developing gonorrhoea and condylomas but none developed syphilis,[13] second group consist of prostitutes of age group between 17–21 years, who were injected with 30 ml of the serum from patients in various stage of syphilis and in time frame of few months they developed syphilis. The study was concluded by Albert Neisser with observation that the development of syphilis infections in the women was due to their exposure to sexual activities.

And not these rum injected to them,[14] the study conducted by Neisser called public attention.

When the same was published as a part of series published on practice of experimentation by daily newspaper, *the munchnerfreiepresse* tiled "poor people in hospitals". The spark of the study did not stop with newspaper article, rather led various rounds of discussion in parliament in context of funding raised for universities and research, with contrary views. The trial carried by Neisser marked history when in 1898, Prussia's public prosecutor began his investigation and presented all the facts and evidence in the court. The court though observed Albert Neeisser to be an authority in medical field and might have a view of the trial not be harmful, however

---

[11] Deepak Vashishtand Sukritibaveja, "*Eponyms in syphilis*", Indian journal of sexually transmitted diseases and aids (2015).

[12] Friedrich h Moll, "*Albert Neisser and the first Prussian directive on informed consent*", Skeletons in the closet indignities and in justifies in medicine (1 American urological association).

[13] *Ibid.*

[14] *Ibid.*

he must have obtained explicit consent from the trial subjects. The court made is explicit that held that its concern was not the experiment rather the consent of the patients who were not informed of the risk and consequences.[15]

Later in 1899, the case was discussed by Prussian government based on a report from the commission comprising of leading German physician concluded that the physician had no right to inject the serum and in any case there was necessity of both; the subject bring informed of about the experiment and obtaining consent of subject before the initiation of any such experiment. The experiment was further categorised to be bodily injury under criminal law as the non-therapeutic research was conducted without the consent of the subject.[16]

In 1900, the government of Prussia issued guidelines, which came to be first state directives on human experimentation including responsibility and free consent and was known as the Prussian code (Also called Berlin Code 1900).

The Prussian code pointed out the specific guideline with respect to consent:[17]

> "... That medical interventions for purposes other than diagnosis, therapy, and immunization are absolutely prohibited, even if all other legal and ethical requirements for performing such interventions are fulfilled if: (1) the person in question is a minor or is not fully competent on other grounds; (2) the person concerned has not declared unequivocally that he consents to the intervention; (3) the declaration has not been made on the basis of a proper explanation of the adverse consequences that might result from the intervention..."

Prussian code was the first code which regulated medical ethics and emphasised on consent in clinical trials.

Nuremberg Code (1947): Doctors Trial

With the extensive medical human experimentations in European countries, Germany formulated the guidelines on human experimentation,

---

[15] *Ibid.*
[16] *Ibid.*
[17] Principle 25 of Helsinki declaration (1964).

1931 which[18] suggested that any innovative therapy must be justified and conducted according to the principles of medical practices and theory.[19] The guidelines mandated additional requirement of unambiguous consent of the subject or its legal representative, called for extra caution in case of experimentation on minors and clearly reiterated that exploitation of social hardships in order to put a subject under clinical trial will be against the principle of medical ethics.[20] The guidelines clearly prohibited the clinical trials in the cases where consent was not received, where animal trial was not conducted first, on minors where the experiment can lead to lethal consequences and in cases involving dying subjects,[21] the guidelines 1931 were followed till 1945.

In 1945, with the end of World War II, international military tribunal was enacted on November 19th, 1945 to conduct the trail of war criminals. Among the various trials, the first trials was that of 23 physicians, responsible for murder, or impairment of the patients who were suffering from mental illness and physical disability, who were tried for crime against humanity for, they carried experiment of the prisoners of wars. The doctor's trials titled as *"united states of America v Karl Brandt"* took place at the palace of justice in Nuremberg, Germany.[22] The indictment was filed on October 25, 1946 and the trial lasted from December 9, 1946 to august 20, 1947. The presiding judges held the 16 of the defendant doctors guilty and seven were sentenced to death. Despite the German guidelines on clinical trials, 1931, no such consideration was given to the freedom of choice and consent to the war criminals.[23]

The trial and conviction led to the Nuremberg code which was published on august 17th, 1947, which provided for the standards to be followed while a clinical trial on human is conducted. The code emphasised on the informed consent of the trial subject and such consent must not be given under coercion, or deception or by way of fraud being played on the

---

[18] Encyclopedia of bioethics, ed. Warren t Reich 2nd edition, appendix, pp. 2762–2763.
[19] German guidelines on human experimentation, 1931.
[20] *Ibid.*
[21] *Ibid.*
[22] Morris low, *"Pathways to human experimentation, 1933–1945: Germany, Japan, and the United States"* Osiris (2005).
[23] Ravindra b Ghooi, *"The Nuremberg code—a critique"* perspectives in clinical research (2011).

subject. The code also gave right to the subject to withdraw his consent at any time and not to continue the experiment. It further lays that the subject of the trial must not be subjected to unnecessary physical and mental suffering and no clinical trial must be carried if there are chances of any harm to the subject; physical or mental. Further the doctor must be ready to terminate the experiment, when and where he fails to apply required professional skill and continuation of the experiment is likely to result in injury, disability, or death of the experimental subject.[24]

Apart from the above principles emphasising on consent and welfare of the subject, the other dictates of Nuremberg code are that the experimental results should be for the greater good of the society, anticipated result should justify the experiment, the risk factor shall not be beyond human control, adequate facilities/precaution must be taken to provide protection to human subjects, the experiment must be conducted in the presence of/by qualified doctors.

The Nuremburg trial resulting to Nuremburg code emphasised upon human life and that no one can be denied of it by lowering them as mere trial subjects. Humans can be subjected to only those procedures where there are no harm and hurt. Though the code defined the concept of consent with ethical, moral and legal satisfaction of clinical trial yet it was silent on what happens, if even after following all precautions, any harm, injury or death was sustained by the subject.

Declaration of Helsinki

In 1964, Declaration of Helsinki was adopted by the 18th world medical association (WMA) in general assembly, in the form of ethical principles for the protection of humans from experiments.[25] **The declaration of Helsinki for the first time, provided binding standards in case of involvement of human subjects in any research.** With the word such as "*a physician shall act in the patient's best interest when providing medical care*"[26]

---

[24] Principle of Nuremberg code (1947).

[25] World medical association, wma declaration of Helsinki – ethical principles for medical research involving human subjects, available at: https://www.wma.net/policies-post/wma-declaration-of-helsinki-ethical-principles-for-medical-research-involving-human-subjects

[26] Declaration of Helsinki: ethical principles for medical research involving human subjects, 1964.

emphasise upon the binding nature of the principles enshrined in the declaration. Further the declaration put the complete responsibility of the safeguards of the clinical subjects on the physician and health care professionals even if the consent has been obtained from the subject. Whereas the declaration permits the adherence to the national guidelines of one's own country, however it stipulates clearly that "*no national or international ethical, legal or regulatory requirement should reduce or eliminate any of the protections for research subjects set forth in this declaration.*"[27]

The declaration part from laying down the protocol for the conduct of clinical trial further provides for the research protocol to provide for "*incentives for subjects and provisions for treating and/or compensating subjects who are harmed as a consequence of participation in the research study. The protocol should describe arrangements for post-study access by study subjects to interventions identified as beneficial in the study or access to other appropriate care or benefits.*" Further the declaration also made a reference to vulnerable groups likely to be exploited and thus, made sure that no experimentation is done to the vulnerable groups and only when there is a necessity of the experiment to be conducted on the vulnerable group, it would be permitted to be conducted. The declaration provides for the constitution of research ethics committee which would approval to the research prior to its beginning, it would keep a check during the trial and check the final report of the trial conducted and concluded. Before the study begins every research, protocol must be submitted to the ethics committee for "*consideration, comment, guidance and approval*".

The Helsinki declaration addressed "the issue of clinical trial and come to be as of the most influential documents and is considered as *the property of all humanity*".[28] It has been an influential in national legislation and is considered as the cornerstone for conduct of human research ethics.

International Covenant on Civil and Political Rights (ICCPR)

The international covenant on civil and political rights (ICCPR) enter into force on March 23rd, 1976 and recognised "the inherent dignity and of the equal and inalienable rights of all members of the human family as the

---

[27] *Ibid.*

[28] Badri Man Shrestha, "*The declaration of Helsinki in relation to medical research: Historical and current perspectives,*" *Journal of Nepal health research council* (2012).

foundation of freedom, justice and peace in the world".[29] ICCPR provides for three non-derogable rights to person; right to life[30], freedom from non-consensual medical experimentation on humans[31], and non-discrimination[32] right ealth being facet of right to life, which is a non-derogable right under ICCPR, ICESCR develops the idea of "core obligations" on the part of the state in the aspect of human rights.[33] The covenant vividly provides the accountability of the state in the words "a state party cannot, under any circumstances whatsoever, justify its non-compliance with the core obligations...which arenon-derogable."[34] The accountability of state extent to regulate the domestic and foreign clinical trials conducted by pharmaceutical companies and hence is the prime ensure of human rights.

Ethical guidelines for clinical trial on human subject by council for international organisation of medical science (CIOMS):[35]

In 1949, "...council for international organisation of medical science (CIOMS) was established by the world health organisation and united nations educational, scientific and cultural organization (UNESCO) for the representation of the biomedical scientific community, which in turn developed international ethical guidelines for biomedical research involving human subjects. The first version of CIOMS guidelines was guideline of 1982 which was revised in 1993 (period which followed the outbreak of HIV/Aids). The ethical issue resulting from the sponsored clinical trials being carried out at low resource setting, resulted in revision of 1993 guideline and the third version of CIOMS guidelines were drafted and finished in 2002 (which was further broadened in 2016 guidelines in light of

---

[29] Preamble, international covenant on civil and political rights, 1966.
[30] Article 6, ICCPR.
[31] Article 7, ICCPR.
[32] Article 26, ICCPR.
[33] Article 12.1, ICESCR.
[34] Committee on economic, social and cultural rights, general comment no. 14, the right to the highest attainable standard of health, un doc. No. E/c.12/2000/4 (2000).
[35] Council for international organizations of medical sciences, *"international ethical guidelines for health-related research involving humans"* (2016). Available at: https://cioms.ch/publications/product/international-ethical-guidelines-for-health-related-research-involving-humans.

major changes and revision of declaration of Helsinki in 2008). CIOMS guidelines have been conceived to facilitate the practical implementation of the wma's declaration of Helsinki and to regulate such implementation in low- and middle-income countries. The aim of the guidelines was to provide internationally vetted ethical principles and detailed guidelines on ethical principles should be universally applied, with attention to conducting research in low-resource settings...”[36]

The reiterations of the guidelines are as follows:

1. *Scientific and Social Value and Respect for Rights*[37]: It presupposes the relations between the scientific and social values in the form of the moral ethics by researchers, scientists, sponsors, and other competitive authorities, which recognise human and respect human dignity. It simply suggests that any scientific advancement cannot surpass the human value and could not open doors to injustice and mistreatment of the human subjects, thus in turn forming the moral ethics of the authorities.

2. *Research Conducted in Low-Resource Settings*[37]: The guideline provides for the pre-requisites to be ensured before research in a community with low resource is undertaken. The researcher and sponsor as part of their obligation must first analyse that the research being carried is for the public good and research has been carried on small population before it being initiated in a human community. It is the responsibility of the concerned authority to ensure that the experiment to be conducted is safe for public health and the research must be preceded by a deep study of the testing. Prior consultation with the authorities engaged in doing that experiment must been ensured.

3. *"Equitable distribution of benefits and burdens in the selection of individuals and groups of participants in research"*[38]: The guideline provide for all the stakeholders (researcher, sponsors, governmental authorities) to ensure that the burdens and the benefits of the

---

[36] Declaration of Helsinki (1964). Timothy J. Doenges, Bryan J. Dik, available at: https://www.britannica.com/topic/declaration-of-helsinki
[37] Guideline 1-2, CIOMS.
[38] Guideline 3-6, CIOMS.

research must be shared equitably. The members involved in the experiment/trial, must be involved with not more than fair share of the risks and burden. The government authorities, researchers, and doctors and human subjects involved in the trials must have full knowledge of the risk and consequences of the trial. Human subjects must also benefit from the trial, hence surpassing the exploitation as cheap human objects.

4. *"Potential individual benefits and risks of research"*[38]

   "To justify imposing any research risks on participants in health research, the research must have social and scientific value. Before inviting potential participants to join a study, the researcher, sponsor and the research ethics committee must ensure that risks to participants are minimum and appropriately balanced in relation to the prospect of potential individual benefit and the social and scientific value of the research." It envisages a two-step process; first *"the potential individual benefits and risks of each individual research intervention or procedure in the study must be evaluated"* and second *"the aggregate risks and potential individual benefits of the entire study must be assessed and must be considered appropriate."*

5. *Choice of Control in Clinical Trials*[38]*:* Whenever the clinical trial is about to start, all the concerned participants must be informed about the consequences and effective risk. The participants (human subject) must not be exposed to danger only because they have consented for the trial. Before inoculation, the study must be conducted completely diagnosing the condition of participants. *"The research ethics committee must ensure that research participants in the control group of a trial of a diagnostic, therapeutic, or preventive intervention receive an established effective intervention."* Hence all risks and benefits must be evaluated as per the criteria set out under this guideline.

6. *Caring for Participants' Health Needs*[38]*:* While conducting a clinical trial effective measures must be ensured to make adequate provisions to address the health need of the participants of the trial. If the health care need of the participants during and after the trial cannot be taken care of by the local health care facility, the researcher and sponsor must ensure prior availability of adequate health care for the participants. *"...the guideline requires a five-fold plan to be undertaken by the researcher and the sponsors:*

- *How care will be adequately provided for the condition understudy.*
- *How care will be provided during the research when researchers discover conditions other than those under study ("ancillary care").*
- *Providing continued access to study interventions that have demonstrated significant benefit; and*
- *Consulting with other relevant stakeholders, if any, to determine everyone's responsibilities and the conditions under which participants will receive continued access to a study intervention, such as an investigational drug, that has demonstrated significant benefit in the study..."*

7. ***Community Engagement[39]:*** The researchers concerned authorities and the sponsors should take into consideration the; local factors while carrying research in a community and must build confidence with the leader of community to negotiate various aspects of research. There must be transparency and disagreement if any must be solved through negotiation. Hence the community must be engaged in conduct of clinical trial.

8. ***Collaborative partnership and capacity-building for research and research review[39]:*** The government authorities, being the guarantors of fundamental rights to its citizens, must review the research and reports from time to time. The independent research organisation and research committees must review the research done by the private sector/institutions involving human subjects so that the implementation of international guidelines on medical ethics and human rights can be followed.

9. ***Individuals Capable of Giving Informed Consent[39]:*** The moral as well as legal obligation of the sponsors and researchers includes selecting potential participants who have attained an age of maturity, are of sound mind and are capable of understanding what is wrong and right. The participants must be informed of the effect and consequences of the trial so that they are able to give free and informed consent for the experiment. There must not be any deception and withholding of information with the participants given enough time to consider their participation.

---

[39] Guideline 7-9, CIOMS.

10. ***Modifications and Waivers of Informed Consent[40]:*** The participant must be free from all obligations before or during the trial to waive the right to consent. However before such waiver of informed consent is granted, the ethics committee should *"establish whether informed consent could be modified in a way that would preserve the participant's ability to understand the general nature of the investigation and to decide whether to participate."*

Waiver of informed consent would be approved if:

"The research would not be feasible or practicable to carry out without the waiver or modification;

- *The research has important social value; and*
- *The research poses no more than minimal risks to participants."*

11. ***Collection, storage and use of biological materials and related data[40]:*** The collection of data and information must be done by the researchers and sponsors in order to provide the information to government authorities. The biological material i.e. Residual tissue is stored for future research with the consent of the patients. All the research data is kept in a record book and some of the research results as a specimen so that it can be shown to the patient and references can be made from it.

12. ***Collection, storage and use of data in health-related research[40]:*** The collection of data is done in the form of research paper and research results, the experiments in the past are used as reference so that failure can be ignored. The reason behind the storage data in health-related research is that the data stored will provide a source to get accurate information and what is the essential part to respond. Data collection and storage must not affect the right and welfare individual. The researcher must obtain either specific informed consent for the use of data for specific purpose or broad informed consent for unspecified future use must be obtained from the person. The collection and storage of data is guided by the guideline 12.

13. ***Reimbursement and compensation for research participants[41]:*** The participants involved in trial must be reimbursed with the expenses of travelling, lodging and time spent in the experiment. The

---

[40] Guideline 10-12, CIOMS.
[41] Guideline 13-16, CIOMS.

compensation must be done if there is loss of any organ or harm to any part of the body. That compensation can be monetary or non-monetary. The monetary value fixed must be reasonable and according to the risk factor at the time of experiment.

14. *Treatment and compensation for research- related harms[41]:* The sponsors and researchers must compensate the participants for any physical, psychological or social harm resulting from participation in the research. The researcher must ensure that the participant receives the required treatment for free along with compensation for loss of wages. The participants must be compensates with reasonable amount and sufficient medical care, wherein the research ethics committee would determine upon the adequacy of the compensation and arrangement for treatment.

15. *Research involving vulnerable persons and groups[41]:* In some trials there is a requirement of some vulnerable group of persons e.g. Children, persons with disabilities or persons suffering from dangerous diseases to be participants. While conducting such clinical trial there must be adequate safeguards and extra protection equipment to neglect any harm to human health of these vulnerable groups. It is the responsibility of the research ethics committee to ensure that human subjects are not exposed to any risk which may result in any kind of loss or death.

16. *Research involving adults incapable of giving informed consent[41]:* The researchers and sponsors must follow the ethical guidelines to conduct a trial wherein the participants are adults who are incapable of giving informed consent. However, such trials are to be carried following the research ethics committee guidelines so as to protect the interest and rights of such participants. The guideline provides that *"before undertaking research with adults who are not capable of giving informed consent, the researcher and the research ethics committee must ensure that:*

> *A legally authorized representative of the person who is incapable of giving informed consent has given permission and this permission takes account of the participant's previously formed preferences and values (if any); and*

> *The assent of the subject has been obtained to the extent of that person's capacity, after having been provided with adequate information about*

the research at the level of the subject's capacity for understanding this information."

17. ***Research involving children and adolescents[42]:*** Children and adolescents must be involved in health research so that requirements for the proper growth can be analysed and development and research can be done in that direction. The researchers must follow the concerned guidelines in order to safeguard the interest, rights and welfare of the children.

18. ***Women as a research participant[42]:*** Women must be included in health related research, however women are usually excluded from these research because of their child bearing potential. When a woman is involved in the trial then only the researchers can know the requirement of the drugs for the disease which are mainly affecting women's health. A woman must be informed of all health risk and it is only the consent of a woman which must be taken into account.

19. ***Pregnant and breastfeeding women as research participants[42]:*** The women who are pregnant and breastfeeding babies have distinct health requirements. The involvement of these women will give new ideas and reasons to understand the dietary needs, medical requirements and data will also build so that the patients suffering from any of these health problems can be treated easily, however research on such women must be carried out as per the guideline 19.

20. ***Research in disasters and disease outbreaks[43]:*** Places where disasters have been observed must be involved in the health related activities for the better understanding of the genomic mutation. Disaster like extreme cold, summer or rain, which requires a good immune system to survive. This all will give a good research point to know better about the conditions of the people living in that area. The research ethics committee guidelines must be followed for the protection of their rights and interest, which cannot be foregone, even during the times of disasters. The ethical principles embodied in the guideline must be followed even during the disease or disaster outbreak.

21. ***Cluster randomized trials[43]:*** Whenever there is any cluster trial, it is the responsibility of the researchers and authorities to identify the

---

[42] Guideline 17-20, CIOMS.
[43] Guideline 21-25, CIOMS.

people and group who will be affected from that trial. Cluster trials result in the large data and information about the experiment.

22. *Use of data obtained from the online environment and digital tools in health-related research[43]:* The data obtained from an online environment is a secondary source and is not reliable until supported with sufficient strong scientific data. This data is related to the experimented data for the reference so that a proper analysis can be done, and a conclusion can be made.

23. *Requirements for establishing research ethics committees and for their review of protocols[43]:* Research ethics committee must establish some guidelines so that researchers can follow and implement them during experiments. The trial process is guided by the ethic committed. Every protocol of a research trial is approved by the ethics committee.

24. *Public accountability for health-related research[43]:* The general public must be involved in the clinical trial by giving them a proper explanation about the experiment. The researchers and sponsors must comply with recognised public ethics and must be accountable to the general public if any harm is caused due to the experiment.

25. *Conflicts of interest[43]:* Each individual may have conflicting interest, however there exist a common welfare for a society and if there is a conflict between individual interest and societal interest, importance is given to the welfare of the society and people. In a clinical trial conflict may arise due to long term benefits of the research. The research ethics committee must review the interest of the researchers and sponsors so that welfare of the society can be observed first.

GLOBAL PERSPECTIVE – GOOD CLINICAL PRACTICE

Good clinical practice is a globally approved quality guidelines for trials, by the international council for harmonisation of technical requirements for pharmaceutical for human use (ICH), an international body generally known as international conference on harmonization of good clinical practice or ICH-GCP. It details the necessity of globally approved standards for the protection of human beings from exploitation of various stakeholders while conducting the trials. It requires strict documentation of every step of clinical protocol and ensures the quality control, protection of basic human rights, and regular inspection for strict adherence of clinical guidelines. It is approved as scientifically authoritative guidelines as it is scientifically tested and proved. However, it is criticised for lack of morality and hence less authoritative in comparison to declaration of Helsinki.

The WHO provides a handbook[44] for good clinical research practice (GCP) reiterating "development of the trial protocol; development of standard operating procedures (sops); development of support systems and tools; generation and approval of trial related documents; selection of trial sites and the selection of properly qualified, trained, and experienced investigators and study personnel; ethics committee review and approval of the protocol; review by regulatory authorities; quality, handling and accounting of the investigational product(s); trial data acquisition while conducting the trial; safety management and reporting; monitoring the trial; managing trial data; quality assurance of the trial performance and data; and the reporting of the trial." The responsibility for GCP is shared by all the parties involved, which includes sponsors, investigators and site staff, contract research organizations (CROS), ethics committees, regulatory authorities and research subjects. Regarding informed consent, GCP involves the summation of the Helsinki declaration, Belmont report, CIOMS guidelines, ICCPR as well as other international guidelines. Not only does the handbook specifically state the information that is required to be given to the trial subject to form an informed consent, but also specifies the eligibility criteria for the administrator of taking the consent. Whereas the handbook states the categories of people as vulnerable groups, it also clears the process of documentation of taking the consent, which cannot be completed just with a signature. Additionally, the WHO also has published international standards for clinical trial registries, which mandates the registration of clinical trials and aims to accumulate the information of all the clinical trials, in order to prevent the repetition of mistakes and to gain the knowledge from the other researches as well. World Health Organization (WHO) aims to state various guidelines already mentioned in the Helsinki declaration and other ethical principles and guidelines and thus formulate a common guideline for all the countries to follow. Moreover, who aims to man date the global registration of clinical trials at one stop and also to provide the results of those clinical trials, so the possibility of errors, harm and injury

---

[44] Handbook for good clinical research practice (GCP), available at: https://www.who.int/medicines/areas/quality_safety/safety_efficacy/gcp1.pdf

can be minimised. As a result, who states four phases of clinical trials, which are as follows:[14]

- Phase I studies usually test new drugs for the first time in a small group of people to evaluate a safe dosage range and identify side effects.
- Phase II studies test treatments that have been found to be safe in phase I but now need a larger group of human subjects to monitor for any adverse effects.
- Phase III studies are conducted on larger populations and in different regions and countries and are often the step right before a new treatment is approved.
- Phase IV studies take place after country approval and there is a need for further testing in a wide population over a longer timeframe.

In European Union, good clinical practice has been regulated by directive 2001/20/EC. European Union has approved the guidelines of ISO 14155 as a harmonised principle. In the United States, ICH-GCP is not statutorily mandated, though it is approved by the food and drug administration (FDA). The national institute of health demands all clinical investigators and staff are to be qualified as trainers of good clinical practice.

The food and drug administration (FDA), a federal agency of us department of health and human services, handles the landscape of clinical tests in us, with an intention to protect the safety, and efficiency of clinical tests and the health rights of trials participant.

There are many conferences being held every year in the realm of clinical trials. The recently held conference on clinical trials in Amsterdam, has mainly tried to handle the "evolution of clinical research in advanced life". There is a patient involvement conference, to be held in the month august 2020 to understand the patient's voice in planning clinical trials.

INDIAN PERSPECTIVE

In India, the clinical trials are governed by guidelines of Indian council of medical research (ICMR), drugs and cosmetics act and rules' 1945, and Indian medical council 1956, central council for Indian medicine act, 1970 and drugs and clinical trial rules 2019. The central drugs standard control organisation (CDSCO) is the national regulatory authority of India, the department of drug controller general of India (DGCI) being the prime licensor. The Indian council for medical research (ICMR) publishes a national handbook of ethical guidelines for biomedical and health research involving human participants, making changes from time to time providing the standard of ethics to be followed for conducting clinical trials and other research.

Ever since, the procedure of conducting clinical trials in India was envisaged in drugs and cosmetic rules, 1945, till the time the need to regulate the policies was strongly felt. In 2012, a Pil[45] was filed by an NGO describing the problems in the compensation granted to trial subjects in case of injury or death of the subject. The 2013 amendment bill[46] to the drugs and cosmetics act was released proposing changes in the regulation of the import, export, manufacture, distribution and sale of drugs, cosmetics and other medical devices as well as to ensure safety, efficacy, quality and conduct of the clinical trials. This was the first bill in India that proposed the penal provisions with regard to the violations of the guidelines formulated by ICMR. However, the bill was not passed due to the reasons that it still needed contemplation on various issues.

The provisions regarding the compensation to the subjects in case of death or injury in a clinical trial is governed by the ethical guidelines of ICMR,[47] which suggests that the sponsor of the clinical trial shall compensate the injured trial subject or the legal heir of the dead trial subject up until the extent of direct relation of the injury to the clinical trial. The direct injury may include physical, psychological, social, legal or even economical. According to the drugs and cosmetics rules' 1945 the decision to decide the granting as well as extent of compensation shall be in the hands of the ethics committee. Despite the provisions for careful regulations and compensation, it was reported that a total of 1443 participants of clinical trial died between 2015–2018, whereas only 88 of them were given compensation suggesting their injury was directly related to the trial.[48]

---

[45] "Swasthya Adhikar Manch, Indore vs. Union of India", W.P (c) No. 33 of 2012.

[46] The drugs and cosmetics (amendment) bill, 2013.

[47] Handbook on national ethical guidelines for biomedical and health research involving human participants.

[48] See Ch. VI, rule 39, draft new drugs and clinical trials rules, 2018 (2017), http://www.cdsco.nic.in/writereaddata/draft%20ct%20rules%20sent%20for%20publ ication.pdf [hereinafter "2018 draftrules"]

In order to overcome the difficulties faced by the existing provisions, to encourage bringing more clinical trials and to promote the indigenous drug development in India, the new drugs and clinical trial draft rules were formulated in February, 2018. One of the significant aspects of the draft rules was the reception of no fault compensation by the government of India, through adding a provision to grant mandatory interim compensation, amounting to 60% of the total amount incurred in the injury, within 15 days of the opinion of ethics committee.[49] However, such provision was realised to be against the objective of the rules which is to encourage the sponsors for bringing in the trials. The new drugs and clinical trial rules' 2019 hence became the most significant legislation promising the favourable and expeditious reception of trials.

Under the new rules,[50] significant changes have been made, which are enumerated below:

1. *Pre and post-submission meetings* – in order to facilitate the process of application for approval to conduct the clinical trials, a provision has been framed for the sponsors to have an advisory pre-submission meeting with the central licensing authority (CLA) or the officers appointed by CLA. Similarly, in case of any further queries from CLA or CDSCO, the sponsor may even apply for a post-submission meeting.

2. *Expedited and deemed approval/licensing* – the rules provide for the time period of 30 days in case of domestic companies to get the license to conduct the trials and moreover, states that in case of no response from DGCI within 30 days suggesting a rejection or deficiency, it shall be deemed to be approved. In case of foreign companies, the time period is of 90 days, provided that the time period of 30 days is to be followed in case the drug is discovered in India or the research and development of the drug have been carried out in India and also the drug is proposed to be manufactured and marketed in India.[51]

---

[49] Rupak de Chowdhuri, "India's new clinical trial rules weaken safety nets for participants" scroll.in, April 4' 2019 *available* at: Https://scroll.in/pulse/918874/new-clinical-trial-rules-weaken-safety-nets-for-trial-participants-to-promote-research

[50] New drugs and clinical trial rules' 2019.

[51] *Id.* At Ch V, Rule 22 and 23.

3. *Local clinical trial waiver* – another provision regulating the market of drugs is the waiver of local clinical trials in case the drug has already been approved by any other country, provided the country is approved by DGCI, who has the authority to approve it on a case-to-case basis.

4. *Fast-track orphan drug registration* – orphan drug is the drug inflicted to cure a rare disease. Under the current rules, it is defined as a drug intended to treat a condition which affects not more than five lakh persons in India.[52] The regulatory pathway, of conducting a trial in case of rare diseases or in the case of unmet needs of India, is fast tracked and less stringent restrictions are applied.

5. *Post-trial access* – the rules tend to deliver distributive justice by requiring sponsors to provide post-trial access to a drug at no cost to the trial participant if the following circumstances are fulfilled:

   (a) The trial relates to an indication for which no alternative therapy is available and the drug has been found beneficial to the subject by the investigator;

   (b) The continued access has been approved by the ethics committee;

   (c) The subject or legal heir consents to post-trial use of the investigational drug; and

   (d) The investing at or has certified and the trial subject declares in writing.

   That for such post-trial use the "sponsor shall have no liability for post-trial use of investigational new drug or new drug."[53]

6. *Accelerated approval for drugs* – the idea behind this type of approval is to render the availability of new drugs in case of serious conditions based on their severity, rarity, high prevalence, lack of alternate treatment and also if the new drug is more beneficial than the already existing one. Under this kind of approval, the surrogate end points are used to gather the efficiency of a new drug, rather than standard outcomes. In other words, rather than relying on the proven results of clinical trials, a predictive opinion is formed anticipating the clinical benefits of the new drug. The 2019 rules provide for the condition of approval in these cases of new drugs subsequent to the phase ii of the

---

[52] Id. At Ch I, rule 2(x).
[53] *Id.* At Ch V, rule 27.

trial and therefore, post marketing trials are required to validate anticipated medical benefit.[54]

7. ***Doctor's predicament in case of life-threatening diseases*** – in case of life- threatening diseases, the rules give away the authority as well as the duty to the doctors and officers of government hospitals and institutions to seek the permission of CLA in order to import the unapproved drugs from different countries, which are approved for marketing in the country of origin. Nevertheless, it also yields power to manufacture in India, unapproved drugs of other countries in case of life-endangering situations.

The patents act' 1970 already provides the power to the government of India to grant compulsory licences to non-patent holders to manufacture patented drugs without any legal implications in case of national emergency, extreme urgency or public non-commercial use.[55]

The Laws of Consent and Compensation in Indian Scenario

It has already been discussed earlier in the research paper that the guidelines related to the compensation and consent ethics are enumerated in the national handbook of ethical guidelines by ICMR, whereas the mechanism to receive the compensation is still debatable in the country. As per the consolidated reading of the guidelines as well as the new rules, every sponsor bears the responsibility to undertake the consent of each subject prior to the clinical trial. In case of injury or death of the subject, the new rules limit the liability of the sponsors to provide medical management as per the discretion of the investing at or till the time it is established that the injury was not directly related to the trial.[56] It envisages the investigator as the final authority to decide whether the compensation or medical management to be provided and if yes, then to what extent. In case of death as well, the compensation may be provided if the investigator discreets the death to be the direct result of the trial as well as the extent of compensation shall also be the investigator's decision. Another change made in the new rules was the report of death to be given by sponsor and the investigator to DGCI, has to be now given within

---

[54] *Supra* at 6.
[55] The patents act' 1970, section 92.
[56] New drugs and clinical trial rules 2019, Ch VI, rule 40(1).

14 days of when the death of the subject came into their knowledge, rather than within 14 days of the occurrence of death in previous rules. In case of post-trial liability, the sponsor holds no responsibility as the drug is inflicted on the post-trial subject after receiving the consent from the subject or the legal heir of the subject ratifying the no responsibility of the sponsor.[57]

India's chief authority on drugs standard control organisation (CDSCO) has published the "rapid response regulatory framework for Covid-19 vaccine development, following which the Indian council of medical research (ICMR) issued national guidelines for general ethical issues, and review proceedings for the covid related and non-related research, clinical trials and issues relating to consent. As per the new rules and regulations, sponsors of ongoing projects shall co-ordinate with investigators and ethical committee, strictly adhere to the approved protocol of clinical in accordance with the good clinical trials practice (GCP) and to maintain complete records and submit the records of amendments if any along with the actual report of clinical trials. It also highlights the importance of rights of patients, welfare, and safety aspects. It is to be placed on record that Indian authorities have appreciated the efforts of various multinational companies' sponsors, local pharmaceutical companies and other stakeholders of clinical trials and amended the changes in the process of clinical trials, striking a balance between the health interests of the people and also the fundamental rights of the trial subjects.

After India becomes signatory to trips (agreement on trade related aspects of intellectual property rights, India is become the hotspot of clinical trials due to various factors like professionally qualified skills, availability of huge population of patients, and existence of variety of diseases. Cost effective Indian market is of course the core reason for the exponential growth of clinical markets in India along with clear cut rules and regulations with timely amendments in the rules and legislations. As per the new law, an online application can be filed to central licensing authority as per the rules via sugam, an online portal managed by the CDSCO. Time lines for approval of application has been cut down to 30 days and a system of deemed approval is assumed if no response has come from drugs controller general of India (DCGI). Most importantly,

---

[57] *Supra* at 10.

if the drugs clinical trial is approved and tested in any other country, which follows good practice procedures of international standards, in similar to Indian standards, the necessity of local trial may be waived.

DCGI, which is the central licensing agency as per the new rules, can also decide the amount of compensation in cases of death and other permanent disability to a trail participant, along with ethics committee. Amount as to how much compensation to be paid is decided with the support of calculation as formulated in the formula of new rules. If the clinical trial is purely for the academic interests, no such prior approval is required, but the result of such trials shall not be made use of, for the purpose of promotion of any drugs or medicines and it shall not be used for medical use in the market.

Authors prefer to notify some of the important references in the areas of clinical trials as it gives glimpse of the new amendments. The most important handwork on guidance is the handbook published by Indian council of medical research and central drugs standard control organisation, which is titled as 'handbook for applicants & reviewers of clinical trials of new drugs in India (January 2017). Another important reference is the gazette notification f. No. DCGI/MISC/2020(104) government of India, director general of health services, central drug standard control organisation, dated 30th March 2020. There are other two guidelines, which are important to mention here is national ethical guidelines for bio-medical and health research involving human participants (ICMR) and also another guideline for gene therapy product development and clinical trials (2019).

CONCLUSION

With the acceptance of democratic values throughout the world, the human rights of freedom of choice, equality among others and right to life and liberty hold the paramount importance in today's world as they are non-derogable rights. Whereas, it is suggested that with every evolving guideline on clinical trials, efforts have been made to clarify the intricacies in aspects of consent and information available to provide the consent, these guidelines being suggestive, the only binding rules upon the countries, especially India are the rules made by the central government of India. In various under developed countries of Africa and other parts of developing countries, clinical trials are part and parcel of their economic policies.

They relax the rules and regulation of ethical code to attract multinational companies for doing clinical trials on their citizens. By the glimpse of the various country's rules and regulations, it seems that rules are relaxed to the effect that the individual rights and fundamental rights have been given unwarranted inflictions in order to invite foreign multinational pharmaceutical companies. It seems rubber is pulled through each side and the individual is stuck in between the financial crisis and health crisis.

On one hand, the world is growing with an aim to decrease the gap between the two, on the other

Hand the instances of unregistered clinical trials, trials without proper information and thus tainted consent, limited liability of the state in case of death and injury, authority of investigators over the quantum of compensation, exploitation of citizens of developing countries, vulnerable groups becoming the targets of atrocities of pharmaceutical companies, etc., are growing up. The supremacy of economics over human rights doesn't seem out of the picture where individuals are just objectified into cheap subjects.

We often observe advertisements in newspapers stating that if you don't observe hair gain; your money will be refunded in a limited time. Advertisements of hair gain oil, body weight gainer, and height increasing tablet or vaccine, and many more are not officially approved by any competent authorities. Participants involved in these trials are unknown to the fact that they are a part of the testing which is going on. In some of the cases the researcher and sponsor may be the same person, so he may not have sufficient funds or resources to compensate, so they independently test the drug on themselves.

It is suggested that the government authorities like central licensing authority in India and medical council of India should review the ethics committee and number of researches done by the laboratory or institution. Timeline has to be set by the organisation so that a well detailed report can be analysed for the approval of any testing. Participants must be qualified and free informed and consent has to be obtained. Time to time the authorities must check the record book of every institution for every research they tested. Final approval shall be given only when a person from that field who has deep knowledge and learning about the subject approves the trial and not on the certificates approved by their own members.

Warning notice shall be issued if any institution found involving participants without their consent and taking undue advantage of the subject. If any institution is found for failing two times consecutively, then their license for testing must be canceled. Guidelines are the framework of the competent authorities, so that development and innovation in the technology must go on, but without losing human lives.

During the last decade, a developing country like India has received impetus in receiving foreign funds for clinical trials from multinational companies as it has relaxed its rules for the purpose of enhancing the number of clinical trials. India is one of major players to reckon with in the conduct of clinical trials and is also one of the largest manufacturing countries of various pharmaceuticals. Various multinational companies have signed joint ventures with local national companies in India to produce drugs and medicines, medical devices and also to conduct clinical trials. India, though tries to make use of all these instrumentalities for the welfare of the people and economic prosperity, also tries to strike a balance in its legal realm between the fundamental rights and economic rights. The Indian democracy and its constitution are fundamentally strong to protect the health interest of its citizens and hence, health is still considered as wealth of the country. India, being a country well known for its yoga, meditation and ayurveda, attaches paramount significance to the health of the people, along with economic interest of the country.

Challenges and Dimensions of Corporate Social Responsibility: Post COVID Pandemic

Mr. Akshdeep Gupta*

ABSTRACT: Corporate social responsibility, also called as CSR, as a word holds little meaning as to contrary to its capabilities and application in real world. It is imperative today to understand what CSR is and how can it be implemented efficiently. The intention of this paper is to explain the role of corporate in this pandemic and effects on near future. The paper will throw light on the areas that are not recession free and how the corporate sector of the society must be governed as it also suffers the same recession. There must be a new dimension which is still unexplored to cope up with all these disputes and challenges. There are however issues related to the introduction of many new schemes and ways to lead a more healthy and environmental friendly lifestyle which leads to environment administration devices into business arrangements and combined with eco-labelling. As companies and corporate were not always environmental friendly it has come to notice that they were the main source of the hazards that has come in the roads of developing nations, nevertheless, the per capita consumption of energy in developed nations will always be in enormous amounts with no considerations on international levels. CSR has always been one of the greatest revolutions of hum kind. With the pandemic lock-down around the world, it has come to notice of many that it is time that CSR becomes thing of priority. This research paper also ranks the main challenges of methodologies CSR. The worth of the paper is prompt to CSR to enhance their methods and techniques in order for greater yield taking into consideration the attest pandemic, effects of lockdown and the level of harm caused on national and international levels to the corporate industry.

INTRODUCTION

For many years there has been a talk about corporate social responsibility, since non-governmental organizations, many companies

* Student, Amity Law School, NOIDA, AUUP.

plus scientific authors participate in its promotion. Many methodologies have been developed to assess CSR activity, affecting the attitudes of stakeholders. The selection of evaluation methodologies is based on criteria such as its acceptance by social responsibility indices and the evaluation of multiple socio-social dimensions. However there are many challenges and dimensions to the CSR, some of which CSR criteria are not specified for each sector, an unacceptable weighting for each dimension or criterion, lack of transparency and ignorance of the most important dimensions of society, more-over, there is a need to find CSR ways to advance its approach, taking into consideration the challenges proposed to assess such social responsibility in a comprehensive approach.[1] CSR increases business accountability not only for shareholders but also or the people of the company. The main areas of the responsibility account for the environmental protection and well being of the employees and community at large, which is very important for the betterment of the humans. However, charitable contribution and involvement of the big corporate in community education does ring a bell to it but it does not comprise for the full dimension that is to the CSR. The main challenge of the present time of pandemic for big corporate would be to fight with the coming depression in the society.

CSR MEANING AND SCOPE

It is well known that people started to be aware of CSR not before 1960. As a concept, CSR found more space in Europe as compared to the United States; whereas, UN has played a very important role in popularising the idea of CSR on a global level.

Fundamental nature for CSR is encompassed by many adjectives, which includes names like strategic philanthropy, social performance, corporate citizenship, responsible and sustainable businesses. CSR is also defined as the procedure for assessing the impact of an organization on society and assessing its accountability. CSR can easily be suggested as a corporate model which regulates and assimilate itself. It defines such activities and functions which help organisations to improve on the level where they were harming their surroundings.

---

[1] Wim Dubbink, *CSR and role of organizations,* (Nov, 2016), https://www.montesquieu/institutional/artschool.

"it will be safe to say that CSR begins home, which means companies have to access the areas of main focus such as:

- Supply chain
- Employees
- Sub-ordinates
- Environmental factors
- Consumers ...."[2]

As it has been discussed earlier, that how CSR is not only a business model, but is an efficient one, which helps any corporate body to hold responsibility for each action that they perform.

By implementing CSR, business owners are made aware and responsible for any harmful activity that they do which indeed affects the environment and people around them. When a business corporation performs CSR, it is affirmative that it will compensate for all the harm that it has caused to the society and will in fact give a positive outlook. It is important that every business has a positive look towards any harm that it causes and tries to reverse it for long-term benefit. *It is widely believed that through CSR programs, philanthropy and volunteer efforts, businesses can benefit society while strengthening their brands.*

Some important points to keep in mind about CSR are:

- Corporate social responsibility holds importance for consumers and businesses.
- Corporate responsibility programs are a great approach to boost morale at work.
- Example: Starbucks is a leader in creating social responsibility programs in many aspects of its business......."[3]

A company which holds responsibility towards its shareholders is a CSR in true nature. It is often believed that companies which get into CSR often try to evolve in such a nature that they are able to provide and give back to the community. As the business grows so does the responsibility

[2] Cécile Renouard, *From CSR to Corporate Responsibilities*, ESSEC BUSINNESS SCHOOL, (Oct 10, 2016). http://knowledge.essec.edu/en/consulting/csr-trans-formation-business-models.html.

[3] Sanne Bruhn-Hansen, *CSR and communication*, TODAY INDIA, (June, 2012), https://www.sustainicum.at.

to elevate the level of return that is being given back and also increases the public expectations. It is a very regular thing that consumers also start to feel quietus towards the brand and feel as if the brands are obligated to give them good service.

In the initial years it was seen as the evolution for the clothing corporations and even today after so many years this paradigm shift has not been successful and completely dependent on the beauty market. Big corporate have a ease when it comes to CSR, be it due to lack of government initiation or lack of public education, the radical study is required.[4]

The purpose of CSR has always been to make companies reliable for what they do and how it affects their surroundings. Today, however, there is a shift in the total regime of company building and it is observed that even small business have CSR on their priority lists. Companies try to administer all the internal and external factors affecting the management.

CURRENT REGIME IN CSR

Today businesses are a very essential part of our communities, it is clear that companies are building themselves as civilizations. The corporate industry plays a very crucial role in overall development of a country; there are many examples where corporate community has solved big financial and material problems like in healthcare, food shortage and many such parts, with the help of CSR. The importance of CSR has been affirmed by UN and even by the European charter and has been promoted he the highest level honour.[5]

According to the Indian Corporate experts, sustainable development is improving the economic condition of the nation, with moving hand in-hand with the civilisation and environment, and CSR occupies support issues related not only to children and women but also related to even the environment.[6] Over time it has come to the notice of corporate that how important it is to maintain harmony with the people around it to grow and succeed in any business in the long-term.

---

[4] Scholten B., *Finance as a Driver of CSR*, JBE JOURNAL (Sep. 2006), Vol. 68, pg. No. 19.

[5] Dr. Tatjana, *CSR & Environment* (2007).

[6] Das Sanjay Kanti, *CSR Practices and Reporting in Indian Financial Sector*, IJBM, (Sept 2012), Vol. 2, pg. No. 9.

If the whole world was to be taken into consideration, India is one of the few countries which has a good CSR regime. However, its history can be divided into four phases mainly, *"However, the phases are not static and the characteristics of each phase may overlap with other phases, to be defining the phases, in the first phase, contributions and humanity was the main contributors of CSR. In the second phase, during the independence movement, there was growing tension on Indian industrialists to demonstrate their attachment to the progress of society. The third phase (1960–80) concerned the element of the mixed economy, which led to the introduction of legislation on corporate governance and the environment. In fourth phase (from 1980 to the present), Indian companies abandoned their traditional CSR commitment and integrated it into a sustainable commercial strategy."[7]*

When CSR was introduced initially in 1960s, it became an annual agenda for every corporate. It came into force due to then introduced economic globalisation and new world technology.

"In a survey, the 82 participating organizations were asked to rate the enterprises on CSR initiatives and indicate their preference for the top three enterprises, in which the TATA group (67%) appears at the beginning of the file, followed by far Infosys (13%), ITC (12%), NTPC (11%) and ADA-Reliance (10%)."[8]

All these expels have been in study since always but even today it is safe to say that CSR is at a very nascent stage in this country and there is need to improve and put a lot of effort by each sector of the society so that it improves and gives CSR opportunity to grow appropriately and efficiently.

"In addition, many factors push businesses to CSR, such as:

1. The Declining Role of Government.
   In the past, governments have relied on legislation and regulations to achieve social and environmental goals in the business sector.
2. Requests for Greater Disclosure.

---

[7] Ghangas Anil, *Various phases of CSR in India*, RESEARCH_GATE (Jan, 2018), https://www.researchgate.net/ publication/323392712_Various_phases_of_corporate social_responsibility in_India.

[8] RBI Notification, *CSR in Indian Banks, Corporate Social Responsibility*, Sustainable Development and Non-Financial Reporting—Role of Banks (Dec, 2007), RBI/2007-08/216: DBOD No Dir.BC.58/13.27.00/2007- 08.

Stakeholders have an increasing demand to be precise.

3. Increased Customer Interest.
   There is evidence about ethical business behaviour is increasingly influencing customer purchasing decisions.

4. Competitive labour markets.
   Market employees increasingly look beyond salaries and benefits and seek employers whose business philosophy and practices are in line with their own principles. In bid to retain qualified employees, companies are forced to improve functioning conditions...."[9]

There are many system which are however, established for the purpose of saving the reputation of the company corporate. "The concept of CSR has different meanings for different stakeholders and depending on the situation of companies, expectations may also differ.

Currently, CSR presents more challenges than those available. Many of these challenges can be addressed on the community level itself, such as:

1. *Zero Community Participation:* The communities here mean local and un-approached group of individuals, which were not communicated with and have no practical idea regarding CSR. It is widely believed that communities do not lack the zest of participating but just lack of knowledge. The far-off communities have no idea about the benefits that CSR activities can grant them. So, it is important to educate everyone with this knowledge.

2. ***Lack of Local Authority:*** There are so many NGOs which are effectively telling the tales of CSR, but in theory there is no need for these NGOs to do any of this work, as there exist some or the other government authority to implement these theories. Therefore there is a lack of evident contribution by any of these local authorities because of which, the local population suffers. This brings a serious strain on the CSR activities and creates an atmosphere of low development, thus limiting the scope of efficient working.

3. ***Lack of Transparency among Community Company Relation:*** It is imperative that the local authority remain truthful to the businesses

---

[9] Finnovation positive impact organization, *latest treads affecting CSR in India, FINNOVATION ORG.,* (April, 30, 2018), https://fiinovation.co.in/latest-csr-trends-and-factors-influencing-csr-in-india.

and the agencies for corporate litigation. Down the road they always think of their own personal benefit. This lack of transparency increases with people and company relation during lockdown and affects the overall growth of CSR.

4. *Lack of Visible Availability:* Not only the public and corporate fails but in some places the media tech also lacks visible availability. In places where media should show the successful business model to increase inspiration among people, they show the negatives only. This practice affects the CSR activities of companies and influences the visibility band of any good company action. The branding facility of these companies in-turn discourages corporate brands to spend less money on CSR and do more for mainstream media.

5. *Lack of CSR Initiatives:* Agencies being government or being non-government always tend to have a very narrow prospective towards CSR initiatives. They tend to provide meaning and define such activities only in theory and lack practical application and means to implementation. As a result, it is found diminishing for anyone to take part in CSR with enthusiasm.

6. *Need for Government Policy Making:* As discussed earlier, even when government agencies form some rules, they are not focused on harmonizing the relationship between company and people but seem to loot the companies and give to people. There is no fair advantage for anyone in this, as companies run out of business people stop getting benefitted and this solution seem good but only in short-term. Therefore it is important to look for long-term and long-lasting solutions rather than short-term benefits.

7. *Want for Implementation and Togetherness:* Lack of government authority over anything is never good. Factors such as company's heath and company's profit never seem to come together. Policies should act like an umbrella which gives shade and as well as saves you on a rainy day rather than being like a divide and rule policy."[10]

PRACTICAL APPLICATION/EXAMPLES OF CSR

There are many examples in India of big corporate helping others even when CSR was not on popular opinions of people. India as society has

---

[10] *Supra* note 10.

always helped the less fortunate in hard times, be it Tata group donating more than 150 million rupees or any Actor donating 50 million, the idea always should be good will and not profits. Global platform has always lacked to see the good natured and as it is famously said that bad deeds of some defame the rest too. There are many examples which are evidence to this practical application of CSR even in the times of Covid Pandemic. *"It provides advisory and technical assistance services for social development and CSR.*

According to a National Geographic survey that surveyed 18,000 consumers in 17 countries,

- Indians as citizens are the most environmentally responsible patron in the whole world. India has the peak of Consumer Greendex, where questions were asked about energy expenditure and conservation, transportation preference, food supply resources, the relative utilisation of green products compared to conventional products, attitudes towards the environment plus sustainability and awareness of environmental issues.

- According to a Nielsen survey availed in May 2009, Reliance Industries with two Tata group companies are the most accepted companies in the nation for their inventiveness in corporate social responsibility.[11]

- *Gujarat Tribal Development:* Department for a development project aimed at raising the tribe in the Sasan region of the Gir forest. The financial services sector is experiencing steady growth. In an attempt to save energy, companies have started to reduce the carbon footprint of their offices. The year 2009 was characterized by initiatives such as the application of renewable energy technologies, the transition to paperless operations and the recognition of environmental standards.

- State-owned Navratna, Coal India Ltd. will invest $ 67.5 million in social and environmental affairs in 2010–2011.

- *Ashok Leyland:* Run a FunBus in Chennai and New Delhi. This bus, equipped with a hydraulic elevator, takes children with different skills and children from orphanages and primary schools of enterprise on a picnic day.

---

[11] Ashwani Singla, *Trust and Corporate Social responsibility: Lessons from India,* Genesis Public Relations Pvt. Ltd. (Jan, 2019).

- *Axis Bank Foundation:* The Axis Bank manages Balwadis, a learning centre for children of urban slums. It also offers skills development programs under PREMA and Yuva Parivartan, in automotive management, welding, mobile repairs, sewing, etc. for young people from disadvantaged neighbourhoods.
- *Bharat Petroleum Corporation:* Boond's storm water recovery project, in collaboration with the Oil Industry Development Council, chooses cities that are harassed to convert them from, scarce to positive for water. Some of BPCL's other social programs include village adoption, HIV/AIDS prevention and care, and rural health care.
- *Hindalco Industries:* CSR activities are concentrated in 692 villages and 12 urban slums, where they reach around 26 lakh people. He built reservoirs, dams and boreholes for drinking water. In the field of education, scholarships are granted to students from rural schools who needed it. His other interests include empowerment and women's health care, in which he treats patients in hospitals, runs medical camps and operates rural and mobile medical cars.
- *Indian Oil Corporation:* It manages the Indian Petroleum Foundation (IOF), a nonprofit trust that strives to preserve and promote the heritage of the country. The IOCL also offers 150 sports grants to promising young people each year. Some of the other initiatives are related to drinking water, education, hospitals and healthcare.
- *Infosys:* Established in 2009, the Infosys Science Foundation awards the annual Infosys Award for outstanding achievements in science and engineering. The company supports causes in healthcare, culture and rural development. In an interesting initiative undertaken by her, 100 Karnataka teachers suffering from arthritis were run for free as part of a week-long program.
- *Oil and Gas Corporation:* It provides community health services in rural areas through 30 mobile health insurance (UMM) units. The CGSB Eastern Swamp Deer Savings Project is aimed at protecting rare species of Easter mushroom deer in the Kaziranga National Park in Assam. The CGSB also supports the education and empowerment of women.
- *Tata Consulting Services:* The Functional Computer Literacy Initiative (CBFL) to ensure adult literacy has already benefited 1.2 lakh people. The program is available in nine Indian languages. In addition to adult

education, TCS also works in the areas of skills development, healthcare and agriculture."[12]

MALPRACTICES WITH CSR

According to the statutory CSR, it was set up in 2016, the funding in social causes would be a revolution, but some parts of India Inc. now abuse it according to money laundering, according to sources using such transactions. Some companies use charitable trusts to fabricate rental expenses on CSR, according to at least two sources that have helped execute and execute such transactions. India is the first and only country to have legally authorized the social responsibility of certain groups of companies. In addition, the financial statements of charitable trusts are also not subject to legal investigation. This combination of factors has opened the new CSR standards to abuse.

"Such abuses are unlikely in corporate trust trusts. But this is possible when they use external trusts," said Mr. Rusen Kumar, founding director of India CSR, a portal that collects information and developments on the CSR across the country.[13]

For example, if ₹ 1000 spent by any one person on CSR, then they directly pay to any such NGO or organisation which works for social benefits. After commission is deducted, the money discreetly returns to the officials or promoters and immediately transforms the amount of white money from ₹ 1000 to black. The middleman also gets a cut in the process. "The promoter often packs the money," said a chartered accountant who also assisted clients in such transactions. These trusts are often created by politicians or wealthy individuals and also serve as a mechanism for illegal money. This money is returned to the promoters and the actual expenses of the institution are covered by the illegal shot by the politician. Spending is then inflated to launder black money.

---

[12] Bhushan Kumar, *latest development in CSR activities,* Hindu, July 34, 2011, at pg. no. 7.

[13] Chaudhury Suman Kalyan, *Banking practices of CSR,* RJEB AND ICT, Vol. 4, 2011, pg. No. 76.

IMPACT OF COVID-19 AND LOCKDOWN

The recent development in Covid lockdown situation has put country or else we can comfortably say the whole world in to sort of a pickle. People are either speculating on what to do or are speculating what their future is going to be. The great depression, after all this is over, is just a tip of the ice-burg. Everyone is scared of losing their jobs and this is a known fact that even before lockdown, jobs were not just lying around.

The biggest question would be that how big corporate are going to deal with the situation. Problems such as pay-cuts and lying-off of workers are not new to the corporate world but the situation as grave as this is something to be given a hard glance at. However, the corporate have been doing great since the last time lockdown started but as it keeps on extended and the days of home-stay don't seem to abyss anywhere. So the CSR is the deal that is going to be the thing of the future. There are many examples where the big corporate have helped either be it financially or be it monetary in the form of material help, big corporate have been doing their part in the world. There has been no pressure from the government till date and there have been no laws which would pressurise the companies to solve any of these problems with money, but we can clearly see that times are tough in the near future and money and material goods will come hard. With the major factories shut down the daily wage workers are suffering, but to the point of homelessness and famine, should not be the thing to swollen eyes. There is a need for stricter rules and stricter laws regarding such conditions of pandemic.

As per the latest news, there have been more than 5 million daily wage workers who have migrated because of reasons such as:
• Shortage of food
• Living condition
• Scarcity of resources
• Loss of money
• Medical emergencies.

These reasons do not account for it all but draw a picture where the entire chaotic situation flashes in front of the eyes. Therefore the laws should be stricter not only to protect nations but to protect the people in it.

CONCLUSION

CSR as a concept is deeply engraved in corporate lifestyle, but it still remains hidden under the shadow of obstacles such as lack of solid actions. Even today after so many years of introduction, it is still a challenge for CSR to see clearly what indicators to use and rely upon. It is still a challenge to mix all the disciples of the society into one and start with a healthy idea in mind. The more aggressive approach towards the topic is to inspire transparency and promote business ethics and discussion and also to raise standards of the working in the corporate work environment. However, there will remain many parts which will act like an inhibitors in the CSR world and with new Covid Pandemic they act like evils of the society. Lack of education and civic manners has always affected the Indian society most but these agents are only helped with more and more ideas by unauthentic and false data whilst policy makers keep relying on them which in-turn further diminish the effects and efficacy of the corporate world. But it would be unwise to say that situation is not capable of changing and in fact many great writers such as David Henderson in his book 'Misguided Virtue' as explained in a great detail that how CSR is more useful and different from traditional business values. He considers CSR as the greatest and highest hour of the corporate lifestyle. *"Furthermore, Times survey has reflected that challenges such as:*

- No community response
- Lack of Local authority
- Lack of transparency
- Data Falsification by NGOs
- Business ethics
- Lack of government initiation.

These factors affect the CSR most in any community. Thus, the Indian encounter with the fate announced over 60 years ago remains to be affected".[14] It is very important to understand the core of any problem before going for hunting of its solutions. Today Indian villages lag behind way back as when compared to urban state affairs. Most of the policies don't even apply on to the villages that have zero capabilities of addressing such problems.

---

[14] *Supra* note 10.

It is said that there is a great opportunity for any business in the rural society as well and companies have not done enough to exploit these opportunities in proper stances. It is well known that CSR can only be successful when there is a proper strategy in place, by corporate and even by the government. It cannot be burdened on only one and be done with it. The responsibility of a well-functioning CSR relies on all the factors as discussed previously. Communities and activist groups have to work together in order to reveal the true nature of any program, their service to the people is the only way people open up to them and tell them their stories in person. It is not a play of numbers but a play of heart. Therefore it is important to understand the problems and address them accordingly. There are day today problems such as food, water, land, education or healthcare, but people today suffer from greater evils which need attention immediately.

The most effective technique is to work together; it is imperative that it will enhance the prosperity and eradicate evils such as poverty all together. It is well sufficient for the companies to understand what is good for people and what is good for their employees to work attentively and loyally, which will indeed benefit them only, especially for big- Indian corporate such as Tata, Birla and Reliance foundations.

Even after all this, it is important to understand that CSR is still on a nascent stage in this country and it is essential that all including big or small corporate dedicate and commit to performance of these functions to improve not only their own profits but to improve the world round them.

Changes Needed in Indian Legal Framework for Tackling COVID-19

Dr. Harshita Singh* and Ms. Priyamvada Jadon**

ABSTRACT: *As citizens and Governments around the universe are struggling to contain Covid-19 dissemination, the calamity that this particular disaster further has led to a nation-wide crisis which has affected the socio-economic sustainability across on wholly levels of society. The real threat, which will hamper all the sections of society, the main focus and the real aim of all the States actors, Civil societies, NGOs, SHGs is to be prepared and focus on the lessening the damages which are expanding the antidote.*

Even with a vibrant legal foundation, this includes the immense powerful constitutional defence, but the current calamity has brought the whole legal structure to crumble and furthermore it brings out the examination of necessitating laws which shall incorporate the dissemination of the plague by emphasizing life over one's personal choice and at the very time we must ensure that the whole society and focus on the movement of supplying essential goods and services.

Keywords: Covid-19, Personal Liberty, Essential Goods.

INTRODUCTION

Under the List System of the Constitution of India, the very aspect of sanitation and managing the healthy life style of public are the essential focus and responsibility which lies on the State and Local Government, at the same time the Union Government focuses on the segregation, inter-state exodus. Furthermore there are only about Union territories and eight of Indian states which have a full functioning citizen healthcare. To illustrate further, the state of Tamil Nadu Public Health Act which is established as a citizen health bench &manages the health of

---

* Assistant Professor, Amity Law School, NOIDA, AUUP.
** Graduate, Amity Law School, Noida AUUP.

the society, the working staff, and also focus on their responsibility of providing a health supply of water, drainage, sanitary satisfaction.

Further, Union Government's main focus lies on engaging in the practice of managing various precautions and responses, while they also use many other legislature measures to sustain and retort pandemic caused by the COVID-19. In January 2020, the Government beseeched its power under the Disaster Management Act, 2005; further the intention was to enhance the viewpoint and to prepare to accommodate the COVID-19 in the various parts of State. Addressing the widespread of virus as a debacle has enabled the States and Union territories to utilise the very adequate amount of funding which is granted from the Disaster Response fund as a medicinal emergency was brought upon by the COVID-19. 2020, March the health ministry had further on recommended that all the states of India shall be implementing section 2 of the 1897, *Epidemic Diseases Act* which aims to protect its citizen and being a very important signatory toward 2005, International Health Regulations, herein a country like India must be adequate enough to further develop more measure to form an effective response toward the wide spread of the disease. These are monitored by a Surveillance program which was introduced in order to be integrated with the disaster furthermore they are also known as IDSP.

1897, EPIDEMIC DISEASES ACT

The 1897 Epidemic Diseases Act is still outlined further to focus on maintain and function the Government machinery into, full front when there is a substantial menace of a threatening virus is a simple code of public healthcare. Furthering the focus shall be diverted towards the provisions of the Act seems to be anodyne. Furthermore it focuses on only four parts which provide immense power for the welfare of the government. Also the State Governments are commissioned to alter the virus, a terminology which is not yet explained or hasn't been described in the framework. The legislature or the government now is delegated to function water bodied vessels which arrive or on the other hand leave the territory of India. Any disobedience to the rules and authority is a punishable offence which is integrated by the legislature, while they are giving an invulnerability of the government officials as they are essential workers and are performing their duties and function under the same framework of government.

Law plays an essential role in this particular pandemic and there is still so much to focus and assess in certain enactments they are historically passed down by the government. Furthermore, to be describing the history of a pandemic disease in India by SL Polu, highlights, when framing the law or the medical strategy to combat the epidemic, the government's main objective is to guarantee and respect international health resolutions or to protect trade and alleviate all fears overseas of a possible wide spread of plague or disease out of India.

To describe the law by David Arnold as *"one of the most draconian pieces of sanitary legislation ever adopted in colonial India."* These precautions include the compulsory arrest of plague suspects, the destruction of infected homes and properties, the bodily inspection or an examination of people and the prohibition of large gatherings, markets or pilgrimages. These situations have aroused mistrust among indigenous communities and resistance to the measures adopted in accordance with the state. Now, Arnold notes that colonial government had diverted its approach in order to favour out any of the moderate measures, such as raising consciousness about promoting charitable actions, sanitation and creating medical research institutions.

Power of States during a Pandemic

After Independence, many states of India and union territories which include Maharashtra, Haryana, Karnataka, Delhi, and Uttar Pradesh they have entreat their dominion with respect to the legal framework. Furthermore this entrusts them to partake Non-Pharmaceutical Interventions (NPIs) to alleviate the pandemic spread in non-appearance of medicinal to treat the disease. These NPIs have included closing of any educational institutions, markets, religious grounds, malls, schools, gyms and furthermore they have advised on social distancing as well as certain new rule and regulations in regards to social isolation and lockdown. While they have further on divided the areas into three systematic zones, which are represented by the government into three respective colours which show the situation of that particular area Red Zone being the most affected area while the Orange Zone to be a moderate affected zone and Green Zone is to be a protected zone from the virus and such is addressed by the central government of India.

Though, there are still some of the supervisory provisions, the grant broad influences the public servants. For illustration, state guidelines like the COVID-19 regulation on epidemic diseases in Bihar 2020, the regulation on epidemic diseases in Uttar Pradesh 2020 and the COVID-19 regulation on epidemic diseases in Delhi have authorized all employees to admit and isolate any sick citizen because of this virus, if the citizen does not regulate them properly, police officers are forced to use physical force to maintain their isolation. Officers were empowered to monitor individuals and enforce certain close areas. The block's chronology depends on the area; in addition, the district magistrate can also issue the blocks. In addition, freedom of expression is reduced by prohibiting anyone from publishing information on COVID-19 without given any before-hand information to the government which is responsible to further on authorize to thwart the wide spread of unreliable bulletin.

Meanwhile, altogether the competent authorities who have power are allowed to perform certain noble functions by protecting the public, whereas the outcome of excessive force can be a disaster to manage.

Records have further hinted that the State has been bestowed with certain power to exercise against any person who is leaking any unreliable or fake bulletin regarding the virus. Furthermore, the public officers are empowered to arrest any citizens who are gathering in a larger numbers without informing the government or those citizens who are not following the rules and regulation set by the government for the lockdown. Any further usage of unwarranted supremacy deprived of any level of transparency has traditionally resulted in a negative bearing on the society which is in participation. But during this difficult time the government has been focusing on obstructing people from gathering in larger number, further being subdued into unsanitary quarantine and problems with the use of essential services reinforced mistrust between the population and the state. Some people have already died of suicide form fear of illness and there are still many more people who are under suspicion of being patients that might have escaped from government hospitals. The existing structure of COVID-19 allows statutes to exercise intimidating tactics which are comparable to violence which was taken by the colonial government. These activities have previously restricted travel from place to place and freedom of expression, religion and privacy.

Assumed the degree and the level of this pandemic, which needs extensive awareness and state investigation and the use of forced, balance obligations need be maintained through appropriate forms and balances in the habit of municipal authority to guard citizens' interest.

Regulation and Right to Privacy

Modulation in COVID-19 affects many aspects of citizens' fundamental rights. Here, we will test the structure in relation to privacy as a right. A right such as privacy incorporates individual self-sufficiency and freedom as a vital precise authorized by the Indian Constitution.

However, this particular right is also subjected to certain rational limitations, such as promoting the civic concentration. In Puttuswamy, the court of law established certain criteria to limit the provisions of the state and affect the central right to solitude, since any action shall take into consideration or shall be sanctioned by the justice system of the country, the anticipated deed is a must or shall be necessary for the purpose of good faith, which if it will extend to such interference and obligation be consistent with the want for such imposition and there necessity be technical management counter to excessive exploitation of such intervention.

There shall be a bona fide review with the aim to satisfy the 1897 Epidemiological Diseases Act, as its' aim is to avert the banquet of calamity, but detailed proportional legislation for an infectious disease such as COVID-19 is unlikely to be described in the law, the main. Therefore, the structure must guide the delegation of legislative power in the states and territories of the union. Though, the original justice does not afford institutional guarantees against state coercion on the privacy of individuals. For illustration, the legal framework does not explain or provide certain guidelines for rationalizing a dangerous epidemic. As a result, citizens are caught between inaction and excessive state power. In the past, citizens were required to move motions in court to order to let the state to take deed or to protect it from unnecessary state actions.

The Municipal bodies can use the legal framework to delimit mass quarantine (both at home and abroad) and take advantage of individuals. In addition, legal immunity is also granted to employees who work there. Therefore, the law focuses on the public interest, ignoring constitutional guarantees against state abuse. Therefore, the law on these particular epidemic diseases cannot license tests of judicious boundaries on the fundamental right to secrecy of citizens.

Changes Needed in Legal Framework

As discussed earlier, the Epidemics Diseases Act cannot properly rationalise between any of the rights of a citizen with the potential of the state. The Administration can, though, still avail insight from its own previous experiences which helps them prevail from the current scenario which guides them into performing better and invoke certain laws. The recent COVID-19 rules and regulations need to be amended in order to function well with the current society, furthermore to also remove immunity against illegal actions done by public officers. In addition, India has a fragmented health policy landscape. The epidemic disease law is one of those elements of multiple interventions in the provision of public health services. The stricture is limited to allowing EU states and territories to takes precautionary measures in the event of a pandemic. It doesn't create any harmonization and communication instrument amongst the government of the Union and the states during a hazardous endemic. The character of the Union government is also not sufficient (as a port quarantine) in this context.

A vibrant, dynamic and proven permitted outline for communicable virus in the interest of public health security is mandatory to enhance the transparency, responsibility and accountability of the State towards its citizens. India as an illustration of a legal framework with such institutional checks and balances is the Disaster Management Act of 2005. This framework establishes authorities at national, state, district and local levels, and explains the role of each stratum of governments under various ministries. The legal framework also contains certain provisions for capacity building through the creation of institutes, funding mechanisms and human intervention personnel. Rather than providing a secure image for public servants/ministers, the law requires them to act legally. Lawful insusceptibility is only granted in explicit cases such as respectable confidence and achievement and for the communiqué of forewarnings.

Furthermore, the checks and balances on the State arbitrariness are set to rest by restricting certain aspects the discrimination caused while on one hand they are providing relief, allowing for payment of any further remuneration to affected people for exertion of establishment or resources and publication of annual reports by the authorities set up under legal framework. While some immediate spruce up in regulatory practices can curb the Indian response to COVID-19, institutional and structural changes are also play a very essential part and are required in order to maintain a balance between health and security with civil liberties. Even when the Indian government has announced that this particular pandemic as a "notified disaster" as mentioned under the Disaster Management Act of India, the main focus remains that the Indian government doesn't possess any fancy or elaborate laws for a pandemic. A legal standing or a legislature which shall govern the health care system for the public in the current way of life

However, 253 article of Constitution of India which grants the Union the power to regulate the legal system which shall give power to International Health Regulations and further require them to set up mechanisms, framework and institutions to prevent, protect, curb and to maintain the welfare of the public and to reply to global viral of disease. Any such legal framework when premeditated for India needs to pass the regress examination of equanimity as set out by the Supreme Court of India.

Recently, a global activist Kashish Aneja who is also in association with the WHO, made a distinction in association with Article 19 and 21, where he had highlighted the problems which are related to the pandemic, where the rights and duties of the healthcare officers and the objective of travel ban is restricted according to the Epidemic Act of India. Furthermore a new viewpoint was also narrowed down by him where a country like India is unable to function well when it is an essential signatory to the WHO, further the legal base and the values of some of India's legal system varies from the regulations of World Health Organization.

Furthering our objective an illustration, there is a restricted barrier on the travelling aspect of this country, where all the major method of transportation is barred by the respective authorities. The essential cause of this barrier is to limit the travel of the people of this country from one place to another, which will further on lead to increase in the number of infected people. But, the main concern is also taken into consideration regarding the reliability of the legal system of this country, where on one hand privacy of an individual should be respected and on the other hand the government should restrict people from carrying any work due to certain potential risk which are still lurking around in the society regarding the virus. Furthermore an inclusive legal framework can provide a proper funding or can either create certain laws protecting the medical emergency in this country. Furthering the concerns regarding this virus the government could operate certain medicinal examination where the healthcare worker and the public are protected to a certain extent and are not much exposed to the public at large.

International Response

Around the globe, many nations have introduced new functioning laws and have also rounded their own healthcare workers by providing them with effective gears and by giving them confidence boost to work for the betterment of the public and protect the interest of the nation by giving a hand in the pandemic. For instance Australia under its own Constitution's section 51, has achieved an amendment where the healthcare officers are delegated with certain amount of power to actively work and protect the welfare of the public. It is an essential and empowered legal framework which is known as National Health Security Act and all the provision are carefully taken into consideration only for the welfare of the public at large and to protect the front line workers, who are risking their own life to work. These laws are also inconsideration with the WHO & IHR and these legal frameworks only respond to the medicinal emergencies in the nation.

In the a huge nation like United States, there Department of Health and Human Services (HHS) has also delegated certain amount of power to the healthcare employees by supporting them during the national emergency and to further avoid the rapid pace of the disease the government has also introduced new guideline and regulations to help cater to the public. The HHS secretary has also introduced new regulations and has also made a valid point in the directions of investigating the virus cases very seriously by further using there national medical emergency regulations for the welfare of the public. They also gave license for only emergency purposes to approve unapproved drugs and many medical measures for these types of emergency. The power of such legal legislature is powerful and is not currently empowered yet in a nation like India.

The European Union, EU Decision 1082/13 is the main holder of all the legal power for treating any national medical emergency as it endorses a compulsory compliance from the IHR. Both the IHR and EU Decision are the major signatory states which will enhance the countries future decisions during the pandemic prevention. All the major nations have concurred their own respective goals and plans which require ban on public meet-ups or quarantine and with this they have also taken into consideration to further take the property into their own accord. In many nations the private sector hospitals are also a front line powerhouse while they are protecting the public and guiding a safe heath system in the public. Meanwhile, all such actions and measures are taken into consideration India is yet not equipped to protect the mass number of people and they have not yet an expert to advocate certain guideline regarding the public-private relationships in the medicinal filed.

Question of Federalism

The Constitution of India under Article 355 has an essential role to play in establishing certain regulations and in empowering federal government officials to protect all requested states from further external violence and other internal disturbances, by promoting their powers to ensure that regulations binding on the government of a given nation are given greater nation as given greater consideration and are also applied fairly, in accordance with the law. Laws are in place to protect the nation as a whole during a medicinal emergency; laws also need to be changed due to the nature of nations' vast borders. The whole issue established by the state and the government of the unit must also be changed due to the rapid changed in the functioning of the nation and the large number of inhabitants.

Since the beginning of the nations' closure, the national government has taken into account the great impact of this disease and ordered the closure on March 22, 2020, because it took the issue seriously and initiated a restrictive closure within the country. NCT had already recited the rules and regulations modified during the shutdown, to be followed by the NCT resident as part of their daily life. The government introduced many offices and travel barriers to decrease the population with less panic, but as soon as the government introduced the shutdown, the public was in chaos and people were unable to comprehend the essential restrictions that were imposed by the government for the welfare and interest of the public.

Reasonably priced shops, municipal services, electronic commerce and internet of essential, water, animal feed, electronic and print media, fuel pumps, Delhi Legislative Assembly, electricity, banks, telecommunications/postal services, food, take-out in restaurants, pharmacy, etc., may operate with certain restrictions. These measures should be in place by March 30, 2020. Likewise, the measures required through notification have also been taken by other state government, such as Maharashtra.

On March 24, 2020, in an attempt to battle the pandemic which surrounds the world at present, the central government implemented a 21 days nationwide lockdown, invoking the law of management 2005, which shall end on April 14, 2020. A decree has been issued to enact the measures bestowed by law to the departments and ministries of Union, central territories and states by the central government. Covid-19 has been categorized as a pandemic situation, disaster or a critical medicinal condition by the central government in order to cope with the prevalent situation.

By invoking the provisions of Disaster Management Act, 2005 central government wielded the power to restrict the movement of general public while maintaining the activities related to essential goods and services. Taking it a step further, in order to ensure that an accumulation of essential goods doesn't take place and supply chain functions well, the central government invoked the Epidemic Disease Act, 1897. This statute enabled the government with provisions to prescribe regulations and take special measures which helped implement government's guidelines to protect against the virus as well as empowered them with penal consequences in cases when they aren't followed, including a maximum prison time of 6 months, keeping in view the nature and severity of the crime.

Under the Epidemic Disease Act, the government has the power to impose temporary regulations or provisions on the general public in order to prevent or combat the onset of disease. It can also give the authorities the power to inspect "people traveling by train or otherwise, and the segregation, in the hospital, in temporary accommodation or other accommodation, of people suspected by the inspector of being infected with this disease". The NCT government, by invoking the provisions of the Epidemic Disease Act, also published regulation COVID-19 on the Delhi epidemic, 2020 for the prevention and containment of the Corona virus.

A quandary may arise when a conflict will be observed between the directions issued by the centre and a particular state. The answer is twofold. First, under Article 254 of the Indian Constitution, in the event of any inconsistency between the laws of state legislature and the Parliament, the laws of parliament will prevail. Second, Section 72 of the 2005, AMD establishes that the provisions of this law will have a dominant effect on all other laws, to the divergence and inconsistency between them.

Without denial the need to avail the essential goods and services are of top priority. However, it is quite plausible that even after invoking the provisions of EDA, 1897 and DMA, 2005 the routine lives of general public won't be a smooth sailing journey. The goal of the government is no easy task; on one hand a nationwide lockdown is necessary to prevent the spread of the contagious virus whereas on the other hand they have to maintain the supply chain while making sure no accumulation of essential goods and services are taking place. In order to achieve this holistic objective and ensure continuous supply and a ban on accumulating essential products, Essential Services Maintenance Act, 1981 and Commodities Act, 1955 has been implemented. The government placed certain items under goods in the CEA and ensured that the provisions of essential services under ESMA continue throughout the nation.

As per the court of Auditors, it is up to the central government to make changes in the supply of essential goods and services if it deems it necessary. They may make it available at fair price, decrease or increase the quantity, prohibit or regulate the distribution, production, sale and supply of such products. Consequently, the central government issues a notice dated March 13, 2020, pursuant to article 2A(2) of the LCE, which classifies "masks (two and three layers surgical masks or the N95 masks) and hand sanitizers" as essential products until March 30th of 2020. This was followed by a notification issued on March 21, 2020 according to which; both 2&3 ply masks as well as hand sanitizers were to be regulated by the centre until 30th June 2020.

The provisions of the Essential Management Services Act, 1968 guarantees the general public with essential goods and services which is required to live a normal life. Under Article 2(1) (a) of the Act "essential services" has been described as any postal, telegraph, telephone services or any transport service like railway, the armed forced of Union, services connected to any main port, or the production of goods, for any purpose related to sanitation, water supply, hospitals or banks, productions, supply, dispensaries or distribution of coal, energy, defence, fertilizers, etc., or any other related matter of services on which the parliament has been empowered to make laws. Therefore, it is evident that the definition of essential goods is very broad in nature and includes within itself many services.

Under Essential Management Services Act, 1968, all transportation services were prohibited with an exception of transports necessary for essential goods, emergency services, public order and fire-fighters. Services pertaining to health care like hospitals and pharmacies etc. were exempted to be operated as well. Any violation if takes place of the abovementioned regulations, Disaster Management Act provides with the penal clause with a maximum imprisonment up to 2 years for various crimes. This is excluding the section 188 of IPC. Consequently, the government took into account the extraordinary requirements of the current situation and therefore adapted the services that can operate during this pandemic. Unfortunately, the gap in the system is still in a well-coordinated implementation of control measures. Although the Disaster Management Act came into effect in 2005, preparation for mitigation efforts and the response mechanism include coordination and communication between different central ministries, state governments and local agencies, like Civil societies, Gram Panchayats, businesses and citizens are at faults. This caused chaos during the first days of shutdown, witnessing a mass exodus of migrant's workers from one state to their home state. The solution which can be derived from these problems, is to be properly coordinated where the effect under an organised structure with participation of state, central and local bodies in decision making for empowering the pandemic and reducing efforts that have been in place for the time being.

REFERENCES

[1] Arnold, D., Science, technology and medicine in colonial India (Vol. 5). Cambridge University Press (2000).

[2] Calcutta High Court, Ram Lall Mistry v. RT Greer (1904). ILR 31 Cal 829, decided on 13 June, 1904.

[3] Gujarat High Court, Devarshi Pragneshbhai Patel v. State of Gujarat, Writ Petition No. 33 of 2015, Order dated 26 February, 2015.

[4] Orissa High Court, Gandharva Jena v. State, Criminal Revision No. 233 of 1965, decided on 18 November, 1965.

[5] Peters, D.H. *et al.,* Lumping and splitting: the health policy agenda in India. Health policy and planning, 18(3), 249–260 (2003).

[6] Polu, S.L. Plague and Cholera—The Epidemic versus the Endemic, Infectious Disease in India, 1892–1940 (pp. 50–81). Palgrave Macmillan, London (2012).

[7] Rakesh, P.S., The Epidemic Diseases Act of 1897: public health relevance in the current scenario. *Indian journal of medical ethics*, 1(3), (2016).

[8] Salunkhe, Subhas *et al.,* Approach Paper on Public Health Act, National Health Systems Resource Centre (2012).

[9] Shah, A. *et al.* Financing common goods for health: a public administration perspective from India. *Health Systems & Reform*, 1–6 (2019).

[10] Sivaramakrishnan, K. The return of epidemics and the politics of global-Local health. *American journal of public health*, 101(6), 1032–1041 (2011).

[11] Supreme Court of India, Anuradha Bhasin v. Union of India and Ors. Writ Petition (Civil) No. 1031 of 2019.

[12] Supreme Court of India, Justice K.S. Puttaswamy v. Union of India, Writ Petition (Civil) No. 494 of 2012, decided on 26 September, 2018.

[13] World Health Organization, International public health hazards: Indian legislative provisions, World Health Organization (2015).

[14] World Health Organization. Ethical considerations in developing a public health response to pandemic influenza (No. WHO/CDS/EPR/GIP/2007.2). Geneva: World Health Organization (2007).

What We Need to Learn from COVID-19 and its Specific Effect on the Lives of Medical Personnel and Daily Wage Workers

Mr. Pratyush Shounikya*

INTRODUCTION

There is, in general, a very vast difference and a long list of disjunctions when clinical trial and biological warfare are concerned and their connections noted. Although, when it comes to noting and trying to find the connection, we tend to understand how one is the offspring of another mingled with the willingness of a human being to gain strategic or tactical advantage over other people, different countries or their critics. But despite the fact that one is a very important milestone in the history of medical sciences, the other is nothing but a biological threat agent.

Although, apart from all the differences that these two hold, we'll talk lesser on what clinical trial or biological warfare are and rather focus on the effects of what the world thinks of the COVID-19 believing it a biological weapon coming out as an effect of clinical trial and what it has taught the general masses and how the world needs to take safety precautions, now be it the laws that needs to be enacted or what the general public needs to learn and take preventive measures as.

Now, it would be too controversial to say, for the least, that COVID-19 was developed in a lab as a weapon by China in order to bring the world down on its knees but is definitely one theory revolving around the world apart from the 'bat theory'. But it is what it is and even if it is not a biological weapon made in a lab, we know that it is a possibility and if China has not done it, some other country can definitely do it and if

* Student, Amity Law School, Noida AUUP.

China has not done it now, it can definitely do it in the future. So we know there's a possibility and that is the possibility we revolve our hypothesis of this paper around from where we need to understand a couple of points. The foremost being, *the world is not safe* in the current scenario and under the present set of laws that we have to protect the interests of the people and countries. All of us know for the least that the Corona Virus is not a strong virus with the mortality rate being just around six percent[1] till 4th of June'20 as per the current statistics. But despite that, the world has not been able to create a vaccine in almost eight months[2] and since then, there have been more than 6.6 million cases.[3] Imagine what a more deadlier virus could have done to the world! The tragedy it would've created, the amount of deaths it would have caused in the whole world and just the picture of it is enough for us to understand how unsafe we are in this world with the countries becoming stronger day by day, hour by hour and minute by minute yet the security and the safety of the world citizens is, in no manner and by no means, increasing and is rather compromised with the multifold increase of power.

So we will talk in detail about what the world needs right now in order to protect its people from the threat of clinical trials and what the effect of this, presumed to be the result of a clinical trial, has already taught us learning from which we can work in making the world a better place to live in and how, in a way, it is also helping the world and earth revive from years of degradation. To understand that the short respite that we have got shows us how poorly we have lived our lives so far, and to also give a brief taste of how it would've been, had we lived our lives differently.

POSITIVE EFFECTS OF COVID-19 AND WHAT WE NEED TO LEARN FROM IT

"The world is certainly a quieter place these days of the lockdown due to the COVID-19 pandemic. Naturalists across India, stuck at home, are reporting wildlife sightings in their backyards. Twitter, Facebook and Instagram videos show us exciting scenes of wild

---

[1] World Meter, Corona Virus Update, https://www.worldome ters.info coronavirus/?utm_campaign=homeAdvegas1?, 16, Jan, 2020

[2] Live Science, https://www.livescience.com/first-case-coronavirus-found.html

[3] Ibid 1.

animals walking down urban streets. Newspapers report that the air is so clean you can see the snow-capped Himalayas from Jalandhar, Punjab; Saharanpur, Uttar Pradesh; Sitamarhi, Bihar hundreds of kilometres away – something not seen in decades. Delhi's air quality this March was the best it'd had in five years for that month."[4]

These are just a few examples of what is happening around and reading it down to Delhi and India gives us an idea what might be happening around the globe, in general. The very basic fact that the depleted ozone layer also started reviving during this pandemic, gives us enough idea of how the earth would be healing in light of not just the pollution level but also slowing down the fast paced lives of the people running a race in every sphere they can in order to achieve what their greediness is pushing them to gain and achieve. This has, indeed, given people an opportunity to live life and spend time with their families and not worry about work or stress out on the little things that people used to stress out and depress themselves upon. The pandemic and the resulting lockdown has actually brought people in front of things in lives that actually matter rather than the ones they have been running after life wealth, fame, etc. while they understood that there can be nothing more prominent than health and wellbeing of an individual and his family members. The consciousness towards hygiene and cleanliness in the fear of getting infected from or spreading the virus has resulted in the development of healthy habits that people, if carried towards the future, will definitely pave way towards making them a better social being. The very basic understanding that the need to improve health and immunity by having a balanced diet while exercising and breathing in clean fresh air can be the easiest way of leading a healthy life, despite being a lesson very well known but very bleakly realised, became the point of consideration for people who started to understand the importance of it.

But there are so many things that it made us realise we should actually focus on, which we are not and hence should strive to improve. The foremost being the investment and improvement of medical facilities, the other one being the stricter surveillance and stricter laws against bio weaponizing. The laws should be in the interests of our frontline fighters,

---

[4] THE HINDU, *Is nature 'reclaiming' the earth in this time of COVID-19? Well... Yes and no,* Published on: 11th April'20, Updated on: 12th April'20.

workers, policies and decisions to improve their conditions from safety standard improvements to accidental recoveries and insurances.

These are some of the basics that we would be talking about, in detail in the coming chapters and paragraphs. But what we also need to understand, that the good things that have happened to us because of the COVID-19 or the resulting lockdown because of it are all short lived and are brief reprieves that we ought to face and we are just delaying it. After the lockdown gets over, there will be vehicles on the road, the factories will start to function full fledgedly, the people will start running after alms of momentary happiness. And hence we need to find permanent solutions to at least, ease off the pressure on the planet earth and work a few steps, if not multiple, to make our lives easier and better to live in.

THE MOST HARD HIT LIVES BECAUSE OF THE PANDEMIC

Although, it's very simple and easy to observe that the present COVID-19 pandemic has affected the lives of all the people one way or the other impacting them negatively, but what is important for us to understand that there are some sectors badly hit, some sizes of population grievously affected and some sets of people ailing because of the present pandemic and they are all differently affected and are hence suffering.

What we need to do is, understand and examine these present situations in order to get an idea of the trends and happenings so as to suggest and frame rules and laws to protect their interests. We would be focusing more distinctly upon these professions, in this chapter, and discuss the abnormalities of what they had to go through while we were sitting comfortably in front of our laptops *Netflixing and Chilling* and enjoying the '*holidays*' while they suffered under the barge of the lockdown affecting their lives and hampering their livelihoods trying to save their and others' lives.

We have seen that the economy is very badly hit and its effects will be observed over a period of time that too for a country like India which, in itself was a staggering economy for a longer period of its past but more recently as we had to go through, India had to slowly reopen its lockdown despite the increasing number of cases which was a completely different scenario than all other countries with a higher contamination rate which is a result of the affected economy. The government, when did not see any source of revival and understood that the virus is going to stay for long until the vaccine for the same comes and because of almost two months of complete shutdown hampering the economic growth and affecting production and export in almost every income generating source, left no option in front of the government to address and answer to.

There are a few fighters who have stood as frontline combatants in our fight against this pandemic but because they have stood in the frontline, we come to realise our failures as a nation, as a sovereign and our incapability to be ahead in disaster management. Although, it is a sense of reprise that we have witnessed and come across people, organizations, institutions who have come up and helped in managing and recovering from the these drastic situations by means of money, food, spread of knowledge, sponsoring kits, etc. but at the same time the incapability of the government to do the same gives us a sense of fear and distress.

Medical Fraternity

Despite the fact that the medical fraternity has stood as a shield against this contamination throughout the world but our incapability to provide them with the means they are supposed to fight with, stand with they them in times of need, respect them, make their lives easier shows how much there is a need to help the frontline workers by means of social support along with strict rules and regulations. Although, as a result of certain mishappenings against the medical frontline workers, the government of India came fast into action by reciprocating by making strict rules and laws to be kept in mind and allowed while dealing with the frontline workers of the medical fraternity. This came to be known as *The Epidemic Diseases (Amendment) Ordinance, 2020*[5] which defined and made punishable any act committed by any person against a healthcare service personnel, serving during the epidemic, which is an act of violence, meaning *'any act of harassment impacting the living and working condition'* or *'harm, injury, hurt, intimidation or danger to the life of'* or *'obstruction or hindrance in discharging of his duties'* or *'loss or damage to any property or document in custody'* of the healthcare service professional *'shall*

---

[5] The Epidemic Diseases (Amendment) Ordinance, 2020, No. 5 of 2020.

be punished with imprisonment for a terms which shall not be less than three months, but which may extend to five years, and with fine, which shall not be less than fifty thousand rupees, but which may extend to two lakh rupees[6]. Along with that, any person if commits *an act of violence against a healthcare service personnel, causes grievous hurt as defined in Section 320 of the Indian Penal Code,* 1860 (definition of grievous hurt under eight grounds) *to such person, shall be punished with imprisonment of a term which shall not be less than six months, but which may extend to seven years and with fine, which shall not be less than one lakh rupees, but which may extend to five lakh rupees.* And hence it was one such relief against the atrocious acts that were taken against the medical personnel on which DS Rana, Chairman of the Board of Governors of Sir Ganga Ram Hospital was quoted saying, *"This was the need of the hour as instances of violence against healthcare workers, including doctors, were on the rise. Not everyone was unruly but a section of people was misbehaving and it needed a regulation to rein it in as this section would not have listened to reason ... There was no other way to check their irresponsible behavior. Healthcare workers are putting their lives at risk in treating patients, and harassment and violence against them is the last thing they want in this crisis situation."[7]*

But honestly speaking, that is not the only issue they were facing and were fighting against. This is one thing that was easily handled and one amendment was enough to address the issue and bring about a change in it but is it the only one? And is the solution to what the general public does to the doctors enough, to solve all their issues and problems? What about the ones which are part of the system. The ones in which the government, itself, is involved or the lack of proper care and check causes the problem to increase and affect more vigorously. Ahmedabad Civil Hospital which is biggest in the state having 1200 beds for COVID-19 patients, complaint of lack of professionalism from staff and senior doctors, majority of faculties in the institute not performing minimum expected duty.[8] Telangana doctors complained to IMCT (Inter-Ministerial

---

[6] Ibid 5.

[7] DS Rana, Chairman of the Board of Governors of Sir Ganga Ram Hospital, Hindustan Times, Updated on 22nd April'20.

[8] DP Bhattacharya, ET Bureau, *Ahmedabad Civil Hospital doctors complain of lack of professionalism*, Economic Times, Updated 12th May'20.

Central Team) for the less number of tests taking place.[9] This was the major concern throughout the country because it was from time and again said that India was doing very few tests and it should actually increase the number of tests it should do in order to tackle the impact of COVID-19. The hospital administration of Delhi's Hindu Rao Hospital themselves were quoted saying on April 1, 2020 that some doctors and nurses had submitted resignations allegedly due to lack of safety and protective gear.[10] This has been the case throughout the country as so many doctors from so many different hospitals of different states complained of not being provided proper medical kits and protective gears to fight against the virus and look at the patients and their well beings. This showed nothing but the failure of the government who sent their front-liners to fight against a virus without giving them enough firearms to do so. And it is not the case that we were not having sufficient resources to provide our doctors with enough PPE Kits by ourselves. It is believed that Indian exported PPE Kits to other countries when it did not have enough cases in its own country but that is one theory which could not see the light of the day and on the other hand we had to wait for the kits to come from China which were later distributed to the doctors in our country.

Workers and Labourers

Whenever there is a situation of crisis, the worst hit is always the lower and the middle class. Although, we would not discuss the middle and the lower middle class because of certain intricacies that they have in their situation which might range from the fact that they are not provided any assistance from the government in the form of food distribution or transferring money into their accounts for certain basic needs to the fact that they can't even take benefit of the social services being done by people, organizations, institutions, etc. because of social stigma revolving around them in the society. Their problem is a very unique one which requires a lot of hypothesis developments and philosophical dwellings which I believe, is outside the ambit and domain of this paper. We would rather,

---

[9] The Times of India, *Telangana doctors complain to IMCT about fewer Covid-19 tests*, Updated on 4th May'20.

[10] Jayashree Nandi, *Lack of PPE, poor infection control put medical staff at risk of Covid-19*, Hindustan Times, Updated on 4th April'20.

instead, talk about the working class that is, the labourers in their struggle during the pandemic and the presumed and prepared struggle for the future because of the change in labour laws around the country in order to attract investment necessary for reviving the economy.

We are all aware of the conditions of the migrant workers during the time of this pandemic which resulted due to complete lockdown of the country with no interstate movement, except essential services. We were introduced to the daily struggles of the workers as we heard the news of people travelling different states by means of autos, motorcycles, cycles and even on foot. There has been news of people travelling from Maharashtra to Bihar on foot. Hundreds and thousands of people have travelled on foot for 1000 kms, 2000 kms because there was no other means to travel as transportation facilities were banned and they needed to come back to their native places, to their families in this state of crisis and the government, both central and state governments had failed to provide these people with the means to transport until the situation became worse and the courts had to intervene and some Film Actors, Social Service Personnel, etc. took it upon themselves to help people travel from their strangled places back to their homes. There has also been news of hundreds of people dying during this course. All these show the incapability of the government and the unplanned actions of theirs because of which the whole system had to stagger and hence affected the whole lot of population which had to suffer. This ineffectiveness is what I have been talking about and having learnt from this experience, the government should work on so we don't have to see these horrifying situations in the near future.

But we all wish this was the end to their sufferings. It, unfortunately, is not! Now, because the economy is on its knees, the government is under pressure to revive it and to bring it back on track as soon as they can. What becomes important in this situation is to attract investment to increase production and that basically will be the major addition to the GDP because time equal to almost one quarter has been lost and there has been almost no production. Hence, what attracts investors more is '*lenient labour laws*' and that is exactly what the government is doing in order to give what the investors need. Now there have been and will surely be repercussions to the actions of the governments not just from internal sources but also from the International Sources. There have already been statements released by the International Labour Organizations that the regimes followed by the governments should be labour friendly and shouldn't affect them badly. But due to the lack of the international organizations' commitment or authority to influence different countries, these averments don't really see any effect on the countries party to it. To get the details of it, we need to quickly get to know what exactly are the amendments or changes in the present labour laws that will be affecting both, a) existing businesses and b) the new factories that will be coming up, that the state governments are proposing in order to revive the economy but will be, by all means, affecting the working conditions of the workers.

- The most important being, the increase in the working hours in the factories from the present 8 hours to the proposed 12 hours. There's also a permission to allow overtime up to 72 hours a week, depending upon the willingness of the employees.
- The major changes being the exemptions from certain provisions of the Industrial Dispute Act, 1947,[11] which are:
  - That, the organizations will be able to keep the workers at service as per their convenience and will be able to terminate the service as per their willingness to do so.
  - That, the Labour Courts or the Labour Department will have no jurisdiction over the actions taken by the industries and will not interfere in the same.
  - The Contractors who will be employing workers lesser than 50 in number will also not be required to register themselves under the Contract Labour (Regulation and Abolition) Act, 1970[12] which was limited to 20 previously under the act.
- The industries will be exempted from the provisions on 'right of workers' which included obtaining the details of their safety and health at workplace, to get better work environment which included ventilations, weekly holidays, crèches, drinking water, etc.
- There's also an exemption from requiring keeping registers and to have usual inspections and be given the right to change shifts as per their convenience.
- And the most important of all, being *'Exemption from Penalties in case of violation of labour laws'.*

---

[11] Industrial Dispute Act, 1947 (Act No. 14 of 1947).
[12] Contract Labour (Regulation and Abolition) Act, 1970 (Act No. 37 of 1970).

Sad part is, it has already started in the major states and will continue for at least the coming 3 years. Madhya Pradesh has already suspended many labour laws for the next 1000 days. Uttar Pradesh has suspended almost all labour laws including The Minimum Wages Act, 1948,[13] temporarily.

Now the point of it is that these changes that have been brought or are being brought in the name of reforms, are not really reforms in true sense because reforms are meant to improve the *status quo* and stripping down all the labourers of their basic rights, is, by no means, improving the *status quo* and making their conditions better but will surely be worsening it. Like, for examples, there will be nothing or no one stopping an industry from throwing away or firing all its employees and hiring new ones, or even them on lower wages. Plus, these kinds of reforms will do nothing but decrease the gap between formal and informal employment, making multiple sets of jobs informal in nature and of informal setup in absence of the requisite laws.

The most hardly hit will be the women employees across all industries because of the huge gender equality gap in our country. Because more women work in our country in absence of labour protection laws than the men and hence a gender perspective can also help us identify the hardship and differences in experience of a more commonly suppressed gender.

CONCLUSION

Although, we started our discussion from the need for better laws in order to not face situations which can be far more extreme than what we have due to Corona Pandemic as a result of Biological Warfare which has full access to be developed and be used by a country against its enemy countries, we ended on the need for better laws for the workers of the society. We also dwelled upon the approach of the government towards two different sets of professions and its commitment towards the recreational structure to improve from what we have gone down upon.

Such unsympathetic perspective of the government against one of the weakest sections of the society and the most prone one to exploitation in times of dire needs during this pandemic is a picturisation of the approach of the governments to tackle the situation and considering the needs of

---

[13] The Minimum Wages Act, 1948 (Act No. 11 of 1948).

the people and hence there is a need for better laws. Not just for the professions but also to check the governments and sovereigns on their actions not just in their action towards their own people but also their approach towards the increased use of clinical trial to not create a biological warfare for the people of the other countries.

Clinical Research: Under the Umbrella of Corporate and Clinical Governance

Mr. Rituraj Sinha* and Mr. Mayank Kapila**

ABSTRACT: Public health is an essential cog in the social mechanism and the State is thereby bound by duty to guarantee standard healthcare facilities for all its citizens. Health-care sector primarily comprises of the hospitals and other allied services such as pharmaceutical industry and healthcare service providers. Health-care industry is one of the few sectors that involves considerable 'public interest' and accordingly has significant impact upon consumer well-being. Moreover, in the past few decades, an exponential growth has been observed in this sector due to the involvement of major private players. These private hospitals are working and are managed like an organization; therefore require integrated governance in order to ensure proper care, quality service and good health to the patients. This chapter emphasizes the role and importance of corporate governance for enhancing clinical governance in the healthcare organization to establish an effective clinical trial procedure. The authors will further discuss certain ethical considerations that are required to be addressed while conducting clinical research so as to ensure protection of rights, safety, integrity and privacy of the participating subjects.

Keywords: Corporate Governance, Clinical Governance, Clinical Research, Clinical Trials, Ethical Concerns.

INTRODUCTION

During the current pandemic era of COVID-19, everyone across the World has realized the importance of having good health. Good health is a product of joint effort of human being and the healthcare organization. A human being maintains governance in his daily routine while a health care organization maintains governance in its management

---

* Assistant Professor, Amity Law School, Noida, AUUP.

** Assistant Professor, B.R. Ambedkar Bihar University, Muzaffarpur.

and different clinical issues. One can envisage a better health only by better governance. In any health organization, transparency and accountability towards care and health of a patient can be achieved only by implementing better corporate and clinical governance. Corporate governance is widely used for corporate organizations whereas clinical governance is used for healthcare organization. However, in today's global world where private hospitals are working and being managed like an organization, integrated governance is the need of the hour to deliver care, quality service and good health to the patients. Therefore, good corporate governance and disclosure principles at the level of healthcare organization make it more structured, transparent and successful.

In simplest term, governance means manner in which any organization entity is managed and governed. Corporate Governance is the manner in which a corporate organization is governed. It is a set of rules which helps in establishing a direct connection between the different stakeholders and the management of the company. It is a key in creating values in the companies. The similar ethical value is also required in the health organization through clinical governance. Clinical Governance is defined as a framework by which healthcare organization improves the quality of service and provides better care to the patients through best clinical care. The best clinical care of a patient can be done by proper clinical researches and trials. Clinical researches are mainly researches which are done on the human beings as participants for the purpose of evolving new treatment and prevention of certain diseases affecting human health.

Through this paper, the authors try to emphasize the role and importance of corporate governance for enhancing clinical governance in the healthcare organization to establish an effective clinical research procedure.

CORPORATE GOVERNANCE: AN OVERVIEW

The concept of corporate governance is not a new concept for academic research. However, it got importance only after the evolution of competitiveness and globalization in the corporate world. The importance of corporate governance was also spurred due to chain of corporate scandals in different countries including United States, United Kingdom, India and several other countries. Corporate Governance encapsulates several disciplines in it ranging from economics to law to management and is thus treated as interdisciplinary field of study.[1] It is basically a set of rules which governs the management and the administration of any corporation.[2]

Corporate Governance is a system which contains an effective decision making rules within legal, political, ethical and cultural framework. According to **Jensen and Meckling**, the purpose of corporate governance is to minimize the total cost in aligning managers and shareholder's incentives and in unavoidable self-interested managerial behaviours.[3] According to **Committee on the Financial Aspects of Corporate Governance** (Cadbury Committee), it is defined as system by which companies are directed and controlled.[4]

According to Blair, corporate governance is the controlling mechanism by set of different institutional, cultural and legal principles which determines how corporation can work. It provides the power to control such work by different stakeholders.[5] **Organization of Economic Co-operation and Development** (OECD) defined corporate governance as a structure which distributes the rights and responsibilities amongst different stakeholders of the company and also determines the rules and procedure of the decision-makings on different affairs of the company.[6] According to **Confederation of Indian Industry** (CII), corporate governance is about ethical conduct of business to bring transparency, accountability and fairness to all stakeholders.[7] According to recently constituted **Uday Kotak Committee**, corporate governance provides a fair treatment to the different investors

---

[1] S. Li and A. Nair, "Asian corporate governance or corporate governance in Asia?" Corporate Governance: An International Review, Vol. 17, No. 4, pp. 407–410, 2009.

[2] C.S.V. Murthy, Business Ethics and Corporate Governance, Himalaya Publishing House, 2009.

[3] Jensen, M and W. Meckling; Theory of the Firm: Managerial Behaviour, Agency Costs and Ownership Structure; Journal of Financial Economics; 3; pp. 305–360. (1976).

[4] Cadbury, A; The Committee on the Financial Aspects of Corporate Governance; London; Gee and Company. (1992)

[5] Blair, M; Ownership and Control: Rethinking Corporate Governance for the Twenty-First Century; Washington D.C.; The Brookings Institution. (1995)

[6] OECD Principles of Corporate Governance (1999). Available at: www.oecd.org , last visited on May 01, 2020.

[7] Available at: www.cii.in.

and stakeholders of the company. It gives power even to the small powerless investors of the company.[8]

In simple terms, corporate governance establishes a bridge between the company and the different stakeholders. It ensures a fair, transparent and ethical conduct of the directors, managers, auditors and other person involved in the decision making process. It restores trust and confidence in the management of the company of different stakeholders including the investors.

CORPORATE GOVERNANCE AND CLINICAL GOVERNANCE

In recent economical world, corporate governance is not limited to only corporate organization but is required in every organization. The healthcare organization is not an exception to that. A hospital is in many aspects not less than an organization. Absence of good corporate governance in healthcare organization can definitely affect the trust of patient and can lead to several scams and scandals and therefore, in several ways it is beneficial for healthcare organization too. Corporate governance in the healthcare organization helps in balancing the financial sustainability on one hand and serving patients on the other hand. Robust principles of corporate governance further establish enhanced clinical governance in the healthcare organization.

Clinical governance is an integrated approach of improving the quality of patient care. It was first used in United Kingdom National Health Service which described it as a mode of creating an environment to make clinical care flourish and make accountable for its quality.[9] It is a framework through which the healthcare organizations are made accountable and responsible to upgrade the quality of their services to safeguard the highest standards of patient care through professional performance, resource allocation, risk management and patient satisfaction. Clinical governance also emphasizes on the proper training of medical and para-medical professionals, research and development in the new field of

---

[8] Report of the Uday Kotak Committee on Corporate Governance, formed by SEBI, Available at: https://www.sebi.gov.in/web/?file=../../../sebi_data/attachdocs/oct-2017/1509102194616.pdf#page=3&zoom=auto,-22,844.

[9] Scally and Donaldson, 1998.

medicine, assessment of services provided to the patients on the basis of expenditure and clinical trials.

In simple terms, clinical governance can be defined as governance of clinical process. A proper care of the patient depends upon the environment and the governance of the healthcare organization in which all the clinicians work together and therefore, it required a commitment at all levels of the management in the organization. It is about creating a culture in the healthcare organization whereby the health care providers are educated regarding the respect, support and fairness towards the patient health and care in order to ensure clinical efficiency and effectiveness.

Corporate Governance and clinical governance are the major co-founders of effective governance in the healthcare organization. Corporate governance and clinical governance should not be treated as two separate concepts but to be treated as faces of a single coin and therefore, it brings to the fore the concept of integrated governance. Delegation, accountability, transparency, fairness, implementation of strategies and other relevant practices not only required in a corporate organization but also in a healthcare organization. Both corporate governance and clinical governance makes the management effective, transparent and fair which enable the healthcare organization to work efficiently with full and prudent utilization of resources.

CLINICAL RESEARCH

Clinical research is considered to be concomitant with the healthcare sector, especially the pharmaceutical research. It refers mainly to those researches which involve human beings as participants and that are conducted primarily with a view to develop better understanding about the diagnosis and treatment or prevention of diseases affecting human health.[10] Every study that is conducted on humans or uses their biological/genetic materials and data with an objective to enhance the wellbeing of the mankind is categorized as clinical research. Clinical research can be defined as the systematic study in human beings conducted in order to generate data for the discovery or verification of the

---

[10] Vasantha Muthuswamy, *Ethical Issues in Clinical Research*, Perspectives in Clin. Res., 2013 Jan-Mar; 4(1):9-13, available at: https://www.ncbi.nlm.nih.gov/pmc/articles/PMC3601715.

clinical, pharmacological or adverse effects on human subjects with an objective of determining safety and efficacy of a new drug.[11]

This research includes a series of clinical trials that are conducted initially on the animals but are designed to test the safety and therapeutic efficacy of the potential drug on the human health. Since these trials involve active interventions on animals and human beings, there are certain ethical concerns about these trials which need to be addressed. Clinical trials are considered to be essential part of the process of drug development and research as they contribute significantly towards the diagnosis, treatments and prevention of harmful diseases that affect human life. These trials are considered to be the fastest, secured and the finest way to determine and assess the impact of prospective drugs upon the life threatening diseases.[12]

Prior to the conduct of clinical trials, certain pre-clinical research is also conducted at the laboratories. In every drug development, a team of scientists and researchers study, evaluate and analyze various molecules or combinations with an objective to find those combinations which can be further developed into a potential drug as an efficacious medicine/ treatment of a particular disease. Once these molecules are discovered, they are tested onto animals in order to analyze its safety and therapeutic efficacy.[13] After repeated tests on animals, the results are analysed which enables the scientists to determine that whether these are fit to be tested on human beings or not. This is considered to be one of the vital steps in clinical research.

ETHICAL ISSUES IN CLINICAL RESEARCH

Since clinical research involves active intervention on human subjects, several ethical issues are involved therein that emphasize upon the protection of rights, safety and well-being of the research participants.[14]

---

[11] Clinical Research and Healthcare, available at: https://www.icriindia.com/industry/clinical-research-healthcare.

[12] Christine Grady, RN, *Clinical Trials*, Hastings Centre Bioethics Briefings, available at: https://www.thehastingscenter.org/briefingbook/clinical-trials.

[13] *Ibid.*

[14] Ahmad W. and Moeen Al-Sayed, *Human Subjects in Clinical Trials: Ethical Considerations and Concerns*, available at: https://www.oatext.com/human-subjects-in-clinical-trials-ethical-considerations-and-concerns.php.

These clinical researches are therefore, required to be conducted in an ethical, transparent and fair manner. Established clinical governance achieved through proper and well-structured corporate governance in the healthcare organization thus becomes important to rule out any violation of ethics or principles involved in a clinical research.

The world has already witnessed the horrific aspect of clinical research that took place in Germany during the Second World War infamously known as the 'Nuremberg Trial'. Such unethical practices adopted by the Germans at the Nazi Cantonment led to the realization about the need for regulation of clinical research.[15] This further led to the development of the 'Nuremberg Code' in year 1947 and accordingly towards the 'Declaration of Helsinki', as adopted by the World Medical Association in 1964.[16]

These ethical concerns relating to clinical research have not been confined to the healthcare sector, but have been considered as another facet of human rights. It is pertinent to mention here that the International Convention on Civil and Political Rights (ICCPR) has also recognized this aspect by expressly providing under Article 7 that no person shall be subjected to the medical or scientific experimentation without his free consent.[17] Further the International Conference for Harmonization was held in the year 1996 wherein certain guidelines regarding clinical research were adopted that are popularly known as 'Good Clinical Practice'. These international guidelines have been developed in order to ensure the design, conduct, implementation, monitoring, audit, analysis and reporting of all clinical trials is done ethically. These guidelines mandate, all experiments/trials shall be performed in conformity with the ethical principles while maintaining objective evidence of research, keeping in view the risk factors involved. The guidelines also emphasize upon formal documentations regarding prior informed consent of the subject and standard confidentiality and adequate remuneration. It further underlines the aspect of qualified and well trained trial staffs. Overall, they seek to protect the basic rights of the subjects while maintaining their integrity and confidentiality intact.[18]

---

[15] *Supra* note 16.

[16] *Ibid.*

[17] Edward J. Mills and Sonal Singh, *Health, Human Rights and the Conduct of Clinical Research within Oppressed Populations*, Global Health 2007; 3:10, available at: https://www.ncbi.nlm.nih.gov/pmc/articles/PMC2174446.

[18] *Supra* note 16.

Prior-Informed Consent

One of the most essential aspects of clinical research is the seeking the consent of the human participants for conducting research. The element of prior informed consent has been incorporated in order to make aware the participating subjects about their basic rights, involved risk and subsequent benefit before involving in any clinical trial. This process is initiated by an oral discussion with the prospective subjects where the 'principal investigator' is responsible to clarify all relevant nuances of the research viz., its objectives; risks and benefits that may accrue to the subject as the result of trials.[19] The investigator has to ensure that all terms, conditions and information have been fully understood by the subject before the grant of his voluntary approval for participation in the concerned trial. Informed consent signifies that it is free from any form of coercion or undue influence. Afterwards, all the terms are required to be formally documented in a language that is well understood by the subject. Everything related to the process of the trials including the role of the subject must be incorporated precisely in clear and unambiguous terms.

Recruitment of the 'Subjects'

Subject recruitment is another vital aspect of clinical research. This process is initiated by a communication between the researchers to the prospective participants aimed at recruiting appropriate participants representing the target population.[20] It is relevant to mention here that determining 'target population' is also equally crucial to the success of the clinical research. Since it depends on various factors i.e. research objective; nature of treatment; nature of disease etc., the researcher has to carefully identify the target population as prospective subjects for his research. Further poor recruitment may lead to wastage of resources, increase in costs of research and may have an adverse impact.[21]

Remuneration for Human Subjects

Payment of remuneration and other pecuniary benefits to the participating subjects is a regular feature of clinical research. The remuneration is being

---

[19] *Supra* note 16.

[20] *Ibid.*

[21] *Ibid.*

paid to the participants as 'fair compensation' for devoting their time and effort towards the research. It is often paid with a view to enhance participation. However, some argue that money cannot be reason for the humans to be subject to clinical trials. Most of the healthy volunteers may desire to participate in the trials out of curiosity, altruism or with a view to contribute towards the advancement of healthcare for the benefit of mankind. It is also argued that monetary compensation as 'driving force' towards seeking participation of human beings jeopardizes the voluntary decision making and rational thinking.[22] Whereas, it is pertinent to mention that financial incentives in the form of fair and reasonable compensation are considered to be an essential facet of the research as it is given as a recognition of the valuable contribution of the participating subjects towards the research. Moreover, it is also considered to be vital in enhancing trust building amongst the investigators and participants.[23]

Protection of Vulnerable Population

'Vulnerable population' mainly comprises of children, minor, pregnant women, differently-abled, old aged persons, prisoners, people suffering from critical-illness and ethnic minorities. Being the most-disadvantaged segment of general population, these people require utmost care and particular attention of the regulatory bodies during clinical research. The issues regarding protection of rights and wellbeing; security; confidentiality and privacy of vulnerable groups is major concern for the regulatory bodies since these people are more prone to be exploited. It is to be ensured that the clinical research that involves vulnerable subjects is designed in such manner while considering all factors essential towards safeguarding their interests. In such cases, the process of prior informed consent must ensure the use of appropriate tools by the investigator in order to enhance the quality of consent process by making the vulnerable subjects well aware about all aspects of the research in hand. Further it is also to be ensured that transparency is being maintained at all levels of research and adequate fair compensation is also provided to the participants acknowledging their contribution towards the research.[24]

---

[22] *Supra* note 16.

[23] *Ibid.*

[24] *Ibid.*

Thus, the above ethical considerations are required to be complied by the healthcare sector in order to ensure transparent process of clinical research while protecting the interest of the participating subjects' vis-à-vis the organization and the larger interest of the mankind. Carrying on clinical research in an ethical and transparent manner can only be achieved if and only if the healthcare organization complies with the principles and components attached to the corporate and clinical governance.

CONCLUSION

During the current era of pandemic due to COVID-19, the importance of clinical research and trial towards the search of potential vaccination has been realized. It is considered as a key tool of research in healthcare sector for proper patient care by testing the safety and the effectiveness of medicines and medical equipment. It is helpful in discovering new methods of diagnosis and treatment of diseases to stop it from spreading and becoming a threat to the mankind. However, any clinical research should not pose a threat to rights or ethics involved of any human being or society at large. Many opine that it is a profit-driven process which is conducted on humans. Perception like this can be countered by showing the full compliance of governance in the healthcare sector. One should understand the importance of corporate governance and clinical governance, rather than integrated governance, in the conduct of clinical research. In order to safeguard the interest of all the stakeholders of the healthcare sector, compliance of principles attached to such integrated governance has now become the need of the hour before every clinical research or else not the disease but the unregulated clinical research can prove fatal to the society and the mankind.

Re-Examining the Ambit of Clinical Trials under Intellectual Property Law in India

Ms. Aarushi Relan*

ABSTRACT: "The scope and opportunities of any field nowadays is incredible and beyond belief. The medicine industry is curing Alzheimer's disease in mice. That is called proof-of-concept study that indicates the drug companies are taking on clinical trials. They are also investing, however, there are many aspects that may work in Alzheimer's patients that don't have access to intellectual property or patentability rights." stated John Trojanowski. This thought indulged great academicians and clinical researchers to explore the scope of clinical trials in intellectual property (IP), per se. The commercialization has led to rebut or debate various aspects of clinical trials in Intellectual Property Rights (IPR).[1] Various researchers and law scholars have explored the dimension of clinical trials within the horizon of Article 39 of Agreement on Trade-Related Aspects of Intellectual Property Rights also known as TRIPs. This paper shall discuss on the role of IP in serving importance to clinical trials which helps to furnish the general public. It shall further state the relationship of clinical trials with benefit sharing which has been explained in fields like biodiversity under Convention of Bio-diversity (CBD). It is necessary that stringent management is enforced for IP rights in context with the clinical trials. In India, this industry has experienced a steady increase in last decade. It has emerged as one of the most renowned global destinations for clinical trials over years. A changed Intellectual Property Regime after the World Trade Organization has led to prime mover of the stated phenomenon and maximization of profits rather

---

* Graduate, Amity Law School, Noida, AUUP.

[1] World Intellectual Property Organization, TRIPS Agreement, Article 39.3 asserts that "Members States of the agreement are required to seek the approval for the manufacturing of pharmaceuticals or drugs, agricultural-based chemical products or novel chemical entities must submit the undisclosed data or test information along with the origination of such considerable effort, in order to protect such data against unfair commercial exploitation".

than serving various altruistic motives and forms in the ideological
underpinning in the rise of clinical trials of the Indian Industry.[2] The research
paper will in determine the meaning of clinical trial, its relation with IPR
and health sector, to what extend the clinical trials be protected by different
forms of IPR and lastly, explain the scope of clinical trials under the ambit of
IPR. The paper concludes with various suggestions and strategies by the
researcher.

DEFINING CLINICAL TRIALS

Any diagnostic experiment which is undertaken to administer or
dispense a pharmaceutical drug can be defined as a clinical trial. Such
an experiment can serve its purpose for one or more human subjects. The
clinical trials are a broader term being classified by a desired set of goals,
audience and phases. It is also concentrated towards goals safety, efficacy,
pharmaceuticals etc. The clinical trials fall within the ambit of clinical
research. The branch of medicine which helps in scrutinizing an effective
medication procedure, safety of general public, symptomatic products
extended and determined towards wide human usage. The clinical research
includes various studies within the purview of clinical research. Safety
studies with regard to clinical trial include testing a drug, duration and
frequency. The other form of study known as efficacy study is designed to
analyze the effects or results of the medicine being manufactured in a
clinical trial. Other forms of studies include Pharmacokinetic, Bio-
equivalency and Pharmacological concepts which further fall under the
scope of Clinical trials.[3]

Clinical Trial falls within the ambit of clinical research which comprises of
observational studies and clinical trials.[4] The clinical research is typically
used to prevent, treat and diagnose the symptoms of a disease. It is
integral to note that clinical research is in complete contrast to clinical or

---

[2] Vikas Bajpai, Rise of Clinical Trials Industry in India, International Scholarly Research Notices (May. 2, 2020, 2:49 AM), https://www.hindawi.com/journals/isrn/2013/167059.

[3] Spilker Bert, Guide to Clinical Trials (1st ed. 1991); Leslie G. Portney, Foundations of Clinical Research (4th ed., 2020).

[4] HSS, *Clinical Trials, What are clinical trials and studies* (Apr. 30, 2020, 1:24 PM), of decision affiliated agencieses the trial.nsor of such clincial right of distrubtion, such generic medicine or drug manu www.nih.gov/health/what-clinical-trials-studies.

medicinal practice exercised by doctors. In the medicinal practice, such experimented procedures through rigorous Research and Development (R&D) are being used in operations and treatments. It is important to establish the clinical research evidence as a form of treatment after being collected.[5] The terminology 'Clinical Research' can refer to an entire bibliography of a drug or pharmaceutical from the scratch i.e. inception in lab till introduction in the consumer market. Therefore, a clinical research can be defined as a branch of medical sciences that helps in determination of safety, effectiveness of a drug or medicine, diagnostic techniques or methods and treatment procedures which are intended for human usage.[6]

The stakeholders involved in the clinical trial procedure include Scientists, academicians, the government, sponsors, clinical research organization (CRO), regulatory agencies of such state, investigators and their staff etc. Sponsors can be regarded as various individuals, pharmaceutical companies, academic institutions, private or public organization especially determined as an artificial person, in order to initiate a clinical trial.[7] The specified duty of an investigator in the clinical trial procedure is to conduct the trial. Such associated bodies or agencies aids the medical researcher to obtain monetary benefits, novel medicinal or scientific equipment, gain reputation, increase the work force involved and publish journals or articles with regard to clinical trials.[8]

In the progression phase, the stakeholders like regulatory agencies assist in serving a very vital role in conduction of a sponsorship for a drug or pharmaceutical. The various causes for restructuration of an activity associated with Research & Development (R&D) ranging from various changes in patent laws to the practices been extended towards an upstream visionary of science. The selection of sponsors by likes of CROs and investigators usually has to be considered by the client population, the study of reputation, cost and expenses, rights of publication, ownerships

---

[5] J.W. Creswell, *Educational research – Planning, conducting and evaluating quantitative and qualitative research,* 2008, p. 300, ISBN 0-13-613550-1.

[6] Pharmatutor, Clinical Research: Trials & Scope (May 1, 2020, 8:05 AM), https://www.pharmatutor.org/articles/clinical-research-trials-scope.

[7] James Lind Institute, *Major Players in Clinical Research* (May 1, 2020, 4:34 AM), https://www.jli.edu.in/blog/major-players-in-clinical-research.

[8] Allison R. Baer, *Clinical Investigator Responsibilities*, US National Library of Medicine, National Institute of Health, 2011 Mar, 7(2), p. 124–128.

related to IP in order to process a clinical trial. It is a very rare situation where CROs and investigators will agree to sponsor the right to publish for study of further results and notions. Moreover, the financial and academic institutions have conflicts for prior IP Rights over such procedures.[9] Eventually, universities and clinical research labs have aided several clinical trial specialists in promotion of commercialization and provide financial innovation.[10]

In United States of America, the imputation and ratification of the medicines or drugs is being managed by the Centre for Drug Evaluation and Research. The Centre is a division under Food and Drug Administration department. Although, it is integral that the novel medication or vaccination is approved in advance by the general public. A duration of eight and a half years is required for the study and testing a new potential drug. In India, the department held chargeable for the clinical trial pretermission, ratification and supervision is called Central Drugs Standard Control Organization (CDSCO).[11]

DEFINING INTELLECTUAL PROPERTY RIGHTSIN CONTEXT TO HEALTH SECTOR AND CLINCIAL TRIALS

Intellectual Property Rights can be defined as a creation of mind which can be literary or musical work, symbol, invention, name, shape, design, geographical indicator or combination of colors. It has been divided into two categories: Industrial Property and Copyrights.[12]IP can be protected through various implementation of laws, these laws include: patents, copyrights and trademarks which not only helps to earn certain recognition but also monetary benefits to the people for the creation and inventions of certain goods and services. TRIPs is considered the most essential and extensive agreement based on IPR. It came into force on 1st January in the year 19995 and was binding on all the members of WTO i.e. World

---

[9] Applied Clinical Trials, *Investigators' experiences cooperation with CROs in Clinical Trials in Finland*, Dec 2015.

[10] I.M. Cockburn, IPR and Pharmaceuticals: Challenges for Economic Research, (Apr. 29, 2020, 8:59 AM), www.wipo.int pubds/en/wipo_pub_10-chapter5.pdf.

[11] NIAID ClinRegs, Regulatory Authority, (Apr. 29, 2020, 9:10 AM), https://clinregs. niaid.nih.gov/country/india#regulatory_authority.

[12] World Intellectual Property Organization, What is IP? (9:45 AM, Apr. 29, 2020), https://www.wipo.int/about-ip/en.

Trade Organizations. The agreement vividly consists of various forms of IP tools like patent, trademark, copyright, plant varieties, geographical indications, trade secrets etc. The agreement helps to govern the laws related to intellectual property rights and also lays down certain standard guidelines for the country members to follow in order to protect effective and adequate protection of intellectual property rights. Intellectual property is basically the intangible assets, which includes inventions, brands, new technologies, source code and other artistic works.

IP has served as a crucial branch in various fragments of the society including science and technology. In context with clinical trials, the IP is making space in the public sector quite steadily. The IP Management has helped in maximizing the opportunity of converting the medications and vaccinations established through R&D into operational tools.[13] However, in IP, it is difficult to strike a balance between the societal and personal interests. It is integral to note that in such situations, commercial interests of the clinical trials must match with the public interests. To harmonize the situation, symmetry must be maintained to attain the confidence of the data scrutinized and commitment to administer an educational dissemination of results from such invention in order to promote the welfare of society at large.[14]As G. Tansey accurately puts it together and states that, *"Health is just one such field or area which is most affected by the struggles over the fact who will control and benefit from the scientific and technological changes as stated".*[15] Tabuman's observation with regard to IPR in 'access and benefit sharing' states that *"the struggle to combat the human disease and promotion of health is inherently an internationalized characteristic, which is an element also recognized for maintenance of peace and security."*[16]

The above stated findings from the renowned researchers reflect that the clinical trials act as an integral tool for the medicinal scholars. Nonetheless, the IP rights have been considered as a barrier. The personal rights favored to the clinical trial specialist have restricted the data to be shared,

---

[13] D.A. Chokshi, M. Parker & D.P. Kwiakowskia, Data Sharing and IP in Genomic Epidemiology Network, Bulletin of the WHO, 2006, Vol. 84, p. 382–387 at 383.

[14] K. Leibowitz and V. Sheckler, Negotiating CT Agreements, The Raj Devices, Sept.–Oct. 2006 at 289–292.

[15] G. Tansey, *Negotiating Health: IP and access to medicines*, 2006, 2.

[16] Tabuman, *The IPS and Biomedical Search*, 10 *AAPS Journal*, 526–536 (2008).

compromised or disseminated to the general public. If such information is circulated, it might result in a contradiction between the trade secret or confidential information and public health care system. In order to attain and achieve 'access and benefit sharing', collaboration has to be shaped and formed. In India, per se, the Clinical Trials have not been reasonably safeguarded by the existing IP tools. Henceforth, it is essential to recognize the Clinical Trials as a new product of IP. As per the recent statistics, the mediocre cost of bearing and progressing a new pharmaceutical drug has reached from 230 million dollars in 1987 to 800 million dollars in 2000. The potential and sliding increase in the healthcare sector is due to inflation, but the increase in clinical trial was, however, acute. It has accelerated its cost almost 5–6 times more than the pre-existing clinical trials.

Just like various modes of IP, clinical trial encourages investment mainly for the reasons of creation, invention, novelty, maintenance, disclosure, development and an effective implementation of clinical trials. It further, aids the general public through the cost effective measures and affordable priced medicines. Moreover, the acknowledgment of clinical trial as an IP grants the commodity to be sold, licensed or transferred. Therefore, it is integral to state that the recognition of clinical trial allows an easy global and international harmonization. While defining current forms of IP, creation of a clinical trial does not adequately protect IP since a sponsor has no set of rights or Redressal established in a clinical trial; secondly, clinical trials provide a limited scope for access to general public; and thirdly, the various kinds of incentives can be compensated with other types of benefits. This research paper pleas to determine clinical trials as new form of IP in order to recognize an increased public sharing or display of important information and access to a sponsor's *quid pro quo* clear and defined rights along with clinical compulsory licensing fees required.[17]

Given the acknowledgeable importance of Intellectual Property Law in order to promote economic growth and technological advancement and expand the benefits of biopharmaceutical research, the provisions found in the Trans-Pacific Partnership (TPP) Agreement in order to protect the

---

[17] R. Kreppel, *Clinical Trials: A new form of IP* (Apr. 29, 2020, 11:00 PM), www.kentlaw. iit.edu//files/academics/honors-scholars/ Kreppel-paper.pdf.

biologic medicines is pretty disappointing and lacks implementation.[18] The most controversial points of the negotiation focused and centered on the provisions for the data exclusivity of newly emerging biologic medicines. The data exclusivity can lead to immense danger to public health due to two reasons. Firstly, such generic medicine or drug manu-facturing industries face difficulty in obtaining a license for manufacture of generic medicines being utilized exclusively for clinical trials. In addition to this, in such duration of exclusivity, the obtainment of compulsory licenses might be extremely difficult.[19]

Co-Relating Access to Benefit Sharing and Health

Access to Benefit sharing is contextually been used in fields like bio-technology and biodiversity. Benefit sharing in a literal sense means that the 'providing access to genetic resources, products and services'.[20] The vital disagreements for Benefit Sharing in context to clinical research are that Benefit sharing is noted as a compensatory activity and based on the principle of solidarity and subsidiary.[21] The basic aim behind extending the concept of Benefit sharing towards the clinical trial may be replied in a widespread belief that the procedure is based on 'altruism'. Moreover, the clinical research and trials have found its way towards the Access to Benefit Sharing by the World Medical Association Declaration of Helsinki where it was construed that it is integral to study the planning procedure and identify the post-trial access by studying the diagnostic and therapeutic procedures involved.[22] The part of managing IP rights over the clinical algorithm and information was to ensure the researchers that the benefit of the clinical research participants have been reserved with the right to publish and research expeditiously. The collaboration so far is construed as most beneficial and essential in public health in particular if such benefit

---

[18] Kristina M.L. Acri Nee Lybecker, *Clinical Trials and Tribulations: Why IP Protection is critical to the future of Biologic Medicine*, IP Watchdog (May. 1, 2020, 11:54 PM), https://www.ipwatchdog.com/2016/05/12/clinical-trials-ip-biologic-medicine/id=69014.

[19] P. Andanda, *Managing IPR over the clinical trial data to promote,* SECO/WTI Academic Cooperation Project, Working Paper Series (2012).

[20] 33 D. Schroeder, *Benefit Sharing: Definition,* Journal of Medical Ethics, 205–09 (2007).

[21] 8 K Simm, Benefit Sharing: its history and ethical concern, 496 (2007).

[22] WMA, Declaration of Helsinki (2004).

sharing has been achieved with success of various synergetic action between regulatory agencies and companies in field of medicine, pharmaceutical, health care, safety, research labs and biotechnology. It moreover, depends hugely upon the developing and emerging strategies in order acts as a managerial source of knowledge and provides information for the benefit of public at large through discoveries and its implementation.[23]

PROTECTION OF CLINICAL TRIALS IN VARIOUS FORMS OF INTELLECTUAL PROPERTIES

According to researcher, the clinical trials can be protected through various forms of IP including patents, copyrights, trademarks and trade secrets. The research paper shall broadly examine the scope and ambit of clinical trials in the forms of IP and extend of protection of clinical trial under IP.

Patentabilty of Clinical Trials

Patents are the form of IP granted to an inventor. An Inventor is a person who invents such a beneficial product, process, manufacture or apparatus. Additionally, it is integral that an invention is unique or novel and non-obvious to a person adequately already skilled in such field of expertise or knowledge. A patent owner is granted an exclusive right over his invention for duration of time. Such an exclusive right helps the patent owner to make, sell, and offer to sell or import such an invention. WIPO states that "a patent is a monopolistic right granted over a novel invention which can either be in the form of product or process, a new technique, procedure or process, a technical solution with regard to an invention which must be disclosed to the general public at large."[24] Therefore, it can be rightly said that the patent holder owns an exclusive right over his own invention for a fixed period of 20 years.[25]

By dominating all such legal eligibilities for grant of a patent are met, the law can protect emerging novel pharmaceuticals, drugs, methods of manufacturing in this IP tool. Therefore, the patents may be obtained

---

[23] OECD, *The Bio economy to 2030,* OECD Publishing House, 152 (2009).

[24] WIPO, *Patents,* available at: https://www.wipo.int/patents/en/ (last visited on September 4, 2019).

[25] *Patent Protection – UNH innovation,* University of New Hampshire, (May 1, 2020, 10:12 AM) https://innovation.unh.edu/patent-protection.

from clinical trials developed solutions which can indicate a novel process, technique or application for the manufacture of such product. Nonetheless, it is integral to note that the primary, basic or factual studies are not protected by the patent law. In addition to this, the law acts as an exception by allowing others organizations or agencies to engage in the research process without its infringement. The term patent can, moreover, be extended towards commercial marketing or promotion of such drug.

The innovative companies dealing in pharmaceutical industries face dilemma when seeking a patent protection for a novel medicinal use. Henceforth, it is advisable to file a patent application as soon as possible due to the principle of prior date of filing and an increased risk of prior art. It is also important to add the experimental evidence in the patent application to increase the authenticity and overcome the objection of novelty by the patent examiner. The acknowledgment of such evidence ensures to recognize an inventive step.[26] Signing confidentiality agreements with the people involved in clinical trials, including the stakeholders must be considered necessarily valid. Various researchers and academicians believe that the clinical trials must not be implemented at home and all unused study of medications must be returned, otherwise it would be difficult to ensure the public member who has possibly accessed to a study medication which could be harmful in nature. Moreover, it is essential to carefully select the patients by studying their history and essential information prior to the clinical trial. By performing a clinical study, the inventor gains clinical insights with regard to correct usage of the medication and invention.[27]

Recently, the pharmaceutical industry is under an outraging fear that the World Health Organization (WHO)'s clinical trials limit the ability of the companies to compete and affects their profitability ratios adversely. The newly added WHO rules provide a compulsion over the companies to disclose the prior art and industry fears that companies might refrain from providing R&D in certain fields since information is sensitive to be

---

[26] Lexology, Clinical Trial Disclosures – An obstacle to Patentability in Europe, (Apr. 29, 2020, 7:48 PM), https://www.lexology.com/library/detail.aspx?g=467ab4da-7401-49d3-a65a-f4b74fe95736.

[27] Lexology, Conducting a clinical trial, (May 2, 6:48 AM), https://www.lexology.com/library/detail.aspx?g=492a5008-c243-4837-8512-432122937f90.

publically announced at an early stage.[28] This lays the researcher's eyes on the competition theory. The theory states that a private company, in general, is competitive in nature. The pharmaceutical companies invest their money and develop new drugs which may or may not be granted a patent protection. However, contrary to the situation, the truth is that patents actually help in prevention of such competition, since patentee gets an exclusive right over a particular medicine which prevents other companies from manufacturing a similar medicine.[29]

The Role of Trademarks in Clinical Trials

A trademark can be understood as a graphical representation of any word, device, symbol or configuration which either one adopts or uses in order to distinguish one type of goods from other.[30] Trademark generally signifies goodwill attached to a brand and to differentiate between same ranges of products in the market. A trademark owner has a right to exclude his product from others by using the mark in connection with selling, distributing or advertising the product by preventing any deception or confusion. However, a trademark owner's right is abandoned when the mark is used fraudulently or the rights have been abandoned.[31]

In clinical trials, the contribution of trademarks stands very limited. The only possible area where trademark would be crucial and necessary is while determining the name of the drug or other services required. However, the researcher observes that the brand name of a drug is often not necessary during a clinical trial. The actual name of the drug also stands undisclosed or unrevealed during the procedure by the investigator. But, post the trial when the drug is marketed publically, the trademark plays a very important and valuable role. It is advisable however, to protect the trademark at an early stage in order to maximize the return of R & D.[32] This also stipulates that the registered mark must be used within 5 years from the date of

---

[28] World Health Organization, Clinical Trials Initiative: Patients or Patents? Bulletin of World Health Organization, (May 1, 2020, 1:05 PM), https://www.who.int/bulletin/volumes/84/7/news30706/en.

[29] J.C. Cohen-Kohler, *Addressing the Legal and Political Barriers to Pharmaceutical Access*, Health Economics, Policy and Law, 229–231 (2008).

[30] V.K. Ahuja, The Law Relating to IPRs, 263 (3rd ed. 2018).

[31] 1J.T. McCarthy, Trademarks and Unfair Competition, 86 (1973).

[32] Trademark Manual of Examining Procedure, Clinical Trials, Oct. (2018).

registration. The trademark owner must prove usage of the drug within such specific time period in order to prevent itself from an office action by the trademark registrant. In the dispute of trademark name 'BOSWELAN', the applicant applied for the trademark in 2007. However, after a duration of 6 years the defendants filed an trademark application against the plaintiff in European Union Intellectual Property Office (EUIPO) and revoked the trademark due to lack of usage of mark by the applicants.[33]

The Extent of Clinical Trials under Copyright Law

Copyrights protect the authentic and original work of an author that is construed as a tangible medium regardless of being published. The Copyright can only protect an expression. However, it does not protect an idea, process, idea, fact, method or a discovery.[34] In a literal sense, it is a bundle of right which is inclusive of the right of distribution, assignment and licensing. In context of clinical trials, the copyrights protect various aspects of a clinical trial data and procedure. Any kind of forms being designed for a working of clinical trial procedure can be copyrighted.[35]

However, copyrights in a clinical trial are considered a problematic arena of study since a copyright cannot protect the underlying idea or principle of clinical trials. It is also difficult to establish the ownership and a control over the clinical trial. Therefore, it is true to construe that copyright protection is unenforceable. In situation like these, sponsors may be capable of retaining the ownership over such works because the sponsor's employee create the work and such control of sponsor with CRO or investigator consists in the hire provision clause. The sponsor is determined as an ultimate owner because he acquires the copyright through monetary funds. Various Contact Research Organizations and inspectors are specifically those that are being united or connected with the clinical research institutions and reject to grant to an employee to sponsor and manage the work with them. A sponsor, moreover, is supposed to maintain an

---

[33] Novagraaf, Clinical trials and the requirement of trademark use (May 2, 2020, 7:46 AM), https://www.novagraaf.com/en/insights/clinical-trials-and-requirement-trademark-use.

[34] Stephen M. Steward, International Copyright and Neighbouring Rights, 20 (1983).

[35] Monika Vance, Rating scales: Mastering Copyright Permissions for Clinical Trials, Santium, (Apr. 29, 2020) http://www.santium.com/rating-scales-master-copyright-permissions-clinical-trials.

ownership and control since they are forced to go on site and are not affiliated with various academic or research institution in order to perform a trial.[36] The enforcement of copyrights can be determined as difficult in nature. Being compelled to use a Contact Research Organization or an inspector which is not related with the research organization again, is a unsettling situation which is only accessible for a specific population and particular institute and industry. Further, the sponsor is required to make a choice between research organization and to a right to hold the copyright ownership.

Protection of Trade Secrets in Clinical Trials and Relation to Trips

A trade secret is confidential information protected by a business enterprise. It is information which can be used for the operation or other forms of enterprises that are construed as sufficiently valuable in terms of actual affordability and to gain potential economic advantage over others.[37] Trade secrets are established as 'information, formulas, programs, devices, techniques and procedures' which act as a part of economic value for the business. Henceforth, it is necessary under such circumstances to maintain secrecy.[38] The trade secret law must be asserted and identified in order to be protected against any sort of misappropriation. Trade secrets can be construed on the basis of two types: Technical Secrets which are strictly related to manufacture and improvement of the quality of such good and services and Business Secrets which are administrative and strategic in nature. Trade Secrets also include designs, drawings, architectural planning, maps etc.[39]

The basic proposition of Article 39.3 is to defend the confidential information which is often referred as 'unfair commercial use' in the article.[40] For further context of the article, the required information shall

---

[36] Katherine R. Leibowitz, The Business of CT: Negotiating Confidentiality, IP Publications, Regulatory Outlook, Medical Devices & Diagnostic Industry.

[37] K.V. Swaminathan, Trade Secrets, The Law of Intellectual Property Rights: In Prospect and Retrosepct, 272 (2001).

[38] 1J. Cohen & A.S. Gutterman, Trade Secrets: Protection and Exploitation (1998).

[39] World Intellectual Property Organization, Trade Secrets Are Gold Nuggets: Protect them, WIPO Magazine, Geneva, Number 4, April 2002, p. 13.

[40] F.M. Abbott. The Cycle of Action and Recation: Development and Trends in IP and Health, Earthscan Publications, 32 (2006).

be 'undisclosed' and shall result in a considerable effort. The Article however, has two exceptions attached in order to provide a balancing action. The exceptions include that information can only be communicated where such information or data is held necessary to protect the general public and protected against unfair commercial usage.

Trade secret law is not reasonably protected in the clinical trials since the law is not practiced in uniformity. Various clashing interests either financial or commercial in nature of various stakeholders within the clinical process are in order to maintain secrecy can be established in difficulty. Particularly stating about United States practice in Trade secrets is already a tricky situation. The law varies from state to state and since few of CROs and investigators are particularly affiliated with the academic institutions and industries. In such situations, court decision could only decide by granting the right. However, such rights are too maintained in secrecy which can further be destroyed by court intervention.[41]The trade secret is required to enunciate the purpose and the value of the study which often across as questionable. By allowing the trade secret as a protection in clinical trials, it can be determined as necessary that the information is kept a secret and confidential. The holder of trade secret henceforth is desired to maintain harony between the disclosed information and secrecy of such data. By encouraging secrecy of information in clinical trials, a disparity is created between the public awareness and substantial available knowledge.[42]

ESTABLISHING CLINCIAL TRIALS AS A FORM OF INTELLECTUAL PROPERTY IN INDIA

Clinical trials can emerge as a new form of Intellectual Property in the world. However, the researcher is of an idea that only if such trials shall be protected and meet the necessary requirement and eligibilities. The eligibility criteria shall include good standards of clinical practice, the detailed credentials of investigators and CROs, history and consent of patients involved in the trial, complete disclosure of the trial to the

---

[41] Douglas Nemec, William Casey & Tara Melillo, Protecting Trade Secrets Disclosed to the FDA (May 1, 2020, 11:34 AM), https://www.skadden.com/-/media/files/publications/2018/02.

[42] K. Lansbery, Protecting Trade Secrets in the Medical Product Process, FDLI (May 2, 2020, 1:00 PM), https://www.fdli.org/2018/04/update-protecting-trade-secrets-medical-product-approval-process.

patients etc. It is necessary to recognize an easy mechanism for the clinical trial which can be implemented peacefully. This helps not only in domestic application of the clinical trial but the international co-operation and harmonization. It is necessary that sponsors and patients have necessary rights when such clinical trials are conducted. It is also essential that the trials performed are cost efficient and effective.

The rights conferred upon the CROs and investigators are right to publish the results or data of such clinical trials. Such publication either negative or positive in nature shall be inclusive of a statement designating the sponsor of such clinical trial and the registration number of the trial. If a clinical trial has been obtained as counterfeit, the clinical trial sponsor shall lose the rights, Redressal or associated privileges and shall be held chargeable or accountable for further reimbursements. It is an idea of the researcher that due to emerging laws in clinical trials, a separate committee shall determine the applications related to the same. Prior to the engagement of the clinical trial, an application has to be approved by the commissioner of such committee. The Clinical Trial shall be purchased by the sponsor of such clinical trial and shall have a right to assign or transfer trial to the third party. By recognition of Clinical Trial as a novel form of IP, the benefit is mostly derived to the sponsor, competitors and the general public.[43]

Generally, a sponsor is benefitted the most out of such established rights and publication by the CROs and investigators. The compulsory licensing fees can also be received by such sponsors. Competitors are also benefitted out of the creation of such clinical trial as publication of a failed trial prevents competitors for investing the time in same. Also, by having access to methodology of expired trials, the competitors shall be able to develop better quality of clinical trials, which will gradually increase.[44] The increase in the clinical trials will provoke other professionals to invest their time in innovating novel trials, pharmaceuticals, drugs, techniques and procedure. Additionally, in India, the pool of scientists and engineering will be encouraged to research on this field which will prove

---

[43] R. Kreppel, *Clinical Trials: A new form of IP* (Apr. 29, 2020, 11:00 PM), www.kentlaw.iit.edu//files/academics/honors-scholars/ Kreppel-paper.pdf.

[44] S. Ross, S. Wood, L. Magee and M. Walker Protecting IP associated with Canadian academic clinical trials – approaches and impact, Trials 13, 243 (2012).

very successful. The public shall be benefitted at large due to a greater admittance to clinical trial information system. The main aim of clinical trials will be to provide India with cheap, tested, safe and better drugs in the market place and easy implementation of clinical trials which is otherwise difficult.

CONCLUSION AND STRATEGIES

The clinical trials must be accepted as a novel and emerging form of IP as Clinical Trials have encouraged the sponsors to invest in clinical trials and minimize the duplicity. It is necessary to increase the escalate flow of information to general public and adversaries in the market. The researcher in addition to this is of the view that it shall assure the rights, privileges, and Redressal to publish research decisions or pronouncements along with supporting evidences. The regulatory authorities shall act and exercise a discretionary power over the data. Moreover, the authorities shall be allowed to apply local laws by relying on the published form of scientific information and approval of the competitor's product. TRIPs Agreement shall be applicable for protection of on domestic level and necessary protection of clinical trials under Article 39.3 would encourage them to be practiced more often. It is necessary that TRIPs act as a model law in such situations at an international level and provide a clear vision in their domestic legislations which shall enable the associated or affiliated agencies in liberty of administrative processes, methods and techniques.

As Adriana Petryna rightly states that "I believe it is accorded as a task of social sciences and natural sciences to produce a people-centered knowledge promote awareness, correct asymmetries of such knowledge in their best ability and be informed with consent, protection and safety in medical and life sciences".

Human Rights Approach to Clinical Trials with Reference to Pandemics like COVID-19

Dr. Ruchi Lal*

ABSTRACT: *A clinical trial (CTs) is defined as "any research study that prospectively assigns human participants or groups of humans to one or more health-related interventions to evaluate the effects on health outcomes."*

The process of CTs is required before a new drug, vaccine or treatment can be successfully administered to patients or can be introduced in the market. Compliance to good clinical practices and safeguarding the rights of human subjects specifically, entitlement to health and informed assent to conduct of CT's, is a globally accepted norm to the ethical carrying on of CTs engaging human subjects. Nevertheless, rapid globalization has permeated biomedical research as well, posing fresh challenges in precluding exploitation of human subjects. These challenges assume new dimensions in face of pandemics crisis like COVID-19. Such medical emergencies place unprecedented demands on global supply chains for healthcare products, clinical research and regulatory infrastructure. As the coronavirus pandemic spreads at unprecedented rates across the globe; sponsors, institutions, and investigators are intensifying their efforts to develop novel vaccines, and thus, beginning CTs in search for potential treatments.

However, it is also true that in a quest to tackle a particular crisis one does not create another. Therefore, it is important that CT's are conducted without violation of inalienable human rights norms and other well recognized ethical principles; otherwise there will have another crisis at our hands to deal with.

This paper begins by examining the several important legal and ethical guidelines to protect human subjects in CT's incorporated in international and national laws. The paper further explores the several international human rights instruments under which obligations to safeguard the rights of participants can be imposed on research organizations, pharmaceutical

---

* Assistant Professor-II, Amity Law School, Noida, AUUP.

companies, etc. engaging in CT's. It also highlights the challenges to human rights norms in conduct of CT's that arises in times of pandemics and concludes with a discussion that in order keep pace with developments in field of science and technology and to deals with any pandemic crisis, regulatory framework will have to evolve to ensure that CTs are conducted without encroaching upon inalienable human rights norms and other well recognized ethical principles.

INTRODUCTION

Metamorphosis and evolution to adapt to new environments have driven the progression of corona viruses that infect animals for thousands of years. They are frequently found to habitat upon camels, cats, and bats, and can sometimes evolve to transmit to human beings, thereby becoming a new human corona virus.[1] Three recent examples of this are Middle East respiratory syndrome-related corona virus, severe acute respiratory syndrome corona virus, and, most recently, severe acute respiratory syndrome corona virus commonly known as COVID-19.[2] Out of these three, the first two were not that severe, however, COVID 19 has caused health emergencies across the world to the extent of it being termed as "Public Health Emergency of International Concern" by the World Health Organization (WHO) Director-Generali.[3] Till May 2020, more than 212 reported to have been affected by COVID-19, and according to WHO data there were more than 3,819,312 reported cases worldwide. More than 265,056 people had died and the numbers were continuing to rise at an alarming rate.[4]

As of now, there are no available specific treatments, in terms of both preventative and therapeutic cure for COVID-19. As the number of individuals being infected by the virus grows exponentially each day

---

[1] Fang Li, *Structure, Function, and Evolution of Coronavirus Spike Proteins*, Vol. 3, Annu. Rev. Virol, 237–261(2016), Center for Disease Control and Prevention (April 26, 2020, 5:30 AM), https://www.cdc.gov/coronavirus/resources.html

[2] J.S.M. Peiris, *Coronavirus* (April 26, 2015), https://www.sciencedirect.com/topics/neuroscience/coronavirus

[3] *Coronavirus disease (COVID-19) Pandemic*, World Health Organization (January 30, 2020), https://www.who.int/news-room/detail/27-04-2020-who-timeline---covid-19

[4] *Coronavirus Cases*, WORLDOMETER (April 30, 2020), https://www.worldometers.info/coronavirus

across the world, national and international research groups, companies are beginning to accelerate their clinical trials for developing effective vaccine and treatment strategy imperative to cope with the pandemic.

Clinical trials (CT's) are a set of imperative practices before a novel drug, vaccine or treatment can be certified as safe and efficacious for being introduced in the market. In common parlance, CT means "any investigation on human subjects carried out by pharmaceutical experts in order to discover or verify the clinical and pharmacological effects of any investigational medicinal product(s) and/or to identify any adverse reactions of such medicinal products(s) and/or to study such investigational medicinal product(s) with the object of ascertaining its safety and/or efficacy."[5] It can also be defined as "any research study that prospectively assigns human participants or groups of humans to one or more health-related interventions to evaluate the effects on health outcomes."[6] Like any other research or scientific activity, CT's are also carried out clandestinely through well-defined procedure.

It is an accepted fact that clinical research and trials are necessary for the development of new medicines and treatment procedures. However, certain requirements have to be met, including steps to ensure that human rights particularly, right to health and informed consent of those taking part in these trials are protected. Nevertheless, rapid globalization has permeated biomedical research as well, posing fresh challenges in precluding exploitation of human subjects.[7] At times, in race to be the market leader, many affluent countries, multinational corporations, pharmaceutical companies and research organizations engage in conduct of CT's in breach of existing legal, ethical and regulatory norms thereof.[8] Apart from profit motive, certain exigencies such as pandemics like COVID-19, demand that relevant stakeholders ratchet up their efforts to

---

[5] Shaurya Singh, *Issues with Clinical drug Trial Cases in India*, https://www.rajras.in/index.php/clinical-drug-trials-india

[6] M.P. Lythgoe and P. Middleton, *Ongoing Clinical Trials for the Management of the COVID-19*, Trends Pharmacol SCI (2020).

[7] F.E. Marouf and Bryn S. Esplin, *Setting a Minimum Standard of Care in Clinical Trials: Human Rights and Bioethics as Complementary Frameworks*, 17(1) *Health Hum. Rights Jour.*, 31–42 (2015).

[8] W. Brown Jr, *Statistical Controversies in the Design of Clinical Trials*, 1(1) Control. Clin. Trials, 13–27 (2012).

fight the disease with accelerated schedules for developing preventive and curative medicines expeditiously, and therefore, CT's are conducted at a fast pace. Such exigencies demand that there should conclusive and reliable evidence before potential treatment can be administered to those affected. Conducting a well-designed regulated CT is the best way to get that evidence. However, to what extent MNCs, research organizations etc.......... are following the legal and ethical regulatory framework for these expeditive CTs, and are they engaging in violation human rights norms, is the focus this study.

INTERNATIONAL LAWS FRAMEWORK FOR REGULATING CLINICAL TRIALS

There are several international instruments and ethical guidelines in place today for protection and guarantee of rights of those individuals who agree to become the human subjects in CT's. This contemporary ethical code in research has emerged from a trajectory of several landmark guiding principles that became a bench mark for human experimentation and research ethics.[9]

The Nuremberg Code[10]

The beginning point of a momentous journey of development of ethical code in human research opened on December 9, 1946, when criminal prosecution was commenced against Nazi doctors who used thousands of prisoners in concentration camps for conducting horrific inhumane medical experiments. Majority of the human subjects of these experiments either expired or were disabled for life, thereby, leading to the establishment in 1947 of Nuremberg Code.[11] This instrument explicitly states that "The voluntary consent of the human subject is absolutely essential." However, due to this edict, it became virtually impossible to carry out research in the area of mental disability and other vulnerable groups.

---

[9] Cheryl J. Erler, MSN, RN, and Cheryl Bagley Thompson, Ethics, *Human Rights, and Clinical Research*, 27(3) *Air Medical Journal*, 114(2015).

[10] R.B. Ghooi, *The Nuremberg Code—A Critique*, 2(2), PICR 72 (2016).

[11] S. Thakur and S. Lahiry, *Research Ethics in the Modern Era*, *Indian J. Dermatol Venereol Leprol* (2017).

Nevertheless, the Nuremberg Code, 1947, even without having the force of law, was first international instrument, which introduced and promoted the requirement of voluntary participation and informed consent in CT's.[12]

Declaration of Helsinki[13]

World Medical Association in 1964 gave certain recommendations for regulating clinical research engaging individuals in the form of Helsinki Declaration. The Declaration provides an international regulatory framework for conducting research ethically and also gives set of guidelines for "clinical care and non-therapeutic research".[14] A prominent departure from the Nuremberg Code made by the Helsinki Declaration was a slackening of the requirement of consent, which was "absolutely essential". This Declaration was reviewed and revised in 1975, 1983, 1989, 1996 with the latest amendment in 2013 emphasizing on "safeguarding the health, well-being and right of the patient are solely the responsibilities of the physician involved in medical research."[15]

Tuskegee Syphilis Study[16]

The Tuskegee Syphilis project is often referred to as "arguably the most infamous biomedical research study in the history of the United States."[17] This medical research started in 1932 when there was no available treatment for syphilis. About 600 male from African-American low-income community were made subjects of this study by giving an assurance of free medical treatment and care. These human subjects were subjected to monitoring for 40 years and were denied treatment; even though by then, penicillin was discovered to be the known treatment for syphilis.

---

[12] Ibid.

[13] WMA, "Declaration of Helsinki Ethical Principles for Medical Research Involving Human Subjects", adopted by 18th World Medical Association General Assembly, 1964.

[14] Ibid.

[15] WMA, "Declaration of Helsinki Ethical Principles for Medical Research Involving Human Subjects", adopted by *18th World Medical Association General Assembly*, 1964, revised latest in 2013.

[16] Elizabeth Nix, "Tuskegee Experiment: The Infamous Syphilis Study", History Stories, 2017.

[17] Ibid.

Furthermore, to assess the disease's full advancement, no treatment was administer to the subjects, resulting in more than 100 deaths, insanity, blindness and other grave health issues in others.[18]

This unethical biomedical research on human subjects, without complying with informed consent requirement caused enormous hue and cry amongst the public. As a consequence, U.S. government setup "International Ethical Guideline for Biomedical Research Involving Human Subjects" which promulgated Belmont Report, 1979.[19] This Report delineated three cardinal ethical principles which are the foundation of regulations concerning safeguarding the research subjects—respect for humans, beneficence, and justice.[20]

International Ethical Guidelines for Biomedical Research

These guidelines were issued in 1982 by the WHO in partnership with Council for International Organizations of Medical Sciences.[21]Revised in 2002, the purpose of these guidelines was to assist primarily the developing countries in incorporating the norms recognized in Helsinki Declaration and Code of Nuremberg. Till that time, numerous organizations and committees across the world had come out with several instruments and guidelines covering the same area. Therefore, all these guidelines issued worldwide were consolidated into one comprehensive instrument to be used universally for one common object i.e. conduct of ethical medical research.[22]

International Conference on Harmonization's Good Clinical Practice (GCP)

In order to reconcile the good clinical practices across the world, the "International Conference for Harmonisation of Technical Requirements for Registration of Pharmaceuticals for Human Use" (ICH) issued the ICH Guideline for GCP. The said guidelines were sanctioned in 1996

---

[18] J. Menikof, "Could Tuskegee Happen Today?"*1 SLU law Journal,* 312 (2008).

[19] International Ethical Guidelines for Biomedical Research Involving Human Subjects were prepared by prepared by the *Council for International Organizations of Medical Sciences and WHO.*

[20] Ibid.

[21] Ibid.

[22] Ibid.

and made applicable to CT's from 1997. These guidelines were formulated by representatives from the European Union, Japan and the USA as well as those of Australia, Canada, and WHO.[23]

The ICH-GCP guidelines when summarized require that ethical norms, thorough scientific principles and clearly defined systematic procedures should be adopted in conduct of CT's. Applying the proportionality principle, the advantages of conducting the CTs should be more than the risk involved. The guidelines also provide that protection of the rights of those participating in CTs is of principal significance and therefore, these should be conserved by seeking their consent before hand and ensuring the concealment of identity of trial subjects. Another important principle in the guideline is that the medical care to the subjects must be administered appropriately by competent practitioners.[24]

The ICH-GCP guidelines today are regarded as a benchmark for conduct of CTs, and have become a global law being followed by countries like European Union, Japan and as well as Australia, Denmark, Finland, Iceland, Norway, Malaysia, Thailand, India etc.

Other Important Regulations and Guidelines Regulating Human Research Standards

(a) "Operational Guidelines for Ethics Committees that Review Biomedical Research, 2000.
(b) Universal Declaration on Bioethics and Human Rights, 2005.
(c) Standards and Operational Guidance for Ethics Review of Health-Related Research with Human Participants, 2011.
(d) Good Participatory Practice: Guidelines for Biomedical HIV Prevention Trials, 2011.
(e) Ethical Considerations in Biomedical HIV Prevention Trials, 2012.
(f) Clinical Investigation of Medical Devices for Human Subjects Good Clinical Practice, 2015.
(g) WHO Handbook for Good Clinical Research Practice: Guidance for Implementation, 2005".

---

[23] ICH Harmonised Tripartite Guideline: Note for Guidance on Good Clinical Practice; 2002, EUROPEAN. MEDICINES AGENCY (1997), https://www.imim.cat/media/upload/arxius/emea.pdf
[24] Ibid.

INTERNATIONAL HUMAN RIGHTS LAW ON CLINICAL TRIALS

The fundamental principles of both bioethical research and human rights is upholding human dignity and precluding exploitation of human subjects. In fact, the genesis of norms regulating the ethical aspect of medical research is the human rights issues arising on account of certain specific cases of exploitation in the past like conduct of horrific experiments on prisoners in concentration camps by Nazi Physicians and Tuskegee Syphilis Study.[25] However, there has been an enormous development in the arena of biomedical research, thus putting forth new challenges for preventing exploitation of principal human rights norms in this field.

This part of the paper explores the several international human rights instruments under which obligations to protect and safeguard the rights of participants can be imposed on research organizations, pharmaceutical companies, etc. engaging in CT's.

Till now, several international human rights treaty bodies have come out with limited guidance or directions for pertaining to the application of human rights principles to CT's. [26] The sole significant report covering informed consent was issued in 2009 by Special Rapporteur on health care entitlement[27] which stated that – "It continues to be questioned whether conducting clinical trials in developing countries can ever be considered ethical, especially when using placebos despite the existence of appropriate non-placebo interventions." On the aspect of informed consent the report stated that there was a requirement to "eliminate double standards applied to developing countries," and towards this end the Special Rapporteur pressed for "the most protective standards if conducting research abroad changes the requirements for informed consent".[28]

---

[25] Supra note 7.

[26] Ibid.

[27] Anand Grover, UN Special Rapporteur on the right of everyone to the enjoyment of the highest attainable standard of physical and mental health, Report of the Special Rapporteur on the Right of Everyone to the Enjoyment of the Highest Attainable Standard of Physical and Mental Health, UN. Doc. No. A/64/272, (2009), http://www.un.org/en/ga/third/64/documentslist.shtml

[28] Ibid.

However, there exists an international human rights framework which provides protective benchmarks for conduction of medical research, including CT's, involving human subjects.

Universal Declaration of Human Rights (UDHR)

This is a landmark document, epitomizing notions which mirrors humanity's most profound and enduring aspirations. The initial lines of the Preamble itself reflect the essence of the entire document: "recognition of the inherent dignity and of the equal and inalienable rights of all members of the human family is the foundation of freedom, justice and peace in the world". Even though, UDHR is a non-legally binding document, yet at an international level, it was first authoritative declaration relating to the inviolable entitlements of all persons.

While UDHR does not explicitly refer to requirement of informed consent in CT's, yet it can very well be read in the text of Articles 3 and 5 of the declaration. Article 3 of UDHR guarantees "the right of everyone to life, liberty and security" and Article 5 provides that "no person shall be subjected to torture or to cruel, inhuman or degrading treatment or punishment". Both these articles can be interpreted to imply that before engaging human beings in CT's, their consent to participation must be there.

International Covenant on Civil and Political Rights 1966 (ICCPR)

This Covenant incorporates three rights which are relevant for conduct of CTs-right to life, freedom from non-consensual medical experimentation, and right to non-discrimination.

Article 6(1) of ICCPR protects the right to life which states that "Every human being has the inherent right to life. This right shall be protected by law. No one shall be arbitrarily deprived of his life." This right is non-derogable in nature from which no deviation is permitted in any situation. Human Rights Committee (HRC) which is responsible for monitoring and implementing the Covenant has stated that "the right to life should not be interpreted narrowly."[29]

---

[29] UN Human Rights Committee, General Comment No. 6, Article 6 (Right to Life), UN Doc. HRI/GEN/1/Rev. 6 at 127 (2003), para. 1.

Article 7 of the ICCPR identifies that absence of informed consent is an abrogation of human rights norms. It states that: "No one shall be subjected to torture or to cruel, inhuman or degrading treatment or punishment. In particular, no one shall be subjected without his free consent to medical or scientific experimentation."

Another right incorporated in ICCPR which is relevant for establishing human rights standards in CT's is Article 2(1) which obligates the nation states to ensure that there is no discrimination against any individual within its territory on the basis of "race, colour, sex, language, religion, political or other opinion, national or social origin, property, birth or other status". This is again a non-derogable prohibition against engaging vulnerable groups in CTs.

International Covenant on Economic, Social and Cultural Rights (ICESCR)

This Covenant also incorporates provisions which have relevance for ensuring a particular standard of care for human subjects in CT's.

The most crucial right in this regard is Art 12(1) which "recognizes the right of everyone to the enjoyment of the highest attainable standard of physical and mental health".

However, towards protection and guarantee of this right, Article 2(1) of the Covenant entails the states to take progressive steps for complete attainment of the Covenant rights. But, in this regard, Committee on Economic, Social, and Cultural Rights (Committee on ESC) has emphasized that the duty "to take steps" is of immediate application.

Furthermore, each right enumerated in ICESCR has a minimum core content which has to be made available to all persons and also imposes corresponding minimum core obligations on state parties which is of immediate effect. In this regard, the Committee on ESC has asserted that "each state party is obligated to satisfy the rights contained in the ICESCR at very least to a basic level of enjoyment except where the State party concerned can show that it does not have the resources to fulfill even such bare minimum obligation." In case of right to health, the minimum core obligation will be non-derogable and thus, provides direction in fixing a minimum standard of care in case of CTs.[30]

---

[30] Supra note 7.

Since ICESCR imposes obligation upon the nation states, issue arises that what will happen in cases where CT's are conducted by MNCs or other private actors. In this regard General Comment 14 of Committee on ESC has clarified that – "States parties have to respect the enjoyment of the right to health in other countries and to prevent third parties from violating the right [to health] in other countries, if they are able to influence these third parties by way of legal or political means."[31]

Further, General Comment 14 states "the failure to regulate the activities of . . . corporations so as to prevent them from violating the right to health of others as a violation of the obligation to protect."[32] Therefore, "violations of the right to health can occur through the direct action of States or other entities insufficiently regulated by States."[33] Thus Article 12 read with Article 2(1) of the Covenant along with General Comment 14 imposes an obligation upon the state parties to ensure that CT's are conducted without any violation of human rights of those involved.[34]

Convention to Eliminate All Forms of Discrimination against Women (CEDAW)

Art. 12(1) CEDAW incorporates the non-discrimination principle in case of access to healthcare services by women. It states that-"States Parties shall take all appropriate measures to eliminate discrimination against women in the field of health care in order to ensure, on a basis of equality of men and women, access to health care services, including those related to family planning."

Having adequate access to health services also comprises the requirement of being informed about the healthcare services such as the risks involved, positive and negatives of particular treatment, which is the core component of informed decision-making. According to CEDAW's General Recommendation 24 the "State's obligation to protect rights relating to women's health requires States parties, their agents and officials to take

---

[31] Committee on Economic, Social and Cultural Rights, General Comment No. 14, The Right to the Highest Attainable Standard of Health, (2000), paras. 9, 47, https://www. refworld.org/pdfid/4538838d0.pdf

[32] Ibid para 43.

[33] Ibid para 48.

[34] Supra note 7.

action to prevent and impose sanctions for violations of rights by private persons and organizations".[35] This is where requirement of seeking prior consent can be read in cases where subject of CTs are women and girls.

UN Convention on Rights of Child, 1989 (CRC)

CRCunder Article 24 guarantee to all children highest attainable standard of health. However, this right cannot be fully realized unless there is available clinically tested evidence in new areas of research. CT's in children are also important since same treatment which is applicable to adults cannot be administered to children since they differ in "physiological capabilities, pharmacokinetic profile and pharmaco-dynamic characteristics". Differences also prevail with respect to "receptor functions, effector systems and homeostatic mechanisms. In addition, age, growth and development influence side effects, and the dose of medications is dependent on body weight or surface area."[36] These difference necessitates that CT's specific to children must be carried out for development of novel treatments. In this regard, Article 3(1) of CRC provides assistance to relevant stakeholders to conduct CT's on children by obligating states to take relevant steps keeping in mind best interest of children. However, it is also important that other ethical guidelines should be strictly complied with in conduct of CTs involving children.

Universal Declaration on Bioethics and Human Rights, 2005

In 2005, United Nations Educational Scientific and Cultural Organization adopted the Universal Declaration on Bioethics and Human Rights. This declaration marks a fundamental phase for locating "global minimum standards in biomedical research and clinical practice."[37]

---

[35] CEDAW, General Recommendation n. 24 (1999), https://www.escr-net.org/node/387809

[36] S. Mollborn, E. Lawrence, James-Hawkins and P. Fomby, *How Resource Dynamics Explain Accumulating Developmental and Health Disparities for Teen Parents' Children*, 51(4) DEMOGRAPHY, 1199–224 (2014).

[37] Adèle Langlois, *The UNESCO Universal Declaration on Bioethics and Human Rights: Perspectives from Kenya and South Africa*, HEALTH CARE ANALYSIS (2008), https://www.ncbi.nlm.nih.gov/pmc/articles/PMC2226192/

The Declaration incorporates certain significant principles relating to bioethics. Of these, there are certain principles which are particularly relevant for CT's. These are:[38]

- "Respect for human dignity and human rights (Article 3.1).
- Priority of the individual's interests and welfare over the sole interest of science or society (Article 3.2).
- Beneficence and non-maleficence (Article 4)
- Informed consent (Article 6)
- Protection of persons unable to consent (Article 7)
- Special attention to vulnerable persons (Article 8)
- Equality, justice and equity (Article 10)
- Non-discrimination and non-stigmatization (Article 11)
- Solidarity and cooperation (Article 13)
- Access to healthcare and essential medicines (Article 14)."

CLINICAL TRIAL IN INDIA

India became fully TRIPS compliant in 2005 and since then number of CT's taking place has grown immensely in the country. There are several reasons for making India an attractive destination for conduction of CT's by various global pharmaceutical companies like large numbers of people with a range of illnesses, availability of qualified medical practitioners and other related personnel; good medical infrastructure and overall existence of congenial regulatory framework.[39]

Requisites of Conducting a Clinical Trial in India

Requisites of Conducting a Clinical Trial in India are:

1. Seeking approval from the Drugs Controller General, India (DCGI).
2. Authorization concerned Ethics Committee where the research is scheduled.

---

[38] Universal Declaration on Bioethics and Human Rights (2005), https://en.unesco.org/themes/ethics-science-and-technology/bioethics-and-human-rights.

[39] Mark Barnes, Jamie Flaherty, Minal Caron, Alishan Naqvee and Barbara Bierer, *The Evolving Regulatory Landscape for Clinical Trials in India*, 73(4) *Food and Drug Law Journal*, 601–623 (2018).

3. Mandatory registration on Indian Council for Medical Research maintained website.

Legal Framework for Clinical Trials in India

Apart from domestic legislations and guidelines, CT's in India are also governed by the international regulatory framework discussed above, like ICH-Good Clinical Practices guidelines, Declaration of Helsinki, and ICMR guidelines amongst several others. Even though these declarations, regulations, guidelines, and opinions are not legally binding, but being soft law, they have persuasive value in regulating CT's across the world including India.[40] In nut shell, the focal point all these guidelines etc. is ensuring that CT's involving human subjects are conducted in an ethical manner, complying with the relevant human rights norms, including informed consent and also that there is constant assessment of balance between risk and outcomes.[41] The regulatory frame work for CT' s in India is also aimed at ensuring that the quality and integrity of data collected in clinical trials is maintained and that human rights, and welfare of research participants are protected. Several important legislations governing clinical research in India are:

Drugs and Cosmetics Act, 1940 and Drugs and Cosmetics Rules, 1945

In India, Drugs and Cosmetics Act, 1940[42] is the primary legislation and Central Drugs Standard Control Organization (CDSCO) is the chief authority for the regulation of CT's. The present act governs the production, circulation and import of drugs and cosmetics for ensuring that before they are made available to the public, these are non-toxic, effective and are in compliance with the existing quality standards. It is comprised of Chapters, Rules and Schedules[43] and is revised whenever required, for meeting the international standards and also to keep pace with development in the field of medical research. Schedule Y of the

---

[40] Priyesh Sharma, *"India: Future of Clinical Trials in India"* (2013). https://www.mondaq.com/india/food-and-drugs-law/2476/future-of-clinical-trials-in-india

[41] Ibid.

[42] Drugs and Cosmetics Act, https://www.rgcb.in/uploads/2014/07/Schedule-Y.pdf

[43] M. Imran, A.K. Najmi, M.F. Rashid, S. Tabrez and M.A. Shah, *"Clinical Research Regulation In India-History, Development, Initiatives, Challenges And Controversies: Still Long Way To Go"*, 5(2), *Journal of Pharm Bioallied Sciences* (2013).

Drugs and Cosmetics Rules, 1945 enlists comprehensive specifications, and abidance requirements relating to CT's conducted. The Act makes it mandatory that all CT's or research covered under the purview of schedule Y complies with necessary requirements of 12 attached appendices, follows the clinical trial protocols, informed consent requirement, seeking sanction of ethics committee and also there is a format for serious adverse event reporting that has to filled by those conducting medical research.[44]

Ethical Guidelines for Biomedical Research on Human Subjects, 2000 and Indian Good Clinical Practice (GCP) guidelines, 2001

Till 2000, numerous instances were reported due non- compliance or violations of informed consent requirement. To prevent such incidents in future, Ethics Committee on Human Research (CECHR) and Indian Council of Medical Research (ICMR) came out with Ethical Guidelines for Biomedical Research on Human Subjects in 2000. According to these guidelines, CT's were permitted to be performed only after seeking approval from Ethics Committees, apart from Drugs Controller in General and informed consent of the persons engaged in CTs was made obligatory. These guidelines were reviewed and revised in 2006 to keep pace with contemporary developments.

Also, ICMR issued the Ethical Guidelines for Biomedical Research on Human Subjects in 2000 and CDSCO developed Indian Good Clinical Practice (GCP) guidelines in 2001 on same line as in line with ICH and GCP.

Amendment to Schedule Y of Drugs and Cosmetics Rules, 1945 (2005)

The Schedule Y was amended in 2005 with the primary objective of placing India at par with internationally accepted ethical standards of research.[45] The amendment enlisted the role and responsibilities of promoters, ethics committees, and investigators and incorporated a checklist of crucial facts to be encompassed in the informed consent form as well as the contents of protocols for conducting CT's.[46] Furthermore,

---

[44] Ibid.
[45] Available at: https://www.researchgate.net/publication
[46] Ibid.

Appendix VIII to the Schedule Y made it mandatory to seek prior approval from ethics committee before conduct of CT's. This amendment also did away with the phase aspect in CT's conducted by international stakeholders, but continued with the previous restriction on Phase I. The 2005 amendments, along with various other steps taken by the government like CDSCO's steps to ensure transparency and accountability, implementation of the Common Technical Document format for submission of applications, mandatory registration of CT's in the clinical trial registry of India, and other parallel requirements, led to an upsurge in the CTs being conducted in India.[47]

Amendment to Schedule Y of Drugs and Cosmetics Rules, 1945 (2013)

In 2013, Schedule Y rules were again amended with the objective to make the norms regulating CT's in India more stringent. The amendment provided for enhanced protection of patients, seeking informed consent from subjects, stringent reporting of timeline of adverse events including deaths of subjects, and in case of death or injury to trial subject, the amendment imposed an absolute liability upon the sponsors to pay compensation to him or his legal representatives. In case of failure of sponsor to provide adequate treatment or to pay compensation, the amendment made a provision for suspension/cancellation of his license to carry out CT's in India. Due to these regulatory changes, the amendment acted as a deterrent on the MNCs and consequently, many of them withdrew their clinical research from the country.[48]

This amendment was made in response to numerous incidents of injury, deaths of trial subjects and other serious adverse events taking place at that time. There was also significant public outrage regarding vulnerable groups like women, children, and person with mental and physical disabilities, being exploited by MNCs as trial subjects.[49] In an effort to stop these flagrant abuse of trial procedures and human rights norms, Schedule Y of Drugs and Cosmetics Rules, 1945 was amended by the government.

---

[47] Krishna Sarma and Manisha Singh, Clinical Trials in India, https://www.fdli.org/ 2018/10/clinical-trials-in-india
[48] Ibid.
[49] Ibid.

National Ethical Guidelines for Biomedical and Health Research Involving Human Participants, 2017

Indian Council of Medical Research (ICMR) is a primary body responsible for preparation, organization and advancement of ethical biomedical research in India. In 1980, it issued Policy Statement for regulating ethical aspects of human research. These guidelines, in order to keep pace with developments in medical research were constantly updated in 2000 and 2006. In 2017, these guidelines were again revised as "The National Ethical Guidelines for Biomedical and Health Research Involving Human Participants".[50] New provisions have been added in the guidelines to cover within its regulatory framework areas like "responsible conduct of research (including publication ethics), public health research, socio-behavioural research, and research during humanitarian disasters and emergencies." The provisions regarding "ethical review procedures, clinical trials, and genetics research" have also been expanded significantly, which will be useful researchers as well as for ethics committees.

Drugs and Clinical Trials Rules 2019

With the objective of promoting ethical clinical research in the country, the government has announced and Clinical Trials Rules, 2019. These new rules will be applicable "to all new drugs, investigational new drugs for human use, clinical trials, and bio-equivalence and bioavailability studies and ethics committees."[51] These rules will override Part XA and Schedule Y of Drugs and Cosmetics Rules, 1945.

Salient features of the Rules relevant to clinical trials are:

- "The primary objective of the rules is to advance 'clinical research in India by providing for a predictable, transparent and effective regulation for CT'S and by ensuring faster accessibility of new drugs to the Indian population.'[52]

---

[50] National Ethical Guidelines for Biomedical and Health Research Involving Human Participants,   2017, http://ethics.ncdirindia.org//asset/pdf/ICMR_National_Ethical_Guidelines.pdf

[51] New Drugs and Clinical Trial Rules, 2019, https://www.iscr.org/wp-content/uploads/2019/05/New-Rules-2019_ISCR-RC_21Apr2019_GMupdates-1.pdf

[52] Swati Jadhav and Ravindra Ghooi, *New Drug and Clinical Trial Rules 2019-Two Steps Forward and One Back,* (2019), https://ijopp.org/sites/default/files/InJPharPract-12-3-209.pdf

- These rules have the reduced the time period required for approving applications to 30 days for drugs manufactured in India and 90 days for those developed outside the country.[53]
- In case of death or disability of trial subject, it will be the duty of Drug Controller General of India to determine the compensation to be awarded to the concerned. Also in case of injury to the CT subject, medical support will be provided as long as required.[54]
- The necessity of conducting local CT may be relinquished for approval of a new medicine if it is approved and marketed in any of the countries specified by the Drugs Controller General with the approval of the government.[55]
- There will be constant monitoring of the CT's by the Ethics committee.[56]
- New drugs approved for use in select developed markets will be automatically allowed in India provided global trials include Indian patients."[57]

These rules become particularly relevant with regard to CTs that are being conduct for developing the novel vaccine/treatment to tackle the existing COVID-19 crisis. If any new vaccine/drugs are developed outside India, these rules will certainly facilitate in introducing the same at a faster pace in the country.

VIOLATION OF HUMAN RIGHTS IN CLINICAL TRIALS ESPECIALLY IN PANDEMICS LIKE COVID-19

Compliance to good clinical practices and safeguarding the rights of human subjects is globally accepted as an imperative requirement to the ethical carrying on of CT's engaging human subjects. [58]The process of CTs is required before a new drug, vaccine or treatment can be successfully

---

[53] Rule 23 of New Drug and Clinical Trial Rules, 2019.

[54] The quantum of compensation is required to be calculated on the basis of the formula specified in the Seventh Schedule of the NDCT Rules.

[55] Chapter IX of New Drug and Clinical Trial Rules, 2019.

[56] Rule 6 of New Drug and Clinical Trial Rules, 2019.

[57] Chapter X of New Drug and Clinical Trial Rules, 2019.

[58] Dipak P. Pandya MD & Jay Dave, "*Protection of human subjects in clinical research : The Pitfalls in Clinical Research*", 2005, https://link.springer.com/article/10.1385%2FCOMP%3A31%3A1%3A072

administered to patients or can be introduced in the market. In these trials, informed consent of the human subjects play a critical part which means that the participants should be categorically made cognizant about certain facts like the conduct of CTs on them, process involved, the possible implications or side effects of trial, etc. However, due to rapid globalization in biomedical research, many a times this requirement of informed consent is unethically ignored by the researchers, thus often leading to adverse impact on the lives of involved human subjects.[59] Certain specific category of persons are particularly vulnerable to being made subjects of CTs without complying with ethical research principles like children, mentally challenged persons, terminally ill patients etc. These persons are administered drugs under the pretext of treating them, however, in reality; they are used for testing medicines which are yet to be introduced in the market.[60] One very good example of human rights violations in conduct of CTs is the Pfizer case, where Pfizer, a pharmaceutical company was accused of testing new medication without obtaining ethical sanction before administering the new drug to children during a meningitis epidemic in Nigeria.[61]

Another case highlighting the abuse of human rights norms in India is the conduct of CT's is Swasthaya Adhikar Manch Vs Union of India & Ors.[62] In this case Swasthya Adhikar Manch, had filed a PIL bring to light the deaths caused by unethical clinical research that was being carried out on children, mentally challenged people, tribal and dalits who were not in a position to give free informed consent.[63] The PIL highlighted several anomalies in these CT's like abuse of ethical guidelines and other

---

[59] Mohd. Humaid, *"Legal issues in regulating the Clinical Drug Trials on human beings in India-Balancing economic opportunities with public health"*, (2016), https://www.indialawjournal.org/article-14.php

[60] Ibid.

[61] Pfizer lawsuit (re Nigeria), https://www.business-humanrights.org/en/pfizer-lawsuit-re-nigeria

[62] Writ Petition (WP) 33 of 2012.

[63] Alishan Naqvee& Abhijeet Das, *"Clinical Research In 2015: The Ghost of Christmas Past, Present and Yet to Come"*, The Financial Express (Dec. 24, 2014), available athttp://www.financialexpress.com/article/pharma/latest-updates/clinical-research-in-theghost-of-christmas-past-present-and-yet-to-come/22744.

regulations governing CT's in India, and also Articles 21 and 32 of the Constitution of India.[64]

In Kalpana Mehta & Ors. v. Union of India & Ors.[65], again a PIL was filed in Supreme Court by Gramya Resource Centre for Women highlighting the deaths of seven persons in Gujarat and Andhra Pradesh, who had met their fate during the 'Human Papilloma Virus' vaccination trials on tribal girls.

It was alleged that researchers (which was an NGO, the Programme for Appropriate Technology in Health and was funded by Bill and Melinda Gates Foundation), had committed a breach of norms by not only allegedly using "unproven and hazardous" drugs but also initiating the project without appropriate license from the Drugs Controller of India.[66]

In both these cases, the Supreme Court commended the work of the NGOs to bring forth the human rights violations that clinical trial subjects were encountering and gave directions to the government to modify the regulatory framework to ensure protection of rights of those participating in CT's.[67]

According to Human Rights Committee, which is responsible for monitoring and implementing ICCPR, right to life as incorporated in Article 6 of the Covenant is "the supreme right from which no derogation is permitted even in times of public emergency."[68] The committee has also stated that this right should be accorded wider interpretation and not be construed narrowly.[69] Here, a more challenging question arises i.e. when there is a life-threatening illness which is highly contagious and for which there is no specific vaccines or medicines but only experimental treatments are available, as in case of pandemics like Spanish flu, Asian flu, Hong Kong flu, HIV, SARS, Swine flu, MERS, and Ebola; to what extent CT's posing threats to human rights of trial subjects should be permitted. On

---

[64] Arpita Sengupta, *Clinical Trials In India: A Way Towards Impoverishment*, NALSAR Student Law Review (2015), https://nslr.in/wp-content/uploads/2019/04/NSLR-Vol-11-No-1.pdf

[65] Writ Petition (Civil) No. 558 of 2012.

[66] Available at http://timesofindia.indiatimes.com

[67] Ibid.

[68] UN Human Rights Committee, General Comment, No. 6 (2003).

[69] Ibid.

one hand, these pandemic diseases results in numerous deaths, disrupt global economy, and drain the global health care systems, particularly in developing and least developing countries having fragile infrastructure. Therefore, combating these effectively is the foundation of the right to health recognized in human rights framework. On the other hand, development of new vaccines and drugs require CTs posing threat to human rights of trial subjects. This is the issue which has assumed prime importance today in the light of the COVID-19 pandemic affecting majority of the countries worldwide.

As the coronavirus pandemic spreads at unprecedented rates across the globe, pharmaceutical companies, research organizations and regulators are intensifying their efforts upon conducting clinical research including CTs for finding new treatments and vaccines to address COVID-19. There is an urgent necessity for unswerving evidence for developing best care for those infected with coronavirus, thus, conducting CT's on infected human are the best way to get that evidence. It is important that those patients who are quarantine or are admitted in hospital should be asked to voluntarily participate in CTs and contribute towards finding effective treatment for everyone. Many countries like India, Australia, USA, and Italy amongst others have already started human trials for a potential coronavirus vaccine. However, in haste to conduct CT's, it is important also important to ensure that rights of human subjects, particularly informed consent requirement, are protected. All subjects of such CT's must receive standard full medical care irrespective of their social, economic or ethnic background. Special protection must be provided to subjects who are women, children, senior citizens, mentally or physically challenged, and other vulnerable groups. To further emphasize, 'due regards of human rights of all' is the basic premise of human rights framework, therefore, it is important that even in pandemic situations, conduct of CT's should be well regulated for ensuring the protection of rights of those participating in these trials.

This approach is similar with the one taken by the Special Rapporteur on the right to health in the report on informed consent, which emphasized that "A rights-based approach to medical research means that special protections must be in place to ensure that the autonomy of potential participants, particularly those from vulnerable groups, is not compromised as a result of power imbalances inherent in the research-subject relationships."[70]

CONCLUSION

Biomedical ethics and human rights are both directed towards "protecting individual freedoms, promote justice, prohibit exploitation, and ensure human dignity."[71] Therefore, human rights norms are often relied upon for establishing and reviewing standard of care in CTs. The most notable human rights principles permeating the international and national regulatory framework and guidelines are right to life, right to highest attainable standards of heath and most importantly, the informed consent principle.

However, CT's are often conducted in an environment where the advancement of science and technology is regarded as having utmost precedence for the greater welfare of the society at large. These results in placing rights in a hierarchy wherein, right to life and health of an individual is regarded as being subservient to the right of the society, to have access to advanced treatment or medicines. Such hierarchy of fundamental, non-degorabale human rights raises concerns over whether the utilitarian principle of "greatest good for the greatest number of people" is an effective reasoning for violation of inalienable human rights.[72]

The issue of precedence of medical research over human rights assumes new dimensions in pandemic situation where due to non-availability of preventive and curative treatments, CTs becomes imperative to generate relevant evidence for developing potential drugs or vaccines.

One such pandemic affecting us all today is COVID-19 which is enlisting unparalleled burden on worldwide supply chains for healthcare products, clinical research and the regulatory framework. Due to the anxiety surrounding COVID-19, a situation has been created where otherwise indispensable precautions and procedures are being ignored in various phases of vaccine development.

---

[70] Supra note 28.
[71] Supra Note 7.
[72] Supra note 66.

It is important that, in these exceptional circumstances, everyone involved in bringing new vaccines and treatments should ponder upon the ways and means to streamline and hasten the required processes. The regulatory practices should be improvised upon for ensuring constant flow of existing medicines and development of novel treatments needed to address all patient needs during the pandemic, while at the same time retaining the integrity of the regulatory framework.

It is true that to keep pace with developments in field of science and technology and, to cater effectively to any pandemic situation like COVID-19 that may arise in future, international and domestic regulatory framework will have to evolve. However, it is also true that in a quest to tackle a particular crisis one does not create another. Therefore, it is important that to develop a regulatory environment which has the potential of ensuring that clinical research and CTs are conducted without encroaching upon inalienable human rights norms and other well recognized ethical principles; otherwise we will have another crisis at our hands to deal with.

International Regulations of Clinical Trial *vis-à-vis* the Ethical Cognizance

Mr. Debarchan De* and Ms. Hardika Kukreja*

INTRODUCTION

There has been an extensive progression in the avocation of medicine. Since the time immemorial the humans have been striving to develop the best possible alternative to cure the diseases or any kind of malady that is harmful to the *homo sapiens*.

The medicines that we use today cannot be ingested or consumed by the patients just after they are sanctioned by the Research and Development (R&D) cells of the Pharmaceutical Companies. Precisely releasing the drugs directly into the market is harmful for the public because many a times it is possible that they would be commercial centric than focused on the public welfare. One of the classic examples of the same is Thalidomide Tragedy. The Tragedy owed its epicenter in the Central Europe. The kids born between the years of 1950s to 1960s era were born with the defect of *phocomelia that* refers to the birth of the child with inherent deformities or retracted limbs. This tragedy enveloped a large area only because of presence of Thalidomide in the medicines. These drugs were consumed by the pregnant women and subsequently the kids born to these women were affected by this which claimed to have no side- effects.[1] The drugs containing thalidomide were used as a sedative and they were released into the market without any trials or tests. Furthermore, the manufacturers of this drug claimed with conviction that this drug was by far safe to use and safe to use even by the women with children in their womb.[2]

---

* Student, Amity Law School, Noida, AUUP.

[1] Dr. V. Pannikar (Medical Officer), *The Return of Thalidomide: New Uses and Renewed Concerns*, World Health Organization, https://www.who.int/lep/research/Thalidomide.pdf

[2] J.H. Kim and A.R. Scialli, *Thalidomide: The Tragedy of Birth Defects and the Effective Treatment of Disease*, Toxicological Sciences, Volume 122- Issue 1, July 2011, Pages 1–6, https://doi.org/10.1093/toxsci/kfr088

There have been several cases like that of the Thalidomide Tragedy which have brought us to the threshold of consciousness that there should be a regulatory authority whose primary function is to test whether a drug should be released in the market or not and if it can be released in the market then what are the restrictions that are to be encumbered on these drugs in order to reduce their accessibility? Moreover, is there a procedure which designates or overpowers the benefits of the drugs over its side-effects?

While answering conundrum of the aforementioned interrogations, the only alternative that can be adopted by the Ministries of Health of every respective state is the testing of "Clinical Trials".

The Clinical Trials unequivocally refer to the medical testing of each and every medicine before it is released into the market and declared safe for use by all the patients.[3] In the technical sense, the Clinical Trials refer to the analytical synthesis of testing the formulation of salts on the humans so as to study the interaction of the medical, surgical and behaviour caused from the use of the said drug.[4] These are considered for two aspects:

1. Whether a drug is effective to cure a harmful disease?
2. Whether a drug has more benefits than the harms caused by it?[5]

There is an imperative need of clinical trials as they encourage the stringent testing of the drugs which highly encourages the global pressure on reduction of diseases and development of safe contemporary vaccines and therapies.[6]

The Clinical Trials aim to test the medical interventions on the human and the facets of this can be measured on the group which voluntary comes to the frontiers for this by taking part in the analysis of drugs on the cells, drugs on the biological processes, effects of drugs on the behaviour, effects

---

[3] Melissa Conrad Stöppler, *Clinical Research and Clinical Trials*, MEDINET, https://www.medicinenet.com/physical_exam_why_does_your_doctor_do_that/articl e.htm

[4] What Are Clinical Trials and Studies?, NATIONAL INSTITUTE ON AGING, United States Dept. of Health and Human Services, https://www.nia.nih.gov/ health/what-are-clinical-trials-and-studies.

[5] *bid.*

[6] Lang, T. and Siribaddana S. (2012). *Clinical Trials Have Gone Global: Is This a Good Thing?* PLoS Med 9(6): e1001228. https://doi.org/10.1371/journal.pmed.1001228

of drugs on the radiological procedures and any other preventive care or treatment.

In Consonance to the opinion of the World Health Organization, the clinical trials can be ramified in four stages. They can be elucidated as follows:

(a) *Phase 1:* It is focused on the study of the drugs on a small group of people so as to analyse their dosage and side- effects. (20-80 people)

(b) *Phase 2:* It focuses on the study of the drugs on a larger group so as to analyse all the adverse possible outcomes. (100-300 people)

(c) *Phase 3:* It focuses on the studies of testing on larger groups on a global level. (700 to 3000 people)

(d) *Phase 4:* It focuses on the study of approval by nations which often lead to the assurance of the safety of the drugs before they are introduced into the market.

The aforementioned deliberation brings forward the exigency of the clinical trials in the global scenario as well as the respective domestic units. Therefore, to understand the clinical trials and its regulations on the international arena it becomes imperative to fathom the historical developments which led to the clinical trials as we see now.

HISTORICAL BACKDROP OF CLINICAL TRIALS

The development in the field of clinical research is a result of a long and fascinating journey. It can be traced back to the biblical times when for the very first time trial of legumes were recorded, to the first clinical test of streptomycin in a randomized manner in 1946,the historical backdrop relating to clinical preliminary contains immense array of uphill tests regarding scientific, regulatory & ethical factors. The acclaimed 1747 scurvy trial led by James Lind had similar components of a clinical trial. The test of "*patulin*" for common cold in the year, 1943 by the UK Medical Research Council's (MRC) was the very first double blind controlled trial.[7]This in-turn led the path for the MRC of the UK to go for the trial of streptomycin in pulmonary tuberculosis in irregular control test for the first time. This is considered as a milestone in regard to clinical trial as it paved the way for more efficient enlistment norm and data compilation related with the specific attributes of other new research.

---

[7] Dr. Arun Bhatt, *Evolution of Clinical Research*, 1(1): 6–10 PMC (2010).

The "Belmont Report", "The Nuremberg Code", "International Conference on the Harmonization Good Clinical Practice", "Declaration of Helsinki Guidance" are considered as milestones made for ethical promotion of human protection.[8] In corresponding to ethical trials, clinical preliminaries began to get exemplified in guideline as government specialists started perceiving a requirement for controlling clinical treatments in the mid twentieth century. As advancements in the field of science keep on happening, there will be new moral and administrative difficulties which would require dynamic updates in moral and lawful structure of clinical trials.

The Book Daniel holds the first recording of clinical trial, according to which the experiment was done by King Nebuchadnezzar, who once decided to order his subjects to follow a diet of only meat and wine which according to him would keep them in sound physical condition. Many subjects objected as they fancied eating vegetables, over meat. The king granted certain subjects to follow a dietary routine consisting of legumes and water for 10 days. At the end of the experiment vegetarians came out to be more nourished than meat-eaters. This was the first time in history that an open uncontrolled human experiment affected the knowledge about public health.

Avicenna put forward certain principles that are mentioned in 'Canon of Medicine'. These principles talk about the provisions relating to clinical trials. Avicenna suggested that in case of a clinical trial for disease without complications the cure should be taken in its ordinary state. He put forward that similar cases of different class should be observed and the findings should be recorded for analysis. This principle looks to target the clinical trials with a more present day approach.

Ambroise Pare is famously known as the surgeon who accidently conducted the very first clinical trial of a novel therapy in the year 1537. He had to look for an unconventional Treatment for the wounded soldiers as the amount of traditional treatment oil was not at all enough for such a huge number of soldiers that were injured in the battlefield. Along with him, James Lind is regarded as the physician who has been successful in

---

[8] Medical Research Council, *Streptomycin treatment of pulmonary tuberculosis*, 2:769 782 BMJ (1948).

conducting a controlled clinical test of the contemporary period for the first time. It was during the time when he was commissioned as a surgeon in a ship; Dr. Lind was astounded by the high percentage of scurvy found among the sailors. He decided to go through a clinical trial to determine the most promising cure for scurvy. Lind's Treaties of 1953 provide a detailed explanation of a controlled trial and its result.

A century had to pass before another milestone was seen in regard to clinical trials. It was Austin Flint, a physician who for the first time carried on the first clinical test analyzing the difference in result between a substitute remedies to an effective treatment this came to know as the 'placebo antidote' for rheumatism. Austin Flint in his book described his observations and takes from the clinical trial to cure rheumatism.

In the year 1943 the Medical Research Council (MRC) UK decided to go through a clinical test to find out the effects of patulin treatment in the case of common cold. The idea of randomized allocation of subjects came during 1923 but it wasn't till late 1946 that the idea was tested for the very first time. The MRC of UK in 1946 carried out a control test of streptomycin in pulmonary tuberculosis that is considered as the first and also a landmark clinical trial in respect to the randomization idea.

The principled system for human protection is found inside the Hippocratic Oath that indicated a vital obligation for a doctor to abstain from hurting the injured are needed person. Howsoever, the oath has a very little relation to human trials and after the result of the trials that were conducted on patients during World War II there was a need to strengthen the rights of the patient.

In International Guidance relating to the morals of clinical study including test patients – the Nuremberg Code was planned in 1947. The Nuremberg Code features vitality of willfulness of this consent. In 1948, UDHR dealt with concern about privileges of people that are exposed to automatic maltreatment.[9] The thalidomide catastrophe paved a way for the U.S. to pass the 1962 Kefauver-Harris corrections, which puts up a need for an educated consent before a clinical trial thus putting a protection for patients that are going for trials.

---

[9] John P Bull, *A study of the history and principles of clinical therapeutic trials*, 10:218248 (1959).

The WMA, "*World Medical Association*" in 1964, at Helsinki explained basic standards along with explicit rules regarding utilization of human test patients in clinical study, known as the Helsinki Declaration. This declaration has been experiencing amendments at regular intervals the recent one being in 2008. Be that as it may, the utilization of fake treatment and post-preliminary access keep on being easy to refute problems.

The International Covenant on Civil and Political Rights in 1964, explicitly expressed, that nobody will be exposed to torment or to savage, brutal or corrupting treatment or discipline. Specifically, nobody will be oppressed without their consent to clinical or scientific study. In the year 1966, Dr. Henry Beecher carried an investigation related to misuses and the revelation of human abuse of Tuskegee subjects during the 1970's strengthened the signal for more strict guideline of government financed human trials. "*The US National Research Act of 1974 and Belmont Report of 1979*" were significant endeavors in molding morals of human tests. The International Conference on Harmonization distributed Good Clinical Studies, which is the general benchmark for ethical direct for clinical preliminaries.

India has as of late been perceived as an appealing nation for clinical preliminaries. However, the nation's excursion in clinical test field has a huge history. The major noteworthy achievements of the ICMR reflect the various perspectives, the advancement and improvement in clinical research for the nation throughout the most recent decade. The CEC of ICMR on Human Research discharged "*Ethical Guidelines for Biomedical Research on Human Participants*" in 2000, which were reconsidered again in 2006.

When "*Drugs and Cosmetics Act*" (*Schedule Y*) surfaced into power and set up the administrative rules for clinical preliminary (CT) consent. This act just allowed clinical preliminaries at a stage lower than its worldwide status. This stage obstructed entry of India in worldwide clinical development. Schedule Y legitimized Indian GCP rules of 2001. This schedule specified GCP obligations of morals board (EC), agent and support and proposed groups for basic reports for example assent, report, EC endorsement, revealing of genuine antagonistic event. These corrections in Schedule Y have been a significant advance forward in course of GCP consistent preliminaries and have given the truly necessary administrative help to GCP rules.

Clinical trial has transpired a long way in sense of development and advancements in its procedures as well as in its provisions. From the first controlled scurvy trial in the early 1950's, it has evolved to focus on the procedure with regard to safety of patients and scientific assessment of success. The field of drug development has seen a major uptake of knowledge from various novel therapies and technologies and has made significant progress, with patient safety as its priority. With ever increasing advancement in the field of science there will be a continuous battle to defeat the ethical and regulatory framework thus making the need for continuous amendments in the legal regime regarding clinical trials.

GLOBAL IMPACT AND REGULATIONS OF CLINICAL TRIALS

In pursuance of Phase 3 of the Clinical Trials, it becomes imperative to analyze the synthesis of the drugs in the group from varied geographical locations, it is beneficial in proving the legitimacy of a drug and the license of trade that can be awarded to such a drug.

The *Good Clinical Practices (ICH E6)*[10] adduces an international quintessential model for the practices with regard to the drug administration and treatment all over the world. These Practices lay down the standard guidelines for the registration, designing, conduct, performance and disclosures of the clinical trials.[11] These principles owe their efficacy to The Declaration of Helsinki.

The Practices enunciate on more than a few topics on the variability and the procedures of trials in accordance with these; every clinical trial has eligibility criteria such as the genders and the medical conditions of the volunteers (human subjects); which impersonates a vital role. The 'Informed Consent Notice' should also be promulgated to the human subjects, in which they are intimidated and informed about all the impediments of the said research and all the policies framed by the Research departments or institutes.[12]

---

[10] Guideline for Good Clinical Practice ICH E6 (R2) ICH Consensus Guideline: ICH Harmonised Guideline Integrated Addendum to International Council of Harmoniation (ICH) E6 (R1).

[11] ICH GCP—Good Clinical Practice, Good Clinical Practice Network, https://ichgcp. net.

[12] Para 4.8 of Guideline for good clinical practice E6(R2).

Anteriorly to clinical trials carried out, it is imperative for all the nations to carry out the pre-testing analysis. This analysis should also contain the data and report of its plausible side-effect. It is usually the testing data before any clinical testing is carried out or any human test subject is involved. It is done to anticipate the reactions or behavioral patterns in response to a drug.[13]

The General Considerations for Clinical Trials E8 also enunciate on the division of the clinical studies as per its approaches. The Table 1 of the document makes this division as follows:

(a) "Human Pharmacology
(b) Therapeutic Exploratory
(c) Therapeutic Confirmatory
(d) Therapeutic Use"[14]

The Clinical Trials are carried on a research question or clinical question, the said research or trial should also be registered.[15] Furthermore, there should be a methodology of data extraction by analyzing the risk for every individual involved and their response to administration of a particular drug.[16]

The ICH Topic E6 (R1) Guideline for Good Clinical Practice executes a dominant disposition in laying down the standards for the clinical trials. The Rule 1.13 of the impugned document bespeaks on the nexus of the clinical trial, it focuses on the necessity of the transparent clinical trial systems by way of therapeutic, prophylactic, or diagnostic agents[17] that reflect on the human subjects and it is represented by way of presentations and statistical data.

Whenever, the clinical trial endeavours to study the effectiveness of a drug by accumulating a novel salt to it, then in that case there is bifurcation of

---

[13] ICH Harmonised Tripartite Guideline- General Considerations For Clinical Trials E8 *International Conference on Harmonisation of Technical Requirements for Registration of Pharmaceuticals for Human Use*, July 17, 1997.

[14] *Ibid.*

[15] Para 4.8.7 of Guideline for good clinical practice E6(R2).

[16] B.D, A.D, Briss PA, *et al. GRADE Working Group, Grading quality of evidence and strength of recommendations*, BMJ. 2004; 328: 1490.

[17] The ICH Topic E6 (R1) Guideline for Good Clinical Practice.

groups. The first group is termed as 'treatment group', this group receives the standard medicine as well as the new drug coupled with it; whereas the second group, receives the standard medicine which is coupled with placebo (identical medicine imitation with no drug ingredient), this group is called the 'control group'[18]. This helps the human subjects in being oblivious to the exposure of the drug and therefore there can be no bias reaction to the administration of the medicine.

The clinical trials are complex as there are several procedure boards involved for review and analysis of the effects of the drugs. The human subjects convoluted in this are also free to exit the research whenever they wish to but the same has to be conferred with the doctors involved as they can draft the exit action plan of the drug trials.

The ICH M3 brings into prominence that there should be diligence in the administration of the drugs. The drugs administered in the initial parts of the studies should be of a meager degree so as to ensure the safety of the subjects. The peculiar thing about these guidelines is that their objectives are two-fold:

(a) The welfare of the public which could immensely benefit from the introduction of drug in the market.

(b) The human subjects involved in the clinical trials so that the least possible casualties are caused while testing of the new drugs.

There is a contemporary form of testing which is done on the patients whereby these patients do not register to be the test subjects of a clinical trial. It is known as Right-to-Try. In the aforesaid arrangement, whenever a patient has a terminal illness and he has exhausted all means of recovery and treatment then he can be eligible for administration of such a drug which is not approved and marketed only if he has the knowledge of all the constituents of such a treatment and subsequently, he has to acknowledge the same by assenting through an Informed Consent Notice. However, this method of clinical trials has only been regularised in the United States of America.[19] It is mandated by way of Right to Try Act,

---

[18] ICH—International Conference on Harmonisation of Technical Requirements for Registration of Pharmaceuticals for Human Use: Topic E 10-Choice of Control Group in Clinical Trials.

[19] Right to Try Act, Public Law 115–176.

2018. It is a part of United States of America's expanded access program.[20] Moreover, the International Covenants are silent on the part of the Right-to-Try.

Correspondingly, the nations, which are a part of European Union (EU) are presently regulated through the Clinical Trial Regulation, 2014.[21] The EU has also established a Clinical Trials Information System (CTIS) for regulating and establishing the systems of clinical trial, it acts as a single-entry point. The Regulations of 2014 ensure that there is safety and transparency in the clinical trial procedures. It is done by the contrivance of electronic assessments and evaluations.[22] Such a structure insinuates an ideal environment for the clinical trials which would reduce the casualties and subsequently grants in effective induction of the medicines in the market.

The aforementioned deliberation candidly brings forward that the standards as demonstrated in the guidelines laid down in the ICH Harmonised Guidelines are effective in illustrative several scenarios of the clinical trials but there is still a long way to go for it to be effective as there are many more techniques that can be covered.

ROLE AND FUNCTIONS OF ICH-GCP

The pharmaceutical companies had a vision to seize the international market but because of the presence of technical dissimilarities in each country they were compelled to duplicate their work before sending it for Investigational New Drug (IND) or New Drug Application (NDA) in different countries. This gave rise to challenges like expansion of research and development costs and delays in marketing drugs, which in turn increased the healthcare cost. Even the patients were faced with problems like delay in getting the required medicine on time. All this resulted in acknowledging the need to rationalize and harmonize regulations regarding the drug development by the developed countries.

---

[20] Expanded Access, U.S. Food and Drug Association, https://www.fda.gov/news-events/public-health-focus/expanded-access.
[21] Regulation (EU) No 536/2014.
[22] *Ibid.*

In 1982, WHO and the CIOMS gave an archive designated as *"Worldwide Guidelines for Biomedical Research Involving Human Subjects"*.[23] The record was discharged for encouraging the nations to follow the code of the *"Declaration of Helsinki and the Nuremberg Code"*. Around the world, numerous associations and boards of trustees gave different records and rules on a similar issue, and a choice was taken to merge every one of these rules.

The ICH-GCP was approved in the year 1996 and was carried out for clinical trial from January 1997. The ICH is an exemplary body for uniting the administrative authorities and pharmaceutical industry to talk about logical and technical parts of pharmaceuticals and create the ICH guidelines.[24] From its initiation in 1990, ICH has steadily advanced, in order to address the issues regarding drug development. ICH's aim is to accomplish more prominent harmonization worldwide to guarantee that safe, successful and top quality medicines are created, and supplied and kept up in the most asset effective way while satisfying high standards.

Since its declaration of hierarchical changes in October 2015, ICH has developed as an association and now incorporates 16 Members and 32 Observers. Compliance with ICH-GCP gives open affirmation of the rights, security, and prosperity of preliminary patients is ensured along the standards of the *"Declaration of Helsinki"*, and also states whether the clinical preliminary information is credible[25]. The ICH-GCP is a fixed guideline that ensures the rights, wellbeing and human welfare, limits vulnerability of humans to unknown risks, improves nature of information, accelerate promotion of new medications.

The ICH-GCP's mission is to make proposals towards accomplishing more noteworthy harmonization in the perception and use of technical guidelines. It also looks forward to achieve the requirements of a pharma-ceutical product registration and also the maintaining such registrations. It also focuses on providing protection of public health for patients from

---

[23] Vijayananthan, A. and Nawawi, O., *The importance of Good Clinical Practice guidelines and its role in clinical trials*, 4(1):e5 PMC (2008).

[24] *Regulatory Harmonization*, https://www.phrma.org/advocacy/research-development/regulatory-harmonization

[25] Vijayananthan A. & Nawawi O, *The importance of Good Clinical Practice guidelines and its role in clinical trials*, 4(1):e5 PMC (2008).

an international perspective. ICH-GCP monitors and keeps the demand for greater mutual acceptance of data and research updated.

The ICH-GCP consist of 13 core principles which are as follows:

- Clinical trials should comply with the ethical principles which have their roots in the *"Declaration of Helsinki"*, and follow the requirements of GCP.
- A trial should only be carried out if the benefit that will be achieved after completion out weights the foreseeable risks and inconveniences.
- The most important consideration should be of rights, well being and safety of the test subjects and it should also beat the interests of science and humanity.
- The information regarding any clinical and non-clinical product should be sufficient to back the recommended clinical trial.
- The whole trial must be described in a scientifically sound and precise manner.
- The trial must comply with the protocols that have been given by the IRB's (institutional review board) decision.
- The responsibility of making the medical decisions of the patients goes to a qualified physician and when required, to a qualified dentist.
- The candidates selected for carry out the trial should have an education qualification, experience and training to complete their respective tasks.
- Consent must be obtained prior to preparation of the trial and the consent should be free and informed.
- The information gathered from a clinical trial should be kept in such a method that it permits its accurate reporting, verification and interpretation.
- The documents, which can identify the test subjects must be protected at all times to meet the confidentiality criteria.
- Every process of drug development should comply with the good manufacturing practice (GMP) and must be taken in conformity with authorized protocol.
- To keep up the quality of every step of the trial, systems with procedures that check the every step of the clinical trial should be in force.

Basically these principles convey that, every single clinical trial ought to be carried out as per moral standards, sound scientific proof and clear definite conventions. The advantages of directing preliminaries ought to exceed the dangers. The rights, security and prosperity of preliminary members are of fundamental significance and these ought to be saved by getting educated assent and looking after privacy. A properly qualified faculty with satisfactory experience will be the one to give out due consideration. Records ought to be effectively open and retrievable for exact detailing, confirmation and translation. Unknown suspicious items ought to be produced by Good Manufacturing Practice.

Presently just European Union, United States of America and Japan pursue ICH rules, anyway as the ICH district controls most of the pharmaceutical market, and since the other nations that are associated with drug advancement and would like to advertise their items in the ICH area, likewise pursue them.[26] Huge numbers of nations (counting India) have altered their respective rules according to the standard of the ICH rules. The facts confirm that numerous nations are not following these rules, however these nations are not engaged with tranquilize advancement.

The function of ICH-GCP is to improve moral awareness, clinical trial idea and strategies, public protection, cost adequacy of innovative work, information acknowledgment and promoting structure. Directing clinical preliminaries as per ICH-GCP rules has decreased the event of frauds and mishaps.[27]

In most recent couple of years clinical tests have developed enormously. There are different, complex investigations in different stages, in different restorative zones going on over the globe. Harmonization guarantees that the prerequisites are orderly everywhere and the information got from various sources can be merged together to guarantee that the investigations have sufficient power.

ICH-GCP is to be followed while carrying out investigation in the ICH region. The data collected by the countries of the ICH area can be from investigation carried out elsewhere but it should comply with the ICH guidelines.

---

[26] Pranali Wandile and Ravindra Ghooi, *A Role of ICH-GCP in Clinical Trial Conduct*, 8:1 (2017).

[27] ICH Harmonised Guideline Integrated Addendum to ICH E6(R1): Guideline For Good Clinical Practice ICH E6(R2) ICH Consensus Guideline:, https://ichgcp.net/2-the-principles-of-ich-gcp-2

By giving uniform guidelines for arranging, directing, observing, evaluating, recording and reporting clinical preliminaries, ICH GCP guarantees that clinical research led in different geologies come up to indistinguishable adequate standards.[28]It additionally guarantees that the patients' right, security, welfare, protection and secrecy are ensured where the investigations are carried out. The GCP rule conveys a solid message to those working on drug advancement to stop doing malpractices since such acts is immediately identified.

The rules give the individuals a confirmation that test subjects are treated with deference and nobility and that their interests overshadow the interests of science and society, this guarantees that the individuals are propelled to take part in clinical preliminaries, without whom no preliminary would ever be led.[29] The rule ensures that preliminaries led at various centers observe similar quality principles and that the outcomes can be hypothesized to all test subjects regardless of race, sexual orientation and so on. There is also an advantage of common acknowledgment of trial information inside ICH nations and even centers outside the ICH areas if the rules are followed.

The century that we live in, developments are occurring at a pace that has been never observed before. Every field, counting the scientific are developing significantly and the clinical field is contributing to make an individual lead a more beneficial life. An enormous reason of this is because of the improvement of new medications. The competition to create more beneficial medications or improve existing ones gives no indication of slowing down.

Earlier, the field of clinical research was carried on by taking moderate step and improvement in an inept fashion. There were numerous irregularities in human care services in all over the world, but these are currently diminishing. The world is yet to become an absolutely orderly society, but we are doubtlessly moving towards it. A life of the individual has unquestionably more importance than it has ever had in our history. Similar rules have guaranteed the advantages of science are not confined to one place and are distributed even over the world.

[28]James Lind Institute, Role of ICH- GCP in Clinical Trials (Nov. 14, 2018) https://www.jliedu.com/blog/ich-gcp-clinical-trials

[29] Harmonisation for Better Health https://www.ich.org/page/mission

ETHICAL INTERFERENCE WITH REGARD TO CLINICAL TRIALS

Clinical researchers have a deep custom of giving warm consideration regarding the physical well-being of test subjects in the research. At the time when research was dangerous, it was basic for the investigators themselves to go through the test mediations. By the turn of the twentieth century, a few examiners had likewise perceived the need to get express assent from patients.

A noticeable model is Walter Reed's analyses on yellow fever that were led in Cuba after the Spanish-American War. Reed acquired assent from test patients, he obtained assent forms written in both English and Spanish.[30] Regardless of this early case of getting assent from volunteers, getting consent from patients was still not made necessary for trials involving patients as the decisions regarding the wellbeing of the patients in a medical research were still taken by the physician themselves. Thus the need to lower the risk was still the main focus here. Through the span of the twentieth century, various kinds of perils were recognized relating to the utilization and testing of medications.

Before the declaration of the current administrative methodology, which was authorized in 1962, drugs were being showcased without sound proof of their efficacy and security. Moreover, experimentation with new medications included testing in doctors' labs in a haphazard manner. In light of such issues and in response to the overwhelming birth absconds brought about by the utilization of thalidomide in pregnant ladies, a complicated arrangement of procedures was instituted to test new medications for well-being and efficacy. Obviously, such methodology was just conceivable once the now-recognizable procedures of leading and breaking down clinical preliminaries had been introduced.

For eliminating biasness from a research, random allocation of assignment to various research groups can be a powerful tool. Biasness can be removed by following any of the three ways of 'Blinding'. In the first way, i.e. Single Blind Trial, the trials are planned in such a way that the test subjects have no idea whether they fall under the study group or controlled group. In the second way, i.e. Double Blind Trial, the trials are planned in such

---

[30] Jeremy Sugarman, Ethics in the Design and Conduct of Clinical Trials, 24, No. 1 (2002).

a way that doctors as well as the test subjects have no idea regarding the group allocation and treatment given. And lastly in the third way, i.e. Triple Blind Trial, it is planned in such a way that even the person studying the data is kept in the dark along with the doctors and test subjects. Double Blind Trial is found to be favoured over the other types.

Removal of biasness from a research is an important step in regard to its design and conduct as its presence might hamper the integrity and put the patients in direct exposure to trials that at the end won't bear any valid results. Although sometimes randomization or allocation of any treatment can be faced with negative prospects if it prevents a patient from getting an effective treatment. Thus, the use of randomization should be justified.

Similar to randomization, there are various positive discussions favouring the placebo control in place of active control groups for application in clinical trial. It is believed that placebo can aid in the manifestation of efficacy when compared to historical and active controls. And, also the trials done with placebo groups are tend to be less expensive and rapid in nature when compared to active groups. Even if the placebo looks desirable from a design standpoint, Freedman said that the need for placebo is a bit exaggerated since it's not correct to opt for placebo group when a more effective treatment exists. The Declaration of Helsinki makes it clear that it is necessary to test the risks, benefits and effectiveness of a new process in comparison to the processes that are being applied in current time. This does not preclude the use of placebo, or no treatment, in examinations where no proven prophylactic, diagnostic or therapeutic method exists.[31]

In case of trial, the collection of data might prove to be a legal and social risk to the subjects. It is highly important to keep this information safe and secure. It is always taken for granted that the assurance of safety of data will lead to higher participation in trials and as well as the authenticity of the data provided. The investigators can lower the chance of abuse to the subjects by taking necessary steps to keep the data collected confidential.

We can very well notice that as the elements of research design put flags on instances related to ethical questions, so does the process of research.

---

[31] Robert V. Carlson & Kenneth M. Boyd & David J. Webb, *The revision of the Declaration of Helsinki: past, present and future*, 57(6): 695–713 PMC (2004).

Obtaining valid consented data, dealing with results, and the responsibility of conduct of research are the few ethical questions that are being raised by the conduct of research.

It can be said that from the view point of ethics, gaining of an informed consent should be taken as a process rather than just completing a consent form. The present way to deal with adverse development from clinical research is very much confusing and tiresome.[32] It can be benefited from streamlining since it will make sure that the data obtained is used accurately.

To achieve the mission to address the ethical obligations faced by clinical research it is important to address the situation not only in respect to the person designing the research but also by the individuals who are responsible for reviewing, funding, overseeing, conducting, publishing and reading.

CONCLUSION

The Clinical Trials undertake to be regulated by a convoluted structure of laws which are governed by the *"International Council for Harmonisation of Technical Requirements for Pharmaceuticals for Human Use (ICH)"*. The guidelines laid down by ICH with regard to the Clinical Trials are enunciated in the form of Efficacy Guidelines which are segregated into twenty segments.

The methodology of the Clinical Trials attenuate a compelling controversy that whether such clinical trials infringe the human subject's basic Human Rights or not? The Efficacy Guidelines have been successful in providing a solution at the threshold of this debate by laying down and subsequently devising the ideal standards by which such clinical trials are to be carried out.

These guidelines commemorate to lay down standards for the clinical practices. The clinical trials and their conducts are primarily and extensively laid down in the E6 of the Guidelines, it precariously deals with the Clinical Good Practices. The impugned document even deliberates upon the acquisition of the sponsorship.

---

[32] Cecilia Nardini, *The ethics of Clinical Trials*, 8: 387 PMC (2014).

The impediments that are usually caused while ensuring the authenticity of the clinical trials are the knowledge and the awareness of the investigators. It is the vital for the investigators to be aware of the said regulations as these regulations govern the ideal conduct of the investigators while carrying out the clinical trials. Any such ignorance can contribute to a solemn menace to the human rights of the human subjects and also the improvidence of the resources invested in carrying out the research as well as in consummation to prove adverse to the people for whose benediction the medicine is introduced in the market.

The induction of these guidelines have been proved effective only if there is a regulatory authority in the federal level or state level ta adjudge the applicability of the guidelines in the various situations. The United States has proved to be the closest to the pinnacle of the mountain of the regulatory authority by giving the prominence and powers of such regulations to the FDA: Food and Drug Association (Department of Health and Health Services). Such a system of a regulatory authority should be adopted by all the countries and time and again the nations should ensure that there is optimum transparency in the procedures of clinical trials.

The aforementioned deliberation can be proved as the support stick to adduce that clinical trial can be seen to be meagre small step in the regulation of medicine before it is introduced into the market but it is imperative as it takes around three to seven years for a person to derive sanction to introduce the medicine into the market. Therefore, it can be undeniably discerned and said that this stage if approval of a drug enacts a major act in the sanction of the said drug into the market for the use by the patients.

The paper has been an endeavour to extensively excogitate upon the terminology of clinical trials but the suggestions that have been adduced on the conjecture of the researchers is that the standards are undeniably old in themselves and the recent amendments have proven insufficient in coping up with the on-going development in the field of pharmaceuticals; for example: the Right-to-try proves to be classic illustration of the incompatibility of the guidelines with the contemporary scenario.

Regulation of Clinical Trials: Controlling Biological Warfare and Promoting Biosafety

Ms. Alisha Sharma*

ABSTRACT: Biological warfare has been in use since time immemorial to win battles stirred because of conflicting ideas. Earlier, the methods of using biological weapons were as simple as contaminating water by animal carcasses and human cadavers but with globalisation and progress in science and technology, biological warfare has refined. From extracting pathogens and toxins out of organisms to altering their genetic patterns, we have come a long way technologically. Developments in science and research deserve significant credit for enhancing the healthcare facilities. A branch of life sciences incorporates dual-use research which occupies an influential role in the engineering of biological weapons. Globalization has granted increased accessibility of technology which has set the stage for the onset of an era that will witness the far-reaching implications of bioterrorism. Biological warfare and bioterrorism are two sides of the same coin and are aimed at causing mass destruction. The fact that biological weapons are easier to transport and cheaper than other forms of weaponry when coupled with complexities in their detection, indicates that the future holds unanticipated dangers. The impact of bio-attacks is not limited to human life and extends to animals, plants, and unimmunized flora and fauna as well. Even though international treaties and agreements prohibit the use of biological warfare, their contribution towards controlling the issue is not satisfactory. Violation of the obligations of the Biological and Toxic Weapons Convention has been a subject of dispute for a long time and member states have indulged in objectionable conduct. Hence, the need for addressing this issue at the grassroot level has come to the forefront. When clinical trials engage in dual-use research, to ensure that the research is not used for destructive purposes, surveillance and regulation are required. Regulation of clinical trials involves licensing from the government and enforcement of biosafety protocols. Enforcing regulation of trials would make them more accountable and

---

* Student, Amity Law School, NOIDA, AUUP.

establish transparency which will promote bio-defense mechanism and alleviate research that is driven towards biological warfare. However, regulation at the national level alone can be rendered inadequate is other countries lack a similar mechanism. The factor obstructing biological warfare in the current scenario is the fear of an attack in retaliation and because most countries possess weapons for defense, the cycle could be endless. Therefore, the establishment of regulatory mechanisms and policies in all sovereign states is required to control the growing concern of threats that biological weapons pose.

This research highlights the impact of biological warfare on mankind, environment, economic conditions of a state as well as the role of treaties in controlling bio-war. It also analyses the existing biosafety and defense protocols and policies with a view to promote regulation of clinical trials.

Keywords: Biological Warfare, Regulation, Clinical Trials, Biological Weapons.

INTRODUCTION

Biological warfare refers to the deliberate deployment of toxins or pathogens originating from living organisms for the purpose of disseminating infectious diseases or death in human beings, plants, and animals. One may associate the resultant effect of such weapons with a high number of casualties but, the intended effect of these weapons also includes disruption of natural equilibrium, economic downfall, and terrorism ultimately leading to widespread panic. Humans have been experimenting with plants and animals for many years, initially inadvertently and with the passage of time, on volition. Perhaps, the earliest instance was when potable water was contaminated to expose unsuspecting humans to infections. Biological weapons can create inconceivable havoc for their detection is more complex than any other category of weaponry such as nuclear, chemical, or radiological. The catastrophe lies in the fact that the agents are devoid of any colour, odour, or a macroscopic physical form which aids their cost-efficient and rapid transmission. With the advancement of biotechnology and nano-technology, the pathogenic or non-pathogenic microbes and viruses are manipulated to improve their survivability rate and spawn unforeseen mass destruction via epidemics. In addition to this, accessibility to novel technologies make the usage of bio-weapons easier. The incorporation of pathogens poses as a threat to national and global well-being. Examples of illnesses used in biological warfare include smallpox, anthrax, cholera, and avian flu.

As biotechnology develops further, mankind stands susceptible to unanticipated threats from agents that can be potential weapons. Dual Use Research Concern falls under the life sciences research projected for a benefit that can be used for detrimental purposes if not regulated. The issue of unregulated Dual Use Research takes under its purview not only scientific research but also, public health, security, biotechnology, ethics, and various societal issues.[1] If misapplied, the research can potentially proliferate bio-warfare. A research conducted in pathology or epidemiology for engineering a vaccine that controls the spread of a disease may be used to produce vaccine-resistant variants through genetic mutations for warfare and attacks.[2] To battle this threat and secure global peace, preventive measures and policies have been deliberated through the establishment of international co-operation. The Biological and Toxin Weapons Convention (BTWC) came into existence on 26 March 1975. It was the first multilateral treaty to specifically prohibit the usage of a class of weapons. The treaty forbids developing, stockpiling, producing, or transferring bioweapons that lack any constructive purpose. The treaty requires member states to make efforts bilaterally and multilaterally to resolve compliance issues.[3] A review conference is conducted every 5 years to devise confidence-building measures and review the convention's implementation. However, due to the lack of an executive body, the past has witnessed blatant violations of BTWC. The episode of Amerithrax in 2001 is one such example that resulted in the death of 5 innocent civilians and illness in 17, making it one of the most frightening biological attacks in U.S. history.[4]

---

[1] *Dual Use Research Concern (DURC)*, World Health Organisation (Apr 27, 2020, 6:11 PM), https://www.who.int/csr/durc/en

[2] E.J. DaSilva, *Biological warfare, bioterrorism, biodefence and the biological and toxin weapons convention*, Electronic Journal of Biotechnology (Apr 29, 2020, 9:36 PM) ejbiotechnology.info/index.php/ejbiotechnology/article/view/v2n3-22/827.

[3] *Convention on the Prohibition of the Development, Production and Stockpiling of Bacteriological (Biological) and Toxin Weapons and on their Destruction*, United Nations Office for Disarmament.

[4] *Amerithrax or Anthrax Investigation*, Federal Bureau of Investigation (Apr. 28, 2020, 8:20 pm), fbi.gov/history/famous-cases/amerithrax-or-anthrax-investigation

Amidst the non-compliance issues, a solution that can combat bio-warfare is solidifying clinical trial mechanisms nationally and internationally. The World Health Organization believes that Clinical trial transparency shall be established at a global level[5] to make the discoveries of healthcare R&D accessible to patient groups and thereby strengthening the reliability factor of tests and treatments on human health.[6]

BIOLOGICAL WEAPONS- MEANING AND EVOLUTION

Biological weapons refer to living organisms and their derivatives which can be employed to cause illness or death of human, animal, and plant lives. Microbes or viruses have been used as weapons since Biblical times and involve human cadavers, animal carcasses, contaminated clothes, plants, and fungus causing toxins.[7] Roman, Greek and Persian literature from 300 BC suggest the same. The utilisation of bioweapons occur in multiple stages. Firstly, scientists research and develop pathogens. Secondly, invasive agents are produced in bulk. This is followed by trials to evaluate the success rate and impact of the pathogen and creation of a delivery system. The storage and stockpiling of the weapons are the last stage. A microscopic pellet containing Ricin, a toxin obtained from plants were ingeniously delivered via the spokes in an umbrella. A widely known instance of incorporating this delivery system is the selective death of foreign nationals in London and Paris in the year 1978.[8]

Biological warfare has its roots embedded in history since 400 B.C. when Scythian archers dipped their arrows with the intention of infecting them, in decomposing bodies or in a mixture of blood and manure. In the

---

[5] R.F. Viergever, R.F. Terry and G. Karam, *Use of data from registered clinical trials in identifying gaps in health research and development,* WHO, who.int/bulletin/ volumes/1/6/12-11454/en

[6] *Clinical Trials,* World Health Organization, https://www.who.int/health-topics/clinical-trials/#tab=tab_1.

[7] Joseph Dudley, M.H. Woodford, *Bioweapons, Biodiversity, and Ecocide: Potential Effects of Biological Weapons on Biological Diversity: Bioweapon disease outbreaks causing the. extinction of endangered wildlife species, the erosion of genetic diversity in domesticated plants and animals, the destruction of traditional human livelihoods, and the extirpation of indigenous cultures* 52 BIO-SCIENCE 583, 583–584 (2002).

[8] E.J. DaSilva, *Biological warfare, bioterrorism, biodefence and the biological and toxin weapons convention,* Electronic Journal of Biotechnology (Apr. 29, 2020, 9:36 PM) http://www.ejbiotechnology.info/index.php/ejbiotechnology/article/view/v2n3-2/827.

12th century AD, "Barbarossa used dead bodies of soldiers to poison wells in the battle of Tortona. In 14th century AD, during the siege of Kaffa, the attacking Tarter force tossed the dead bodies of those who died of plague into the city to attempt to inflict an epidemic upon the enemy state. In the 18th century, English forces in North America distributed blankets contaminated with small-pox to naive civilians."[9] In the 20th century, usage of biological weapons started to become sophisticated, thanks to developments in life sciences and biotechnology. In recent times the only factor inhibiting biological warfare is the fear of the response from the targeted state and disturbing international diplomacy and relations. Presently, several countries possess the resources to carry out a biological attack. The United States disposed of its biological weapons in 1970 subsequent to the presidential executive order, the reason being a declaration of such weaponry as non-essential for defense.[10] The former USSR funded elaborate research on the plausible implementation of bio-weapons on food crops such as rice and wheat through fungal diseases, on livestock through viral and bacterial illnesses such as anthrax and disease-carrying insects through mosquitoes, fleas, and ticks.[11] These were tested to accomplish the aim of damaging the agricultural sector to disturb the food production of national economies. The Scientists of the Soviet Union purportedly used advanced genetic engineering methods to produce the vaccine and antibiotic-resistant variants of anthrax, plague, and smallpox for attacking the civilians and military forces.[12]

---

[9] A. Hunsicker, Understanding International Counter-Terrorism—A Professionals Guide to the Operational Art (2006) 188–190. https://books.google.co.in/books/about/Understanding_International_Counter_Terr.htmlid=K4XefrTlSygC&printsec=frontcover&sourcekp_read_button&redir_esc=yv=onepage&q&f=false (Apr 28, 2020, 9:30AM).

[10] T.V. Inglesby, Toole, A. Henderson, *Preventing the Utilisation of Biological Weapons: Improved Response Should Prevention Fail,* 30 CID 926, 926–927 (2000).

[11] Gulbarshyn B., Yerlan K., Dastan Y., *Former Soviet Biological Weapons Facility in Kazakhstan: Past, Present, and Future,* Monterey Institute of International Studies (Apr 29, 2020, 9:02 PM), http://www.nonproliferation.org/wp-content/uploads/2016/10/op1.pdf

[12] Ibid.

IMPACT OF BIOLOGICAL WEAPONS

The by-products of biological warfare are seldom measured in terms of harm caused to the biodiversity and endangered species.[13] While containing epidemics caused by biological weapons that affect humans, it is imperative that endangered species kept in consideration to preserve bio-diversity. Certain rare species such as D. stephensi, may have a greater probability of being eradicated;[14] hence, restricting their habitats in isolated and urbanized lands where there is minimum foreign interaction elevates the chances of their survival. For this purpose, the US military lands serve as a habitat for endangered animals and plant species even though they comprise just 3% of the total US federal land.[15]

Canine distemper is a generic disease caused by viral pathogens that affect domestic dogs. The disease can be transmitted to wildlife species and unfavourably impact the wild fauna. The disease has proliferated disturbing symptoms in the vulnerable species of carnivores that find habitat in the wilds. As shocking as it may seem, canine distemper is one of the many diseases that is being cultured and tried in laboratories to be released as biological weapons. "Another such example is in the context of ecology and evolution, the effect of the Rinderpest epidemic on African unimmunized faunas has been superseded by the impact of chestnut blight fungus on the deciduous forests in North America." The widespread exposure of chestnut blight fungus adversely affected the eastern North American forests. Preservation of domesticated livestock is crucial for retaining the unadulterated genetic trials for physiological and biological engineering to study improved immunity from insects, parasites, infectious diseases, and instability of environmental factors such as climate, altitude, solar radiation. "Globally, 4000 breeds exist of domesticated livestock species which include cattle, water buffalo, pig, horse, sheep and goats, etc."[16]

---

[13] Daszak, P., Cunningham A. and Hyatt, A.D., *Emerging infectious diseases of wildlife-threat to biodiversity & human health,* Science's compass, https://www.scienceinthe classroom.org/sites/default/files/related/443.full_.pdf.

[14] Ibid.

[15] L.M., Meffe K., Hardesty J., Adams L., *Conservation of Biodiversity on Military Lands: A Handbook for Natural Resources Manager, 1996,* The Department of Defense Biodiversity Initiative (Apr 28, 2020, 8:34PM), citeseerx.ist.psu.edu/viewdoc/download?doi=10.1.1.161.3094&rep=rep1&type.pdf

[16] Joseph Dudley, M.H. Woodford, *Bioweapons, Biodiversity, and Ecocide: Potential Effects of Biological Weapons on Biological Diversity: Bioweapon disease outbreaks causing*

Pathogens that are usually harmless for their natural hosts have proven to be fatal for other species. It is suggested that Avian Malaria and Avian Pox contributed towards the extinction of a local bird species in Hawaii. "Epidemics of infectious diseases are a major factor that influenced mass extinction in Madagascar and North America.[17] The impact of biological weapons on livestock or crops could prove to be destructive through a trickle-down effect on wild species of animals and plants."[18] This is because humans may become resistant or immune to certain diseases but the defenceless wildlife does not evolve similarly. Researches need to emphasize the importance of protecting the endangered from bio-weapons as it is an extreme form of human intervention that disrupts the natural balance.

Most of the prevalent pathogens and toxins used as bio-weapons cause broad-spectrum illnesses that boast a high mortality rate in humans and domesticated livestock. 75% of the genetically altered microbes used against humans cause zoonotic diseases which are dangerous to the environment once released. These include anthrax, plague, tularemia, etc. Viral pathogens like rinderpest, FMD, and brucellosis are identified as cultured biological weapons against livestock which can affect unimmunized wild species.[19]

As an advanced species, we have expanded our understanding of the control of infections and disease. However, our response and defence mechanism remains inadequate when it comes to the protection of bio-diversity.

---

the extinction of endangered wildlife species, the erosion of genetic diversity in domesticated plants and animals, the destruction of traditional human livelihoods, and the extirpation of indigenous cultures 52 BIO-SCIENCE 583, 583–584 (2002).

[17] D.B. Wake, V.T. Vredenburg, *Are we in the midst of the 6th mass extinction? A view from the world of amphibians,* PNAS, https://pnas.org/content/pnas/105/Supplement_1/1146/6 .full.pdf.

[18] Daszak, P., Cunningham A. and Hyatt, A.D., Emerging infectious diseases of wildlife-threat to biodiversity & human health, SCIENCE'S COMPASS (Apr 29, 2020, 7:24PM), https://www.scienceintheclassroom.org/sites/default/files/related/443.full_.pdf

[19] Joseph Dudley, M.H. Woodford, *Bioweapons, Biodiversity, and Ecocide: Potential Effects of Biological Weapons on Biological Diversity: Bioweapon disease outbreaks causing the extinction of endangered wildlife species, the erosion of genetic diversity in domesticated plants and animals, the destruction of traditional human livelihoods, and the extirpation of indigenous cultures* 52 BIO-SCIENCE 583, 583–584 (2002).

Apart from affecting living organisms, a biological weapon can take a heavy toll on a country's economy if it evolves into an epidemic or pandemic. The FMD outbreak in Britain is an instance that resulted in a loss of $12 billion to $14 billion in 2001. Similarly, the estimated cost involved in the eradication of the FMD outbreak in Taiwan in 1997 was Fifteen billion dollars.[20] The financial implications of any epidemic disease are intense, the situation demands investment in healthcare, medication, production, and medical research. The loss is manifold in countries like India where the population density is extremely high and involves drawbacks such as poverty, poor sanitation, and hygiene.

The current pandemic has caused a critical economic downfall worldwide by stunting all economic activities and disturbing global supply chains. "According to the United Nations Department of Economic and Social Affairs, the global economy is likely to shrink by 1%."[21] COVID-19 has also caused the most drastic fall in global equity since the Great Depression followed by a 60% dip in oil prices, hitting an all-time low.[22]

CLINICAL TRIALS AND GENUS OF BIO-TERRORISM

Clinical Trials are defined as the research that analyzes the effects of novel treatments and drugs on human health. These studies involve trials of medicines, equipment, cells, and other biological material, surgical and radiological methods along with preventive care.[23] However, the research used for health-care has the potential of defeating its own purpose. This scenario can be manifested in two ways-intentionally and inadvertently.

---

[20] Joseph Dudley, M.H. Woodford, *Bioweapons, Biodiversity, and Ecocide: Potential Effects of Biological Weapons on Biological Diversity: Bioweapon disease outbreaks causing the extinction of endangered wildlife species, the erosion of genetic diversity in domesticated plants and animals, the destruction of traditional human livelihoods, and the extirpation of indigenous cultures* 52 BIO-SCIENCE 583, 583–584 (2002).

[21] *Global economy to shrink by almost 1% in 2020, due to COVID-19 pandemic,* THE ECONOMIC TIMES, (Apr 29, 2020, 11:40 AM), www.economictimes.indiatimes. com/news/international/business/global-economy-could-shrink-by-almost-1%-in-2020-due-to-covid-19-pandemic-united-nations/articleshow/74943235cms?from=mdr......

[22] *Five charts showing the global economic impact of coronavirus,* World Economic Forum, weforum.org/agenda/2020/04/take-five-quarter-life-crisis

[23] *Clinical Trials,* World Health Organization (Apr 28, 2020, 8:45 PM), https://www. who.int/health-topics/clinical-trials/#tab=tab_1

When science is used to produce weapons from natural elements, an obvious inference aims at the rise of bioterrorism. The US National Intelligence Council via its unclassified report in 2004 suggested that the first biological terror attack is likely to occur in the year 2020.[24] With the current pandemic and the theories suggesting that COVID-19 was a pre-planned biological attack,[25] it is only crucial that transparency and accountability are established in clinical trials that cannot be achieved without their regulation. Novel coronavirus has resulted in brutal casualties and crashing economies worldwide. The crisis is such that some nations may take several years to revive themselves. With the progress in scientific acumen globally, the prowess of biological weapons continues to grow stronger and unpredictable. Even in a country like India, which is anticipated to be the host of more than 20% of global clinical trials[26], the threats remain unpredictable without regulation and safety protocols.

Biotechnology and nanotechnology have created methods for gene-alterations employed in dual-use research which enable mutation is strains of plants, animals, and vector insects.[27] Developments as aforementioned have prompted the need to establish regulations, protocols, and mechanisms to have surveillance over research activities aimed at terrorising humanity and damaging the ecosystem.

Another factor instrumental in the spread of biological weapons is the disposal of waste from the healthcare industry. It is estimated that 15% of the waste from the healthcare industry includes toxic waste that can contribute to biological hazards, infections, and drug-resistant micro-organisms. Biological waste takes under its purview transgenic plants and animals that are cultured with recombinant DNA. Since this waste is not managed due to a lack of regulations and enforcement agencies in many countries, they become a source of advertent harm to the environment and living organisms.[28]

---

[24] *Globalisation, Bio-security, and the Future of the Life Science*, Institute of Medicine & National Research Council, https://www.nap.edu/read/11567/chapter/3.

[25] *A bio-weapon or Effect of 5G? Seven Conspiracy Theories that are Around Coronavirus That Will Shock You*, The Economic Times.

[26] J.S. Srivastava, *Need for ethical oversight of clinical trials in India*, 99 Current Science 1505, 1505-1506 (2010).

[27] D. DiEuliis and J. Giordano, *Gene editing using Cas9/CRISPR: implications for dual-use & biosecurity*, 9 Protein Cell 239, 239-240 (2018).

[28] *Health-care waste*, World Health Organization (Apr 28, 2020, 6:22 PM), who.int/news-room/fact-sheet/detail/health-care-waste

BIO-SAFETY: INTERSECTION OF CLINICAL TRIALS AND SECURITY

Before the relevance of bio-security is discussed, it is imperative to understand its meaning and scope. Bio-safety refers to security in order to prevent inadvertent or intended *malafide* use of pathogens or toxins which can be used as biological weapons. Laboratory bio-security and bio-safety function on principles of containment in order to ascertain the minimum risk factor associated with the studies conducted in the laboratories.[29] An extensive bio-safety policy is ideally based on procedures, practices, and habits that restrict exposure to bio-hazards and bio-weapons arising from dual-use research. However, if these safety measures are to be used to achieve their objectives, nations need to cooperate and realize their responsibility in this regard. Since countries continue to indulge in negligent conduct, governance of clinical trials has been a constant subject of debate in the past.[30]

In order to alleviate the concerns surrounding the safety of the environment, a holistic bio-security and bio-safety protocol must be established, nationally, and globally. Implementation of these safety policies requires the creation of a well-connected channel of health officials, research institutions, hospitals, doctors, and the general population.[31] Since biological warfare is capable of causing irreversible damage, the bio-safety mechanism serves as a preventive measure against bioterrorism through domestic and international transparency and surveillance. Countries have been indulging in dual-use research for malevolent reasons behind the facade of trials carried for benefit of society.

The Geneva Protocol ratified in 1925 and the Biological and Toxin Weapons Convention (BTWC) ratified in 1975 were the early attempts at

---

[29] *Bio-risk management: laboratory bio-security guidance*, WHO, (Apr 29, 2020, 12:21 PM), who.int/csr/resources/publications/biosafety/WHO_CDS_EPR_20066.pdf

[30] Smyth, Rosalind L., *A Risk Adapted Approach to the Governance of Clinical Trials: The Research Community Needs to Support a New Initiative to Reduce the Regulatory Burden*, 344 BMJ 10, 10-10 (2012).

[31] Kewal Krishan, Baljinder Kaur and Anshula S., *India's preparedness against bioterrorism: biodefence strategies and policy measures,* Dept. of Defence & Strategic Studies, Punjabi University, Patiala, India (Apr 30, 2020, 6:12AM), https://www.currentscience.ac.in/Volumes/113/09/1675.pdf

the international level to perpetuate solidarity against the use of biological weaponry. Even though the Soviet Union was a signatory to BTWC, it allegedly violated the principles of bio-safety and carried out the production of the largest bio-weaponry complex. Purportedly, in 1979 anthrax was accidentally released by the Soviet Institute of Microbiology and Virology in Sverdlovsk. The accident resulted in the death of 67 civilians and an infection in 33. The Union attempted to mask the true picture involving the military research and trials by claiming that the cause of the outbreak was the ingestion of contaminated beef.[32]

Bio-safety protocols in simple terms are regulating the conduct of clinical research and trials. Where bio-safety focuses on the protection of environment and civilians, a parallel aspect encompasses laboratory bio-security which focuses on the safety of the researchers. Even though both factors are complementary, there are inconsistencies that exist when it comes to their implementation. Safety protocols would suggest restricted access to the premises but the restriction may compromise the emergency response with respect to lab bio-security.[33] In order to diminish the risk associated with clinical trials, it is essential that harmony is ensured through a connected communication channel between researchers and policymakers.

Dual-use research is conducive to modern healthcare especially when the world is susceptible to biological warfare and hence, a balanced approach needs to be adopted to facilitate the constructive purpose of clinical trials. It is undeniable that misgoverned clinical trials have gestated events of blatant terrors but they have also proven to be useful in identifying safe and effective treatments in times of despair. During the outbreak of the Ebola Virus, FDA discussed clinical trials and their roles extensively. FDA recognized that if conducted for the prevention of epidemics and pandemics, clinical trials could have mitigated the damage caused. Admittedly, clinical trials are not a substitute for public health measures yet they have the potential to stunt the transmission of biological weapons.[34]

---

[32] *Globalization, Bio-security, and the Future of the Life Science*, Institute of Medicine and. National Research Council (Apr 28, 2020, 7:56 PM), https://www.nap.edu/read/11567/chapter/3

[33] *Bio-risk management: Laboratory biosecurity guidance*, WHO (Apr 29, 2020, 12:21 PM), who.int/csr/resources/publications/biosafety/WHO_CDS_EPR_20066.pdf

[34] Erin Durkin, *FDA Weighs Practical, Ethical Issues For Clinical Trials During Epidemics*, Inside Washington Publishers (Apr 28, 2020, 6:45 PM), https://www.jstor.org/stable/

A successful clinical trial contributes towards better preparation against bioterrorism and biological warfare the inferences from clinical trials play a vital role and are conducive to controlling the outbreak of a disease. However, unregulated clinical research, therapies, and drug trials render the risk of producing a biological weapon. Whether inadvertent or intentional, clinically altered viruses, pathogens or microbes present a threat to biological safety and sustenance of bio-diversity.[35] A regulated surveillance mechanism can ensure that research is not carried out for giving effect to malicious motives.

REGULATION OF CLINICAL TRIALS

Global Stance

The World Health Organization's initiative to incorporate transparency and coherence in clinical trials worldwide is named the International Clinical Trials Registry Platform (ICTRP). It is aimed at building a platform that records progress globally and creates a single point of access to eliminate any vagueness by making this information available to the public.[36]

Clinical Trials in the United States are guided by "The Centre for Drug Evaluation and Research, Centre for Biologics Evaluation and Research and Centre for Devices and Radiological Health." The 2018 draft of Guidance Documents reflect the approach of Centres towards the conduct of trials and good governance. The documents iterate technicalities of identifying those who fail to register their clinical trials and other data

26700281?Search=yes&resultItemClick=true&searchText=regulation&searchText=of &searchText=clinical&searchText=trials&searchText=and&searchText=epidemics&se archUri=%2Faction%2FdoBasicSearch%3FQuery%3Dregulation%2Bof%2Bclinical %2Btrials%2Band%2Bepidemics&ab_segments=0%2Fbasic_SYC-5152%2Fcontrol &refreqid=search%3A82f4641da0782cef3b87827d287d51d7&seq=2#metadata_info _tab_contents

[35] Joseph Dudley, M.H. Woodford, *Bioweapons, Biodiversity, and Ecocide: Potential Effects of Biological Weapons on Biological Diversity: Bioweapon disease outbreaks causing the extinction of endangered wildlife species, the erosion of genetic diversity in domesticated plants and animals, the destruction of traditional human livelihoods, and the extirpation of indigenous cultures* 52 Bio-Science 583, 583–584 (2002).

[36] *Clinical Trials*, World Health Organization (Apr 28, 2020, 8:45 PM), https:// www.who.int/health-topics/clinical-trials/#tab=tab_1

relating to their results, those who furnish falsified data or fail to submit FDA certification in violation of the Public Health Service Act. "It also discusses the civil money penalties in case of violation of the Federal Food, Drug, and Cosmetic Act." However, the Guidance Documents hold no authoritative value and lack legal enforceability.[37] The guidelines are framed considering the legal interpretation of words and incorporate the word "should" to imply the absence of any mandate. This implies that the Centres have wide discretionary powers that dilute the value of guidelines to mere recommendations.

The conduction of clinical trials is expected to change soon with the application of Clinical Trial Regulation which will repeal the EU Clinical Trial Directive of 2001. The Regulation aims to synchronize assessment and surveillance procedures through the European Union via Clinical Trials Information System (CTIS). The CTIS will maintain a record of all clinical trials with the collaboration of the European Medicines Agency, Member States, and the European Commission. The Regulation seeks to achieve transparency by making the records available to the public unless the data involves commercially confidential information, sensitive communication. The CTIS is being developed and is expected to be audited by December 2020.[38]

Pharmaceuticals and Medical Devices Agency (PMDA) is a body within the Ministry of Health, Labour, and Welfare in Japan that supervises the clinical trials. In 2018, Japan enacted the Clinical Trials Act to legally enforce the ethical guidelines which lacked the sanction of the law earlier. The change was implemented to make the system of research more reliable and transparent.[39]

---

[37] *Draft Guidance for FDA Staff, Responsible Parties, and Submitters of Certain Applications and Submissions to FDA,* U.S. Food and Drug Administration (Apr 30, 2020, 10:21 PM), https://www.fda.gov./regulatory-information/search-fda-guidance-documents/ civil-money-penalties-relating-clinicaltrialsgov-data-bank

[38] *Clinical Trial Regulation,* EUROPEAN MEDICINES AGENCY, (Apr 30, 2020, 10:57 PM), www.ema.europa.eu/en/human-regulatory/research-development./clinical-trials/ clinical-trial-regulation#transparency-rules-section

[39] Kenichi Nakamura, Taro Shibata, Regulatory Changes after the Enforcement of the New Clinical Trials Act in Japan, 50 JJCO 400, 399–404 (2020).

India's Regulatory Mechanism

In 2019, the Ministry of Health and Family Welfare notified the New Drugs and Clinical Trials Rules (NDCT Rules) which finally codified the rules pertaining to clinical trials and their conduct in the country. The Rules ensure greater reliability as they require the establishment of an Ethics Committee that has to be registered with the Central Licensing Authority. The Committee permits the conduction of trial and examines all material facts if any adverse event occurs in the process. The report of the Committee's findings is sent to the Central Licensing Authority which examines its further.[40] This two-tiered scrutiny aids in facilitating transparency and accountability.

ROLE OF TREATIES

The first attempt at restricting biological warfare was the Geneva Protocol ratified in 1925. The Protocol prohibited use of gaseous and bacteriological methods as weapons however, it did not impose restrictions on their productions, stockpiling, and development. Additionally, it also exempted the states that reserved their right to retaliate in case a biological attack is inflicted on them.[41] Therefore, the debates surrounding the protocol paved the way for the Biological and Toxic Weapons Convention (BTWC).

The Biological and Toxic Weapons Convention came into force in 1975 and became the first multilateral treaty aimed at prohibition of the development, production, stockpiling, and transfer of biological pathogens for unjustified purposes. The Treaty obliges member states to dispose of such biological weaponry so as to render them futile for future use or redirect the employment of the weaponry towards the establishment of peace and harmony. It is understandable that the existence of co-operation at a global level is a utopian theory due to compliance issues. Even though the convention in spirit suggests coordination at the bilateral and

---

[40] Ashwin Sapra, Biplab Lenin and Kartik Jain, *New Drugs & Clinical Trials Rules, 2019 – A Regulatory Overview,* Cyril Amarchand Mangaldas, (Apr 30, 2020, 8:23 PM), https://corporate.cyrilamarchandblogs.com/2019/07/new-drugs-clinical-trials-rules-2019-regulations-india

[41] *Protocol for The Prohibition of the Use in War of Asphyxiating, Poisonous, or Other Gases, and of Bacteriological Methods of Warfare (Geneva Protocol),* NTI, (Apr 28, 2020, 7:47 PM), nti.org/learn/treaties-and-regimes/protocol-prohibition-use-war-asphyxiating-poisonous-or-other-gases-and-bacteriological-methods-warfare-geneva-protocol

multilateral level and also provide a portal for complaints to the UNSCR in case of suspicion or actual violation of the treaty, BTWC lacks an executive body that enforces the obligations and resolves compliance issues.[42] Despite all the shortcomings, BTWC through its confidence-building measures has been successful in recording acceptance of its obligations by 173 states by 2015. The review conferences held every 5 years underline the scientific and technical progress in life-sciences and attempt to promote transparency and fortify BTWC's endeavours through additional agreements.[43] One such agreement is the Mendoza Agreement which was signed in 1991 by Argentina, Brazil, and Chile. The Agreement imposed restrictions identical to the BTWC on the signatories with respect to biological and chemical weaponry.[44]

Factually, BTWC has not been able to contribute substantially to its cause. One of the reasons for its failure is that the scope of the convention does not take within its ambit basic research or the actions of an individual. In the last few decades, acquiring and producing biological pathogens has become more economic. The member states which had not considered the use of biological weapons may now develop novel microbes in the garb of dual-use research for defensive purpose. Similarly, obtaining equipment and devising technology to cause bio-warfare has become easier with globalization. Security experts have expressed their concerns regarding the potential of mass-destruction that is associated with bio-warfare. Especially when clinical trials are conducted in the absence of surveillance and without safety protocols, organisms capable of reproducing outside the premises of laboratories can create unprecedented mayhem.[45]

---

[42] *Convention on the Prohibition of the Development, Production and Stockpiling of Bacteriological (Biological) and Toxin Weapons (BTWC)*, NTI, (Apr 28, 2020, 8:20 PM), nti.org/learn/treaties-and-regimen/convention-prohibition-development-production-and-stockpiling-bacteriological-biological-and-toxin-weapons-btwc

[43] Kewal Krishan, Baljinder Kaur and Anshula S., *India's preparedness against bioterrorism: biodefence strategies and policy measures,* Dept. of Defence and Strategic Studies, Punjabi University, Patiala, India (Apr 30, 2020, 6:12AM), https://www.currentscience.ac.in/Volumes/113/09/1675.pdf

[44] *Mendoza Agreement,* NTI (Apr 28, 2020, 8:42PM), nti.org/learn/treaties-and-regimen/mendoza-agreement

[45] *Globalisation, Bio-security, and the Future of The Life Sciences,* Institute of Medicine and National Research Council (Apr 28, 2020, 7:56 PM), https://www.nap.edu/read/11567/chapter/3

CONCLUSION AND SUGGESTIONS

Biological warfare and bioterrorism are at their onset and the competence of treaties in effectively controlling and inhibiting the concerns is as bleak as it gets. The history has witnessed alleged violations by the USSR once, and the possibility of a subsequent violation cannot be overlooked. The fast-paced growth and accessibility of transportation facilities along with up-gradation of technology and life sciences are sowing the seeds for germination of epidemics and pandemics that are created by the human for destroying the human.

Realistically, the probability of mitigating bio-warfare is not very high. However, this does not weaken the impact of a biological attack. Therefore, the researcher suggests that in a nation like ours where poverty, poor hygiene, and sanitation has been a detrimental factor to public health, investments made in the acquisition of pharmaceuticals are not enough. Containment and healthcare infrastructure should be an essential facility that is accessible to all. India is already a population-dense country and the numbers continue to rise, in such a situation it is imperative that containment and quarantine centres attract greater importance.

Further, the control on the use of biological warfare cannot be achieved without the support of clinical researches and trials that consistently work at upgrading the efficiency of the health-care industry. The regulation of clinical trials ensures the peaceful use of dual-use research to propagate agendas of bio-safety. Scientists, researchers, doctors, paramedics, and government agencies need to combine their forces and create a network chain to ensure that the nation is equipped to battle biological warfare.

Albert Einstein said, *"I know not with what weapons World War III will be fought, but World War IV will be fought with sticks and stones."* If the destruction caused by war continues to outgrow the efforts directed at controlling the damage, the foresight will indeed come to a realization.

International Guidelines on Clinical Trials and its Global Impact

Ms. Vanshika Jha*

INTRODUCTION

Pandemics have always been significantly capricious events in history. As to the advantage of the diction of health & purity in relation to the concept of modern rationality in the due course has approved and administered in idea of the creation of demarcation line, wicket gate and quarantines. As the concept of tries to identify the set of guidelines that have been set out to establish the relation and the set-out guidelines that have been meted out for the concept of clinical trials. The impact that the clinical trials are forming at the global arena. It is important to understand that modernity, coupled with globalization has created a dark side of its own: pandemics such as of the coronavirus pandemic, global terrorism and modern technological disasters such as of Chernobyl and Fukushima that have gone ahead and provided with a worldwide impact.

CLINICAL TRIALS AS AN CONCEPT

The concept of clinical trials is required and are seen to stated and comprehend a global perspective that is needed in order to create the reduction of disease that help into burdening the countries through the spread of viruses with the virtue of creating safe and efficacious new therapies and the production of vaccines. Developing countries seen to be underrepresented at the arena of research because of absence of the commodities that are required to bring an efficacious system and the need for the working of the trained researchers, but as it shows that in some of the poorest regions where the need of research based results that can help in the attainment into bringing the greatest impact towards the increase of the early mortality. Shown by the researched data that the adaptability of

* Student, Amity Law School, NOIDA, AUUP.

the concept of clinical trials are fundamental in nature that look forward in bringing towards the range of developing the newer solutions as products through a process of gaining evidential material needed by the individuals that work forth the attainability of the desired results, which can either be for the product license gaining the extensions or the need for pre-established therapies in the pre-established ailment that are for the same forth newly established techniques of therapies and the vaccines to the approval and acceptance that is to be put in use. Then again it has been seen that there is requirement of the "clinical trials". In concept of "clinical trials" have gone global as an whole it all an all an greater development and requirement in the global arena, as the conduction of clinical trials helps in the multiple variations of trials in the developing countries which can also be categorised as the low middle income countries (LMICs) are seen to relate as the greatly accepted and positive experience as of which the research sites gain by stating the operating in the profit oriented mechanisms or the (NPS) non-profit sponsors raises the research levelers that bring forth the haleness into the improvement of the countries that are gaining to reach above the minimal standards with the greatly requiring the investments that are to be needed to the various research centers to attain the working mechanisms.

The outer paid for trials are also bringing forth the above level accomplishment looking forth the research thorough grunt work & involvement of the consented parties in the course of product burgeoning with the various sectors of the global public health initiatives.

As in relation to the Global research functioning all in all requiring of building the efforts to substantiate and bringing forward the encouragement towards the investigations from the LMICs to establish and run their own trials, that are required as the provision into the creation and for an incentive and the possible ordinance in order to designate and attain their own research & development to help in recreate beyond the concept of the outer paid sponsored trials. One of the examples that can be put forth is a local-investor led clinical trial that has been set out in Sri Lanka that went on to address the local relevant issues of the area. The concept of clinical trial looks forward in bringing in the certain aspects of the developing counties in order and usage in order to curb any biological warfare in the global arena. There have been certain widespread dipartites that have been prolonged in the global aspect in relation to the "clinical care, scientific and health literacy, economic and social care development" that is seen to be existing between the developed and the countries that are breaking from the barriers of the countries with the less attainable methods of trials. The presented variations that carry among an array of issues that are taken advantage of and aggravated by the issue of the power gap. The World Health Organisation (WTO) and various other journal editors have seen to explain the concept of the clinical trials in the words of "the assessment of the research that arises from the designated assigs individual involvement or group if individuals in more than one research corelated interventions to research and to asses on the possible health outcomes .Patients that are to be picked without an selection from the pecking order to an intervention that consists of any of the under examination of any new branded supplement or the standard-of-care solution, or that might consist an individual patient being that might be picked at the random are to be taken in due care by the hospital staff that have been pre-taught in more than one alternative modes.

INDIAN PERSPECTIVE OVER CLINIAL TRIALS

The Central Drugs Standard Control Organization (CDSCO) is the National Governing Regulatory Authority in India. That is correspondent to the that of the equivalent to that of the United States Food and Drug Administration (US FDA). CDSCO an arm of the Ministry of Health and the Family Welfare, Government of India. Their agenda is work towards the governance the propounding of the safeguard that are working for achieving over the enhancement of public health by the way assuring in for the safeguards and volatility over the quality that the drugs are being produced in and of the medical technologies and the cosmetics that are to be used in for the due course of the project.

The Drugs Controller General of India (DCGI) is an official of the CDSCO which for one is to be stated as the final regulatory authority that works in order over the acceptance towards the conduction of clinical trials that are to be taking place round the globe. The ambit in its working pertains to the addition, and also elongate to the careful examination of the sites where the trials are to be conducted and the careful examination of the of financial aiders in the clinical evaluation and the production and the prerequisite that works in the country, the outgrowing with an oversight of the Central Drugs Testing Laboratory (Mumbai) with support of Regional Drugs Testing Laboratory that are headed by the "Indian Pharmacopeia Commission" plays among various other roles, responsibilities into the governance of its functions.

"Biological attacks, both state-sponsored and otherwise, are a real threat despite the many treaties prohibiting them. Though the Indian Army is trained to prepare for chemical, biological, radiological and nuclear attacks, the program are on the back burner due to lack of resources," as stated by the internal station for Joint Warfare Studies Director Lieutenant General Vinod Bhatia who is now to be retired from the force and of, who was earlier designated post of the Director General, Military Operations. India, over the vast variation of individuals in the population, forlorn health related issues that arise due the lack of connectivity, is to be seen upon the virus as an ticking clock. Even with the presented catastrophic events that are in relation to the infection and recovery rate of Covid-19, as the novel coronavirus is called, is comparatively seen to be low, experts that re-working into the curtailment of the virus, go on to say that the complete and available date is not to be sufficient to draw conclusion or comparative solutions. As stated with the face of Covid-19 crisis, the "US President Donald Trump" pitched America as a state of panic putting forth the vacillate, discharging for the subjected action of the subject to an outright fabrication. Many political leaders are to be situated in quarantine indicating that nobody in the current scenario at the global level is safe. Many of the states and nations that are in the state of shut-out due to the massive spread of the virus. Stated by the former Indian Air Force Commander-in-Chief of a key Air Command, "The actions and the desired capabilities that are to be required to tackle bioterrorism are identical to the ones required to curtail and contain the spread of corona-virus. Large medical facilities that are needed to isolate, treat, and decontaminate patients before discharging them. Require the need of special clothing for personnel operating in contaminated zones and not just the usage of masks." Major of the lethal non-conventional warfare danger that has begun to torment the global arenas security are stated as to be:

- Biological weapons that are to be assembled by various terrorist organizations.
- Chemical warfare agents that are to be used by totalitarian governments in order to kill or exterminate the dissidents at home and abroad.

THE BIOLOGICAL WEAPONS COVENTION (1972)

The convention in relation to the biological weapons is regarded to be the enunciation of the beginning of the multilateral disarmament treaty which was focusing on the matter concerning the curtailing the progression and the production of stockpiling as an complete classification over the weapons that would lead into the mass destruction, it is by signatories the 10th April 1972. BWC came in force the 26th march 1975.

In the above explained analysis was to help in accordance to assess parties that resulted in being the members of the convention was held in 1986 in which agreement that state parties were in order to set out the guidelines create a large forum of confidence building measures (CBM) an authoritative instruction was to intercept or curtail the occurrence of ambivalence in contrast to uncertainty and over the surmise which are working in order to improve and put forth the international collaboration over the field in the course of creating the need for peaceful biological activities.

It has been seen that the concept of the CBM were to proliferate over into the third conference, as states over into the agreements, state parties that look forth to embark on the provision of the concept of annual reports utilizing the agreed notions that were seen & overtook on the specific activity related to the BWC which can be categorized into date research institutions and scientific laboratories, the data relating to the vaccine production facilities, and over the collection of data upon the national biological defence research and development program stated in accordance to the declaration in relation to the past activities, as in for the parameters of the offensive and of the defensive, the stated model of the biological research and of the developmental program, contains the information pertaining to recrudesce of the infectious diseases that are to be similar accounts of similar repeated episodes that are to be seen and are caused by toxins.

As for the fourth review conference (1996) that took forth the enunciation look forward to the welcoming of the decision of the Ad Hoc Group worked in order to broaden the completion of task at hand and adapting ideas before. Fifth Review Conference that was in 2001. Ad Hoc Group was incapable towards bringing forth conclusion of the discussion over negation of the drafting of a legal protocol/ procedure.

Due to on-going differential ideologies that centered out different views and suggestions over the working of certain key suggestions lead towards, Fifth Review Conference (2001) that went on for presiding over its adjournment into its working order and continue over their findings into November 2002 Geneva. The discussion was brought forth again in November 2002 and finally taken in for the Final Report that would include a decisive decision over into the generation of annual meeting of the states and in adherence to those putting of the professional meetings between the states that were to be meted out in the fourth coming of the next 3 years resulting in for an review of the conference in 2006.

Sixth Review Conference (2006) brought forth an success in over the meticulous review over the final draft that was laid out into the conference, accepting of final document over by mutual consensual decision of the state's parties acceptance to an total adherence of the detailed plan in for the promotion over the universal adherence, and votes and for the active role in for the streamline of the working of its guidelines over the submission and distribution in for the Confidence-Building Measures (CBMs). It has attained to establish an meticulous internal program spanning from 2007 to 2010. In forth to the significant development, the Conference accepted to establish an Implementation Support Unit (ISU) for the required support to the States parties working over the accordance and adherence over the Convention.

RECENT GUIDELINES FROM GLOBAL REGULATORY AUTHORTIES

- The Medicines and Healthcare products Regulatory Agency (MHRA) works in accordance with the issuance of the guidance over the working into the management of clinical trials into current scenario pertaining over the COVID-19 pandemic. Over the other things, the working and the adaptability of the guidance takes an usage of the broach the matter for the states are seen to rise in the rate of deviations of the set out guidelines that are responsible into the repercussion of the COVID-19 and are not to be seen of grave danger until the patients are seen to be a greater danger/threat to them or the society.
- "Netherlands' Central Committee on Research Involving Human Subjects (CCMO)" has seen to be meted out an issuance of a guidance allowing for exceptional usage of the amendments or

deviations that are for the usage of the gaining of knowledge without the due consent that are working in the allowance over establishment to understand the better usage study drugs that are seen to be sent-off straight away to trial subjects. The CCMO has also put forth the attainability of a speedy track of approval process or the procedure in relation to the clinical trials are related to be meted out into the growth of vaccine for COVID-19.

- Italy, Italian Medicines Agency (AIFA) has propounded the number of guidelines that are containing the numerous suggestive measure and countermeasure that are to be meted out for the due persistent usage of the clinical trial operations seen to be in the shift of the global arena under the umbrella of COVID-19-issues that are to be seen are in order to contain the virus from spreading and creating a mass amount of deaths round the globe. As in for the other guidelines: a study sponsors are to be required to have hematological analyses that are to be meted out in public usage and the facilities that close to the individuals habitation; clinical trials with the usage of trial sites that are shut down for the usage of society are to be unavailable or suspended or shifted close by trial facility; sponsors that are seen to be first hand reimburse any upper ended costs of damage that are incurred to by the individuals in the state of certain situations. The sponsors are required to first-hand provide for the investigational medicinal products straight away for the patients rather than to the hospital or the treatment facility, a delay in chain can lead to a greater liability.

Companies may need to quickly opt for the greater opportunities over to the drastic shift of the factors that might be in relation to the institutional review boards' (IRBs) levying the newly imposed policy and the containment and suggestions towards the in process study. Such as, various sites are curtailed any foreseeing visits over the clinical trial fund sponsors – including over the process of an on-site monitoring – over the levying of any further notice to avoid lack of the lacking of the spread.

- Companies have been using the method over by proposing to the alternative approaches, such as that of relating to the usage of web camera conferencing or other distance calling modes that are to be performed and the tasks that are generally to be taken in account by the individual, by the individual or the company. These changes are required to fall within the instant adherence towards the protocols and/or revised informed consent forms to regulators and the IRB that investigate the purview of the study.

- Into the currently working of the clinical trials are being seen as the upcoming studies, the concept that has been seen of the study sponsors is for the understanding which seeks towards the usage of any of the additional screening required towards the study of subjects before the enrolment or it is to be done along the ongoing on site procedures. the mode to an additional usage of the testing kits & measures that have seen to be available, companies that may seek to additionally adapt to whether screening for COVID-19. Once again, such additional testing would seem to likely not fall into accordance with the guidelines and may result into the amending of the inclusion/exclusion criteria and other aspects that are to be assessed over into the of study protocols.

- The Companies works in regulations as to whether the study subjects who have been reported tested positive for the detection of the virus, that has been currently surfacing COVID-19 either removed from the ongoing studies, especially in the course the when where the study drug that is to creation, may lead towards the difficulty in the provision of the treatment of the viral infection. This may lead to an scenario, the companies are due to understand and imply over the safety with due accordance and understanding the study drug using in the individual patients, which is also a way to assisting of the required regular insight, for any of the selected individuals. It can also be said that to make instant to make changes in accordance or curtail the understand the protocols for especially look into the addressing what desired steps are to be taken for the study staff that should take part in the event of any of the subjects that are accepted into the study of the COVID-19 patients.

- Vendors that are into the course of performing clinical trial-relating to the services often may come to encounter an issues that can lead to impact their operations or the project of their working, such as it might be in relation to an a rise in the cost effective measures or the labour, any relation to an decrease in the working of the available employees or contractors that are working for the project.

- The Companies that are working often seem to hope in forward towards the working of proactively contact the working of the vendors that are in order to seek permission around the anticipated risks or difficulties that are to be seen and might fall upon over into the carrying out of the pre-decided upon services, risk that is often to be seen for the seller or the buyer who might bring forth an clause of force majeure towards the termination of rendition under the various buyer/seller agreements that are to be meted out.

- While searching for the EUAs in regard to the vaccines and other modes of the therapies, sponsors should Hedley consider into the working for the health care providers to promulgate the feasible plan in over the collecting data which will be able to be interpreted by the FDA. They are also required to should consider another long-term plans over for the studying their theories what are to be seen in relation to the IND programs which follow up an agreeing upon the permission to bring forward a product license or working in accordance to the approval.

- March 15, FDA lead to an refusal as for not granting EUA towards the production or the manufacturing of any biological drug or the vaccine for the COVID-19 infected individuals, has also been seen that, however, that FDA is known to be working in accordance towards the consideration of the untraditional approaches to creating a speedy trial over into the development of the required therapies. There have been reports that FDA is not to agree upon measures for clinical trials to be able to strive right for the in adherence to the sponsor's decision over the developing.

- FDA is due to acceptance of the substantive measures that are presented over the sponsors in order to pursue with the accelerated approval and the acceptance over by portraying an effect on surrogate endpoints—proxies are to be present for showing that it is a product can that works in order to contain or curing of an infectious disease. That may consider an fruitful denouement.

CONCLUSION

Clinical trials have been the mode for the growth of research work and the levelling of the data collection in order, towards the proper collection of data and conduct the working, as the Covid-19 and other addons of the biological warfare continues to attain measure. This will also lead to an a gregarious collision over onto the operations of the research communities, pharmaceutical, biotechnology, other medical options into the context of their clinical development activities. The put forth guidelines help into the brining forth a positive change into the aspect of clinical trials in the global spectrum. It brings forth several platforms for the usage of clinical trials.

Legal Impacts of Medical Experimentation and Clinical Trial

Mr. Kush Kalra* and Ms. Anita**

ABSTRACT: India is emerging as an encouraging destination for medical research. To make sure that the universal brilliance of standard and uprightness of data accumulated in medical research is conserved and also to make certain that the privacy, dignity, individuality and welfare of research subjects are within shield of legal frameworks are safe.

To respond to questions relating to the apt cure of prospect, patients with a particular medical condition. Clinical trial is a considered experiment designed. Researchers test recent medicines, devices, vaccines and therapies on volunteers in clinical trials before the treatments are permitted for use in the general population. Few cases have been recently highlighted in India where medical practitioners were found to be occupied in "illegal" drug trial, being conducted on female children and youngsters. The issue of Medical experimentations is basically concerned with Human Dignity.

Projects to India are outsourced by Global Pharmaceutical companies for several reasons: cutting the cost of medicine development, profit enhancing and speeding controlling acquiescence, and, fostering a environment that is less unfriendly among the world's impoverished ill. As compared to developed countries clinical trials are 50 percent cheaper.

Multinational companies are being encouraged by Government of India for conducting clinical trials in order to draw foreign investments for technological and financial gains in this sector.

INTRODUCTION

Researchers test new medicines, devices, vaccines and therapies on volunteers in clinical trials before the treatments are accepted for use in the general population. To respond to questions regarding the most

---

*PhD Scholar, Sharda University, Greater Noida.
**UGC NET, PhD Scholar, CSS University, Meerut.

suitable treatment of potential patients with a particular medical condition, clinical trial is considered as a premeditated experiment.

In medical research where human beings are involved India is being considered a favourable destination. To make sure that general excellence of standard and uprightness of data accumulated in medical research is conserved, the legal frame works as safe devices to make certain that the dignity, individuality, privacy and welfare of research subjects are safeguarded.

Three types of authoritarian frame work and measures are there in India which may be categorized as Law, guidelines and regulations. We have the legislation in the group of Law expressly for the Drugs and Cosmetics approved in 1940 and axillaries regulations passed in the year 1945 as a necessary behaviour to be followed and enforced by a controlling authority.

In Y Schedule given with Drugs and Cosmetic Act, which is issued by the CDSCO, administered by DCGI, Delhi the implementations of these laws are specified. The guidelines are neither invariably accepted nor mandatorily pursued.

Authority for managing, protection, safeguarding and ensuring standard is included in the 'Drugs & cosmetics Act, 1940' and to experiment the capacity to produce an anticipated result of drugs and medical research outcome. Rules and regulations which are compulsory measures and legal framework have been formulated under rules for Drugs and Cosmetics, 1945.

Few cases have been recently highlighted in India where medical practitioners were found to be involved in "illegal" drug trial, being conducted on female children and youngsters.

The issue of Medical experimentations is basically concerned with Human Dignity. The Human Dignity as defined by L'Heureux-Dube, J. is a complex notion to capture in precise terms.[1] At its smallest amount, it is obvious that the constitutional shield of dignity requires us to recognize the worth of all persons as members of our society.

The definition of Clinical experimentation is as follows "any experimentation research that prospectively assigns human participants or

---

[1] (1995) 29 CRR (2nd) 79 at 106, Egan vs. Canada.

groups of humans to one or more physical health-related interventions to evaluate the effects on physical health outcomes." Not only Interventions consists of medicines but also cells and other organic commodities, radiologic actions, devices, behavioral treatments, preventive care, etc.

Medicine discovery process worldwide is done through clinical trials. To cure number of persistent diseases Medical experimentation in common is a excellent thing and extremely compulsory.

CLINICAL TRIALS: AN INDIAN PERSPECTIVE

Charka Samhita and Sushruta Samhita, two ancient scripts written near the beginning of 200 B.C. and 200 A.D. respectively, demonstrate India's old skills in medical testing. However, a lot has transformed in the clinical testing situation since then.

Projects to India are being outsourced b Global pharmaceutical companies for several reasons: attractive profit, cutting the cost of medicine development and speeding controlling acquiescence, and, fostering a less unfriendly environment among the world's impoverished ill. As compared to urbanized countries clinical trials are more than 50% cheaper in India.

Multinational companies (MNC's) are being requested for conducting clinical trials in order to present foreign investments for financial and technological gains in this sector. Clinical experimentation central ideology is that it should be of wider assistance to society. There cannot be two societies—one that take risk whilst the other reaps the benefits.[2]

In India, Drug & Cosmetic Act, 1940 (amended in the year 2005 & 2008) and Drug & Cosmetic Rules 1945 (amended in the year 2005), has defined a 'clinical trial' as follow "Clinical trial means a systematic research of recent medicine(s) in human subject(s) to generate data for discovering and/or verifying the clinical, pharmacological (including pharmacodynamic and pharmacokinetic) and/or adverse effects with the objective of determining safety and/or efficacy of the recent medicine".

Clinical trial can be broadly categorized as either sponsored (e.g. by a pharmaceutical or device Company) or investigator initiated (e.g. an

---

[2] Most of the concerns were looked into detail and recent instructions and laws were introduced to strengthen the existing rules. Thus, a balance between the ethics and trade has been created for both the government and the private sector.

investigator plans & Conducts a experimentation research). In both type of experimentation, imaging staff will encounter acronyms and terms with which they may be familiar. Learning the "language of the Clinical trials is one of the first task of technologist, investigator or scientist who is asked to participate in or desire to be involved in clinical experimentation.

Regulations are mechanism to make certain that the quality and integrity of data collected in clinical trials is maintained and to make certain that the privileges, safety and wellbeing of participants.[3]

WHO CONDUCTS CLINICAL TRIAL AND WHERE THEY ARE CARRIED OUT?

Clinical trial can be broadly characterized as either sponsored or investigator. Sponsored clinical trial might be sponsored by pharmaceutical companies, academic medical centres such as university based or privately operated university, individuals or group of individual who are willing to take on sponsorship.

If trial is investigator initiated, then such clinical trial is led by an investigator. An investigator (sometime referred as the principal investigator or primary investigator), is an individual under whose authority the Clinical trial occurs.[4] For example in an oncology Clinical trial, the investigator may be an oncologist who delegates the control and administration of radioactive material to a nuclear medicine physician as a sub investigator and a nuclear medicine pet technologist for injection and scanning.

Researchers conduct clinical trials in different settings. Clinical examination can take place in many location, including hospitals, universities, doctors' offices, and community clinics. The place depends on who is conducting the research.

---

[3] Like any experimentation or commercial activity in India, clinical trials are also supposed to go through a very lengthy procedure before they can be carried out. The clinical experiments are put under Schedule Y to the Drug and Cosmetics Rules of 1945, which were amended keeping in mind the increasing number of foreign pharmaceutical companies who are using India as their experimentation base.

[4] The role of investigator is significant as stated in the FDA definition. An investigator is entirely responsible for conduct of clinical trial, and he or she can delegate research task to other individual.

TYPES OF CONTROLLING MECHANISMS

Regulatory mechanisms to govern clinical trials in India are available in three forms:

1. *Law:* A rule of way enforced by a controlling authority e.g., Drugs and Cosmetics Act 1940 and Rules 1945.

2. *Regulations:* An explanation regarding the implement of law. For instance, Schedule Y issued by CDSCO is the Indian regulation for clinical experimentation.

3. *Guidelines:* Guidelines are interpretation of rules which do not have legal obligation and are not universally accepted. Though these guidelines are accepted as Industry Standards. For example, Indian Council of Medical Research [ICMR] instructions, Indian GCP instructions. For conducting clinical trials in India there are quite a few laws, rules. Regulatory bodies and instructions to plan and observe trials in a fair and ethical way.

FUNDAMENTALS OF CONDUCTING A CLINICAL TRIAL IN INDIA

1. Drugs Controller General, India (DCGI) consent required.
2. Approval from respective Ethics Committee where the research is intended.
3. Compulsory registration on the ICMR maintained website www. ctri.in.

Regulatory Bodies Involved with Clinical Trials in India

The high cost of medicines limits access to physical health care around the world. The role of controlling bodies in clinical trials is to ensure quality medicine supply and maintaining physical health and well-being of trial participants. In India, the central government's agency names Central Drugs Standard Control Organisation (CDSCO) under the aegis of Ministry of Health and Family Welfare develops standards and controlling measures for medicines, diagnostics and devices; lays down controlling measures; and regulates the market authorisation of recent medicines as per the Drugs and Cosmetics Act. The Department of Chemical and Petrochemicals of Ministry of Chemicals and Fertilizers (MOCF), through National Pharmaceutical Pricing Authority (NPPA) sets the prices of medicines; maintains data on production, exports and imports; and enforces and monitors the supply of medicines and also gives opinions to parliament on the related issues.

Judicial Discourse on Regulations of Clinical Trials

Due to dearth of medical jurisprudence in India, one is duty-bound to analyse India's most assertive organ[5] i.e. judiciary. Indian judiciary being "the sanctuary of Indian humanity"[6] had in past decided on number of cases directly or indirectly dealing with the subject-matter. The Supreme Court disposed of a writ petition[7] dealing with ban on sale, creation and produce of Quinacrine in shape of pellets, on the grounds that the Government was progressively taking steps in this regard under Sections 10-A and 26-A of the Drugs and Cosmetics Act, 1940.

This judgment illustrated the Supreme Court's viewpoint of intolerance towards clinical malpractices and its protective altitude in this regard. The Government, however, languidly notified such change, and it was urged to move swiftly in Lok Sabha. Also, despite Quinacrine being banned in India through judicial orders, its continued prevalence is still reported in various parts, thereby reflecting the need for a stronger regulatory mechanism. Major critics of the drug regulatory mechanism came out to be the Parliamentary Standing Committee (PSC) on 'Ministry of Health and Family Welfare', remarking in its 59th Report, the lack of perceptions and "skewed priorities" of the organisation Central Drugs Standard Control Organisation (CDSCO) leading to excessive "propagation and facilitation" of the drug industry players, neglecting the interests of consumers. Further, it concluded that the drug regulatory jurisprudence in India was not in proportion to the standards in US, UK and Australia. It reflected India's lack of awareness for its infrastructural shortage, jeopardising the whole licensing phase. Further, the Allahabad High Court, took cognizance in a pending writ petition relating to proliferation of illegal medical experimentations and related it to violation of fundamental rights i.e. right to life and criminal liability especially Sections 302, 304 of

---

[5] See A.M. Ahmadi, "Judicial Process: Social Legitimacy and Institutional Viability", (1996) 4 SCC J-1, pp. 4–5.
[6] See V.R. Krishan Iyer, Legally Speaking, pp. 167, 171.
[7] A.I. Democratic Women Ass. vs. UOI, (1998) 5 SCC 214.

Indian Penal Code.[8] The Court considered awarding damages to the unaware research participants being used as "guinea pigs".

In another case[9] Ss. 26-A, 5 and 7 of Drugs and Cosmetics Act, 1940 was in question. It was contended before the court that the notification based on recommendations of experts committee set up by Drugs Consultative Committee was issued under Sec. 26-A totally eliminating produce and sale of fixed dose combination of corticosteroids with any other medicine for domestic use for treatment of asthma. The validity challenged by placing before the Court various studies and reports on the subject in support.

The court held that, it is the Central Govt. in exercise of powers under Sec. 26-A and not the Court which is competent to make comparative evaluation of relative merits of the studies and reports. Whether comparative chemical trials were required to be conducted before issuance of the notification is also a matter to be decided by the experts and if necessity of such trial is not felt by the experts, it cannot be held that there was no proper assessment of the material submitted by the manufacturers. Notification is also not in consonance of Art. 19(1)(g) of the constitution as the complete prohibition forced thereby on the basis of expert advice was a reasonable restriction. Less drastic course of permitting manufacture and sale of the drugs with a caution about its use would not be adequate to protect general public from the injurious consequences.

The Supreme Court[10] has made it clear that it would not interfere with the evaluation made by expert bodies in technical/scientific matters. The Court observed that, the notification under Section 26A of Drugs and Cosmetics Act, 1940 is completely ruling out the manufacture and sale of a particular drug combination, issued on the basis of opinion of expert committee, regarding difficult effects in case of its consistent use, is a restriction rational and not in consonance of Art. 19(1)(g) of constitution of India.

---

[8] Rahul Dutta v. Union of India, decided on 26-2-2014 (All).

[9] Systopic Laboratories (Pvt.) Ltd. v. Dr. Prem Gupta and Others, 1994 Supp (1) SCC 160.

[10] Ibid.

International Conventions on Clinical Trials

Past 1947, "there was no generally accepted code of conduct governing the ethical aspects of human experimentation, although some countries, notably Germany and Russia, had national policies. One of the darkest episodes in the history of medical experimentation – the horrific experiments carried out by doctors on concentration camp victims in Nazi Germany – was exposed at the Nuremberg trials of 1947. Emerging from the Nuremberg trials was a code of ethics setting out standards to which physicians must conform when carrying out experiments on human subjects".

There are a lot of global instruments that bestow and maintain the privileges of participants in clinical experimentation. Current principles in human experimentation principally emerged after World War II, when Nazi doctors used jailed persons for "inhuman experiments. This resulted in the creation of the Nuremberg code in 1947, which clearly stated voluntary assent as an absolute requirement for human subject experimentation.

Nuremberg Code 1947: The Nuremberg Code was the first modern effort by the international community to create instructions governing experimentation on humans. The standards on medical experimentation laid out by the Nuremberg Tribunal in United States v. Karl Brandt115 (Nuremberg trials) have come to be known as the Nuremberg Code. In Nuremberg trials, Nazi doctors were convicted of the crimes committed during human experiments on concentration camp prisoners.[11]

Declaration of Helsinki 1964

The Declaration of Helsinki was the first international regulation written by physicians for physicians. It is, indisputably, a remarkable document. In less than 2000 words, the World Medical Association (WMA) spells out a set of ethical instructions for physicians and other participants in medical experimentation." It widely regarded as the keystone document on human experimentation ethics. At smallest amount for clinical

---

[11] Clear rules were given as to what was legal and what was not when conducting human experiments. Although not a binding international treaty, the Nuremberg Code became the first international standard defining permissible medical experiments.

experimentation, it is necessary that the results of laboratory experiments be applied to individuals to supplement scientific awareness and to assist distressed humanity.

Council of International Organization of Medical Sciences (CIOMS) Guidelines 1982

International Medical Sciences council was acknowledged in cooperation by the World Health Organization (WHO) and the United Nations Educational, Scientific and Cultural Organization (UNESCO) in 1949 as an worldwide, nongovernmental, not for profit organization and now includes forty five international, national, and associate member organizations. CIOMS goal is to ease and encourage international activities in the field of biomedical sciences, in partnership with the United Nations and WHO.

Convention on Human Rights and Biomedicine (CHRB) 1997

The Human Rights and Biomedicine convention, adopted by Europe in 1997 is a transnational mechanism meant to defend human rights in the explicit pitch of biomedical experimentation, genetics, and physical health care. An exceptional legal mechanism, with authority to seize accountable the ratification states that do not fulfill with the lowest amount of level of security conferred to human rights regarding biology, medicine and physical health care.

Clinical Trial Rules in U.K.

No medicine can be sold in UK without establishing the safety and effectiveness and obtaining a marketing authorization. To collect the data regarding the safety and effectiveness Clinical trials are carried out. The effect of the clinical trial should be submitted to the controlling authorities while obtaining marketing approval. These regulations ensure that clinical testing is undertaken to the highest ethical, scientific and financial standards and guard the rights welfare and dignity of the experimentation participants. Guidance from the European Medicines Agency states that the request for marketing authorisation should include reports of clinical experimentation carried out with the medical product, regardless of whether they are: 1) Completed, 2) Relating to the same medical condition or 3) Conducted by the applicant for the marketing authorisation or some other organisation.

Medicinal devices placed in UK market must fulfill with appliance specific legislation i.e. The Medical Devices Regulations 2002 (Statutory Instrument 2002/618). "The Medical Devices Regulations 2002 (Statutory Instrument 2002/618) came into force on 13 June 2002 and implement the provisions of the:

- Medical Devices Directive 93/42/EEC.
- Active Implantable Medical Devices Directive 90/385/EEC.
- In Vitro Diagnostic Medical Devices Directive 98/79/EEC.

These Regulations establish systems under which a manufacturer must submit to the UK Competent Authority, statistics about clinical investigations of medical devices to be carried out in the UK".

CONCLUSION

Clinical trial industry in India is estimated to be worth approximately around 170 million dollars. A million-dollar query is at what rate it will grow up. Some estimates suggest that it will grow to between 500 million and 1 billion dollars by 2010, others foresee a size of around 250–300 million dollars, assuming that India captures about 10 per cent of the global Clinical Research market. But admittedly, the pace of change has been rather sluggish. When just a few pharmaceutical companies venture into using India as a salvage country around 1990S India's journey into clinical research started (i.e., bringing in those studies which were not doing well globally).

Clinical trial is a subject which is necessary for new frontier of medicines and research; whereas on the other side we have also seen the health activists and petition in Supreme Court to ask whether the norms and guidelines while conducting clinical trials are properly followed or not? And whether the informed consent of the people who are part of these trials is in fact being taken in the way that is necessary? For those who are often terminally ill and desperate for a solution, clinical trials are imperative but for many when they sign, they don't really understand what they are signing up for.

Till 2013, there were no specific regulations to control and supervise the clinical trial, and this resulted into unethical practices. Foreign drug companies steadily started approaching to India in order to carry out clinical trials for their medicinal products and devices. Initially it was seen as a positive for India as it gave employment to the Indians and boosted economy.

Clinical trial exploit poor and vulnerable. Later, it was observed that drug companies are treating participants as Guiana pigs and taking un-due advantage of illiterate people of India. An initiative was taken up by one NGO and a petition was moved to Supreme Court regarding the uncontrolled and unregulated clinical trial. Plea was also made against the new chemical entities. Multinational pharmaceutical companies generally have patent over the new chemical entities.

They used to develop the drug in their country but for the trial they come to India. Phase 2 and Phase 3 are the riskiest phase of the clinical trial. After the clinical trial they return return to their country for marketing approval of the medicine. This was the clear exploitation of Indian human subjects. Companies were getting cheap labour and subjects but in return India was getting nothing except the deaths of innocents and serious adverse events. According to the government data, 2500 deaths were reported during the clinical trial of new chemical entities between 2005 and 2012. During this period, total 475 clinical trials of new chemical entities were carried out of which only 17 were approved for clinical trial. Hon'ble Supreme Court announced its historical judgment in 2013 and banned such uncontrolled clinical trial. Supreme Court also directed the Government to enact effective laws to govern the conduct of clinical trial.

Indian regulators say that India follows global guidelines to conduct clinical trial. Most of the countries like US, UK, Japan etc. have the guidelines as laws but in India they are just recommendations. In country where laws aren't followed where the recommendations would be followed. And it's not only about deaths or serious adverse effects, what about the violation of different kinds?

ETHICAL REVIEW OF TRIALS

For the permission to be accurately well-versed, the information imparted to possible participants must obviously describe study procedures, make a distinction investigation from cure, standard state care and interchange available treatments and practically depict the potential for medical and other payback from participation. Carefully it is to be explained that the potential for restlessness, toxicity, and other risks that may come with the member in the research and clearly demarcate the member's rights concerning departure from involvement. The ethical committee must guarantee that permission is required for the respect of patients and their authentic apprehension.

- To manage the susceptible population a severe need is for the government. For those Phase one trials that are official, the regulators must create a special set of guard and regulations. The making of a Department of 'Human Research Subject Protection' (HRSP) with the Ministry of Health and Family Welfare is suggested.

- It is necessary to draft nationwide strategy regarding reimbursement for research injuries which highlight the tasks of each stakeholder. Probable research injury should be measured based on risk assessment, severity and genuineness of the injury. There is a necessity to have arbitration committees to settle on the degree of damages.

- For all trial participants post-trial condition should be offered in India, due to the necessary ethical principles as long as participants need and are still able to enlarge assistance from experimental interventions, but have no substitute access. Attempts should be made by sponsors to verify that trial participants have access to established interventions outside the research period.

SUGGESTIONS

- Human resource preparation should be done cautiously to deal with the quantity of clinical experiments in future. Instant need is to teach clinical professionals in monitoring, research design, and analysis of clinical trial data.

- To achieve meticulous monitoring and reconsideration of clinical examination data may be with the assistance of "consultants" which is a pioneering way. Consultants may be from academic world. Their answerability is for inspecting facts and figures at sites and support organizations and ensuring global ethics are met. Partnerships with industry experts and professors in the long run will be supportive, particularly in the preparation of Standard Operating Procedures (SOPs) for regulatory inspection.

- Syllabus should be designed to include more on-the job education and there should be more training institutes to improve the number of students.

- In the Indian context guidance should be given to a group of professionals who focuses on the issue of knowledgeable consent. Professionals will confirm that rights of trial subjects are protected and that assent is controlled and educated.

- Enlightening likely participants about clinical experiments play a great job in enrolment success. Patient focussed resources might need to be in numerous languages depending on geographic locations.

- Educational resources should understandable and subject friendly in order to be of worth to individuals of all levels of analysis capability. In addition to improve readability of papers, teaching concerning clinical experiments should include a tough sense of cultural ability. Simply presenting truthful information to potential subjects about a clinical experiment without the suggestion of engaging them in a way that makes them relaxing will do slight to progress enrolment and retention. Therefore, it is significant to recognize and welcome cultural differences, to be responsive to how a subject's healthcare faith scheme influences observance.

Waste Management under COVID-19-Disrupting Lives: The Challenges and Solutions

Ms. Superna Venaik*

ABSTRACT: India's waste administration emergency has genuine ramifications for its environment, economy and general well being. The Biomedical Waste Management & Municipal Solid Waste Management being one of the foremost ecological issues of India. Improper managing of biomedical waste and solid waste causes threat, danger to community. Numerous research, investigations uncover, about 90% of BWM & MSW are discarded informally in open dumps and landfills, making concerns for the general wellbeing and nature.

With COVID-19 insights exhibiting an upward concave trajectory, challenges relating to the generation and management of waste has become disturbing and alarming at this point. The family unit squander is blended in with residential perilous waste for example used needles, mask covers, gauzes, sponge, bandages and so forth. The recyclables such as, cardboards, plastics which may be tainted with COVID-19, represents a genuine hazard to the sanitary workers. It can be asymptomatic transporters who can cause transmission also.

Perceiving these difficulties, the Indian Ministries on Environment, Forest & Climate Change and Urban Development have given a few strategies to improve the circumstance by proclaiming the Solid Waste Management Rules and Biomedical Waste Management Rules. In this paper, an endeavor has been made give an exhaustive survey of the attributes, age, assortment, transportation, removal and treatment innovations of waste rehearsed in India. Looking for advancements that can limit squander age and convert all loss into valuable items, which advances a circular economy through resource asset effective and cleaner creation in enterprises and boost asset recuperation and reusing, recycling for landfill free urban communities. Inspite of the fact

---

*Assistant Professor, Amity Law School, NOIDA, AUUP.

that, it is difficult to ensure widespread access and all-inclusive wellbeing inclusion without a creation bases organized to go to the present and future social needs.

Keywords: Used Masks/Plastics, Environment, Corona Virus Disease, Strategies.

INTRODUCTION

The present COVID-19 a pandemic of the novel coronavirus brings up issues, raising questions and poses challenges relating to the municipal waste management policies and techniques, for example, security and wellbeing measures for workers, squander treatment necessities, unique methods due to coronavirus for squander part. While the waste disposal has been unmistakably rehearsed in different structures. Waste management is a significantly a late action which is intended to recognize and oversee the squanders all through as long as they can remember cycle with solid accentuation in decrease, re-use and reusing exercises. The spread of COVID-19 has expanded public consciousness of the results of an absence of flexibility and readiness to manage such a pandemic infection. Environmental Climate change, water pollution and the drivers of biodiversity misfortune, for example, deforestation and illegal wildlife trade, may expand the danger of further pandemics, for example, vector-borne or water-borne infections.[1]

Inappropriate removal of harmful waste can pose genuine perils to human beings health and to environment, earth. In an instance, the squanders that are disposed inappropriately may drain into the groundwater and it will cause extended defilement of a local's water flexibly. It will have genuine results in rural communities, which rely upon groundwater springs for irrigation and self-consumption.[2] In urban areas also, on improper disposal of hazardous waste, if an unprocessed waste discharges into open drains, which enters the water distribution system, then it can be very

---

[1] Towards recovery- Environmental responses to Corona Virus Disease, Pandemic cited at OECD; Available at https://www.oecd.org/coronavirus/containment-recovery-environmental-responses-covid-19; last accessed on 01-05-2020.

[2] Ravleen Kaur, "Toxics in Your Background." Down to Earth 2008; Replicated – Environmental Law Institute & NL School, India – Environment, Occupational, Safety & Health Compliance Handbook, 2009.

harmful.[3] At same time, an introduction to unsafe waste through self-consumption, breathing contaminated air or direct contact with skin may cause numerous intense, extended or haul wellbeing dangers.[4] Such dangers change incredibly relying upon the kind of unsafe waste at issue, however may incorporate carcinogenesis, regenerative variations from the norm, and focal sensory system issue.

National laws and statutory frameworks are always some essential pre-requisites for controlling transboundary movements and removal of squanders and explicitly solid waste, biomedical and hazardous wastes. The law and policies are needed to provide a guideline/system for outlining the procedures, techniques illuminating obligations for every individual connected with administration of hazardous or dangerous squanders/wastes to guarantee the protection of environment and wellbeing from conceivable harmful impacts of movements/transboundary movements, treatment and disposal or removal of squanders i.e. wastes recovery.

COVID-19[5]

Novel coronavirus Disease – these set of viruses "Coronaviruses (CoV)" are an enormous set of contaminations, which causes affliction running from a normal flu to progressively serious ailments, like, *"Middle East Respiratory Syndrome* (MERS-CoV)" & *"Severe Acute Respiratory Syndrome* (SARS-CoV)". The virus, Corona (COVID-19) is another strain, found in year 2019, which is not being distinguished in the people. This virus is zoonotic, which means it is transmitted among living creatures and individuals. On carrying on extensive research, investigations and examinations, it came to knowledge that SARS-CoV got communicable from civet cats to human beings & MERS-CoV from dromedary camels to human beings. A very few known coronaviruses are already flowing in creatures that has not yet tainted people.[6] A calamity isn't limited by political, social, economic or geographic limits. At a point, when it

---

[3] B.C., Vandana 7 P. Dhar. "Urban Water Supply & Sanitation" Economic Instrument, Environment Sustainability; O.M. Prakash, National Institute of Public Finance & Madras School, Economics, N. Delhi, 1998.

[4] "Scope, Extent of the 'Harmful substances and hazardous wastes' sub-program." Harmful Substances, UNEP 2013, online accessed at WWF.

[5] Causative specialist for COVID 19: SARS-CoV-2.

[6] United Nations, Department of Economic & Social Affairs on COVID-19; Retrieved from https://www.un.org/development/covid-19.html; last accessed on 01-05-2020.

happens, it impacts all. Universally there has been an expansion in the number of reported cases.[7]

As the COVID-19 pandemic carves its dull section into the historical backdrop of humankind, causing serious, genuine disease, illness and death, and upending every day's life. As the pandemic difficulties, challenges national systems, shutters businesses huge and little and limits millions to their homes, it leaves the public's most vulnerable groups exposed to its most ruinous impacts.

Persistence of COVID-19 on Substance

The most recent report printed in *"New England Journal of Medicine"*[8] stated, about virus infectious persistence level upon wooden materials is around 24 hours, lasting period for the plastic & stainless steel is nearby 72 hours. An anxiety, concern, stress and worry arises for employees who are engaged in sanitation jobs, health labourers and casual subdivision waste workers, which cannot be neglected. In India, ragpicker labours strength, on an estimation may be of 1.5–4.0 million, who performs waste assortment, arranging and reusing or recycling the hazardous waste[9]. Undoubtedly, if this is not taught or workers safety issues are not addressed, their wellbeing will be laid down in danger. Subsequently, it is a pressing requirement for every individual to be sensitized on isolated and secured removal segregated and protected disposal of household waste. Beyond what many would consider possible, dry waste ought to be isolated inside the premises for a fitting timeframe before removal, in this manner permitting the infection to bite the dust. Natural waste must be managed through in house treating the dirt procedures.

COVID-19 – A Challenge for Municipal Solid Waste Management

1. Susceptibility of Virus.
2. Asymptomatic – COVID-19 can be a carrier and cause transmission.

---

[7] P. Chidambaram Message on Disaster Management Act, 2005; Retrieved from https://www.undp.org/dam/india/disastermanagement-india.pdf.

[8] Study uncovers to what extent COVID-19 stays irresistible on cardboard, metal and plastic; University of California- Los Angeles; available at https://www.sciencedaily.com/2020/htl; last accessed on 02-05-2020.

[9] *Rajanya Bose & A. Bhattacharya:* Rag pickers, Un-recognised & Unpaid-Critical for Management of Waste in India cited on 12 May, 2017 in India Spend Online Journal; available at https://archive.indiaspend.com.

3. Chances of mixed waste handling – Waste reviews & audits headed by Institute "*The Energy and Resources Institute*" in year 2019 uncovered, about places in Delhi of area East, North and South zone, that nearby about 88%, 89% and 95% family units respectively were giving over household hazardous waste with general municipal solid waste.

Introspecting – The Facts

With the limited accessibility of just 198 "*Common Bio-Medical Waste Treatment Facilities* (CBMWTFs)" and 225 "*hostage incinerators*", the most difficulties, challenges which India's going up against the social insurance facilities, that needs to deal with the ascent in squander, the waste quantities foreseen from the COVID-19 outbreak.[10] On specific address to this, coronavirus focal point, the epicentre Wuhan, China has observed increase of six times, the biomedical squanders in this pinnacle of its outbreak. CBWTFs treated the bio medical waste in approximation of 78% Nation's full quantity of 2,00,000 tons as per the 2017 year assessment. The rest of remaining untreated and discarded wastes were dealt by captive treatment facilities and certain wastes were profound burials. Several parts of the States, Districts do not have any CBMWT facilities. Whereas, in addition to, non-harmful wastes, similar to dry reusable waste (waste which has prompt money related worth) should likewise be dealt with most extreme consideration in the wake of interacting with Covid-19 patients. Alongside infection loaded waste from artificial treatment centre, the diagnostic and quarantine facility centre, the greater issue emerges from the household or family unit, misuse of those displaying minor or negligible symptom.

The National Pandemic Preparedness Plans (NPPP) were developed by all countries between 2005 and 2010 in anticipation of influenza pandemic.[11] These are extraordinary resources which can be modified with regard to encounters and gaps identified in the COVID-19 pandemic.

---

[10] **Sourabh Manuja:** Waste administration frameworks to handle Covid-19 pandemic; Cited online at live mint on 9th April, 2020; available at https://www.livemint.com/can-waste-management-handle-covid-19-pandemic/html.

[11] Bhatia and Abraham: Time to Revisit Response to Pandemics, Indian J. Med Res 151, February & March 2020, pp 111-113; Available at http://www.ijmr.org.in/temp/IndianJMedRes1512111-4858397_132943.pdf; last accessed on 01-05-2020.

Accordingly, foreseen innovative technological advances can be implemented in the immediate future.[12]

NATIONAL LAW AND POLICIES FOR GOVERNANCE OF WASTE MANAGEMENT

The Environment Protection Act, 1986[13]

The legislation targets in setting up an adequate, appropriate protection system, by conferring authorities to the Central Government to regulate the provisions with respect to discharging of all types of waste on land, in stream. The EPA, 1986 is one of the essential law making bodies for protection of the environment and for regulation of waste management. Section 7- Environment Protection Act, puts a main forbiddance on environment with a provision that – no one as an individual/healthcare facility, conveying any activity, which should emit or discharge or release some environmental contaminants as impurities in abundance of listed gauges. Further, another provision of Section 9 mentions, *"If any occasion takes place, which hurts or harm the environment through any predicted or unanticipated occasion, the individual liable for the damage is compelled by a sense of honour to forestall or mitigate the toxin released because of such occasion."* The individual is additionally obliged to report the Pollution Control Boards of State/Central Governments concerning the instance, which may affect the natural environment.

The Rules for Hazardous Wastes (Management, Handling and Transboundary Movement) Rules, 2008

Another essential guidelines or directions for regulation in India, tending to the dealing of hazardous waste. The Rules gets enforcement through the Environment Protection Act 1986 which authorizes the Central Government to "take every such measures, as it deems vital or expedient with the end goal of assurance and improving the quality of the

---

[12] World Health Organization; Basic strides for making or refreshing a national pandemic flu readiness plan. WHO; 2018. Available from: https://www.who./influenza/preparedness/pandemic/steps-influenza; accessed on March 25, 2020.

[13] The Act was enacted vide Article 253 – Indian Constitution on the aftermath of Bhopal gas catastrophe. It tries to actualize the resolutions made at the United Nations Conference at Stockholm on Human Environment 05/06/1972.

environment and preventing, controlling and abating environmental – ecological contamination, the pollution[14]."

The Rules puts a commitment on an occupier of hazardous factory, industry, unit- to deal with handling of environmental waste in safe and sound manner. The occupiers are required to send the untreated wastes which is dangerous, hazardous, harmful waste for the treatment of reprocessing or reusing or recycling in a safe manner to the recognized/ approved facility centre by the Central/State governments. Every individual, occupied with the trade of professing the treatment of hazardous process in storing, packaging, collecting, destructing, transforming, processing etc. has to obtain license from the State Pollution Board. The aforesaid occupier as recyclers, an occupier, the re-users or the re-processors are allowed to store the waste for as long as ninety days[15].

The Municipal Solid Waste Management Rules, 2016[16]

The solid waste defined under Solid Waste Management Rules 2016 as "solid waste incorporating solid or semi solid household left-over, the sanitary, commercial, organizational, food preparation, shops waste and another nonresidential litters, the street sweepings, silt removed or collected from the surface drains, horticulture waste, agriculture, dairy waste, treated bio-medical waste excluding industrial, the bio-medical and electronic, battery waste, the radio-active waste all generated in the region under the local authorities and other entities being cited in Rule 2;[17] They are of

---

[14] The Environment Protection Act, 1986.

[15] The SPCB - State Pollution Control Board can prolong the allowed period of capacity storage duration.

[16] The Central Government, enacted these Rules through statutory authority conferred through Sections-3, 6, 25 – E. Protection Act, 1986.

[17] The Solid Waste Management Rules 2016–Rule 3(46) defines the term Solid Waste; Rules applicability to the urban local body professed by Registrar General & Indian Census Commissioner as modern industry townships heavily influenced by Railroads, Air Terminals, Airbases, Ports and Harbours, Defence Establishments, Special Economic Zones, State and Central Government Institutions, spots of shrines, religious and historical importance as may be notified by respective State government from time to time and to each household, institutional, business and any other non-residential solid waste generator arranged in the regions with the exception of mechanical squanders, hazardous squanders, unsafe synthetic substances, bio medical squanders, electronic waste, lead acid batteries beside radio-active waste as mentioned in The Environment Protection Act 1986.

various sorts such as Biodegradable waste, Non biodegradable waste and Household hazardous waste.

Adaptations to "The Management of Municipal Solid Waste"

1. Civic amenity sites, reuse and repair centres have either close down or their services are reduced. On request benefits, the services are likewise intruded.
2. Sorting the specific standards at home for masks, gloves, tissues and disposable cloths not to be blended in with the recyclables, bio waste, residual-lingering waste.
3. Frequency for waste assortment has been adjusted according to explicit needs because of staff lack, wellbeing and safety measures which decreases the proficiency.
4. For Waste Treatment, disparagement to the obligatory preliminary blended waste treatment before its removal or disposal might be required either by incineration or controlled landfill.[18]

Biomedical Waste Management Rules 1998

The terminology defined under Biomedical Waste Management Rules 2016, "Bio-medical waste means any squander, generated in the process of diagnosis, treatment or immunization of human beings or animals or research activities pertaining thereto or in the production or testing of biological or in health camps." It further mentions all wastes generated at health care facilities, which might have adverse effects on individual's or on environment if the untreated wastes are not disposed properly.[19]

---

[18] The Association of Cities & Regions Organization for sustainable management issued Rules as The Municipal Waste Management rules during COVID; cited at https://www.acrplusorg/waste/management-covid; last accessed on 01-05-2020.

[19] Every single such wastes, which may cause harm to the environment or individuals health adversely, considered as infectious and such wastes are to be treated according to Bio Medical Waste Management Rules 2016.

Classes of Bio-Medical Waste Segregation

Types	*Nature of Waste*	*Management Facility for Artificial Treatment & Removal Options*
Beige colour	(a) **Human beings Functional Wastes:** tissues, organs/body parts & fetus.	Ignition or Plasma Pyrolysis/ profound funeral.*
	(b) **Animal Anatomical Waste:** New investigational creature corpses, parts of body- organs, tissues, animals waste used in investigations or in research in animal clinics, laboratories of schools.	Burning or Plasma Pyrolysis/ interment.*
	(c) **The Dirty Squander:** Substances tainted with lifeblood such as bandages, dressing casts- cotton swabs & bags encompassing remaining/discarded blood constituents.	Burning/Plasma Pyrolysis/deep interment.
	(d) **Perished or Rejected Drugs:** Medicinal left-overs antibiotics, cytotoxic pills & things polluted with cytotoxic medicines, glass/plastic ampoules, containers.	Lapsed cytotoxic medications has to be returned to the manu- facturer/supplier. Everything additionally disposed drugs shall be sent back to manufacturer or to be disposed by ignition.
	(e) **Element Wastes:** Substances used in production of biological or discarded antiseptics.	Incineration disposal/Plasma Pyrolysis/Encapsulation.
	(f) **Chemical Liquid Waste:** Fluid wastes created from substance usage on production of biological, discarded disinfectants. Another X-ray film developing liquid, Formalin, infection ridden secretions etc.	Waste shall be pre-treated prior to the mixing with other wastewater as given in Schedule-III.
	(g) Excluded cotton, mattresses, bedcovers polluted with lifeblood or body fluid.	Non-chlorinated chemical disinfection tracked by incineration or Plasma Pyrolysis for energy recovery. In absenteeism of overhead facilities, shredding, mutilation sterilization. Squander to be sent for recovery, incineration, Plasma Pyrolysis.
	(h) **Microbiology – Biotechnology and other medical laboratory waste:** Blood packs, Lab cultures, stocks or specimens of microorganisms, live/attenuated vaccines, human/animal cell cultures used in research, industrial laboratories, production of residual toxins/dishes & gadgets used for cultures.	Pre-treatment for castration, fumigation with non-chlorinated synthetic substances as per National AIDS Control Organization or World Health Organization guidelines thereafter for Ignition.

Types	Nature of Waste	Management Facility for Artificial Treatment & Removal Options
Bloods hot Colour	Recyclable polluted waste generated from throwaway matters – tubes, flasks, intravenous cylinders and sets, catheters, urine bags, vacutainers with their needles cut) and scarves, syringes (without needles and fixed needle syringes).	Autoclaving, micro-waving/hydroclaving by destroying, mutilation or combination of sterilization and shredding. Treated waste shall be sent to government approved licensed recyclers for energy recovery or plastics to diesel/fuel oil/for road making, whichever is possible. Plastic waste ought not be sent to landfill sites.
Transl ucent colour	Metal wastes – Used prickles, syringes with fixed needles, needles from needle tip cutter or burner, scalpels, blades and any other polluted sharp object, which may cause puncture and cuts. It includes both used, discarded and contaminated metal sharps.	Autoclaving, Dry Heat Sterilization by shredding, destroying or mutilation or encapsulation in metal container or cement concrete; combination of shredding cum autoclaving; and on the permission of the State Pollution Control Boards or Pollution Control Committees to send wastes for its final discarding on iron foundries/sanitary landfill or designated concrete waste sharp pit.
Navy colour	(a) Glassware-polluted glasses or broken/ discarded of medicinal flasks and bottles excluding those, if contaminated with cytotoxic wastes. (b) Metal form Implantations in human beings.	Disinfecting on soaking washed glass wastes after cleaning with detergent and Sodium Hypochlorite through autoclaving, microwaving or hydroclaving and lastly it is to be sent for recycling.

Source: "The Bio-Medical Waste Management Rules, 2016."[20]

The Manufacture, Storage and Import of Hazardous Chemical Rules, 1989

For applying upon the individuals who are manufacturing, storing and importing of harmful unsafe chemical substances. Its primary reason for the MSIHC Rules, build up necessities for occupiers for recognizing,

---

[20] Notified in the Official Gazette of India, Retrieved from http://www.indiaenviron mentportal.org.in/2016.pdf; last accessed on 01-05-2020.

forestalling and limiting the effects of potential significant mishaps. Occupants should have crisis layouts, will be asked to give reports in regard to proposed exercises before they start tasks, to give point by point reports following any significant mishaps and keep up exact names on compartments of hazardous chemicals.[21]

Batteries (Management and Handling) Rules 2001

The application of is on using the batteries & its constituents. Batteries are explicitly demarcated in the Rules to incorporate the lead acid batteries containing metallics and are wellspring of electrically powered energy. The producers, traders, compilers and reprocessors have extensive, explicit obligations in the Rules, comprising the stated procedures on collecting, reusing, reprocessing and transportation.[22]

The Chemical Accidents (Emergency Planning, Preparedness and Response) Rules

It tends to cover the ambit of the mishaps "including a fortuitous or unexpected or unintended event occurrence while taking care of any perilous – hazardous chemicals concoctions bringing about ceaseless, irregular or rehashed presentation to death or injury or damage to any person or harm to property."

The Plastic Waste (Management and Handling) Rules, 2011

A set of governing directions for controlling the utilization, assembling, manufacturing, reusing and reconditioning the plastic left-overs. The plastic squander which is disposed off after its utilization of completion of the items lifespan. The Rules have an unchanging applicability for every wholesaler, distributors, customers, retailers/manufacturers of plastic products. The reusing, reprocessing of plastic items is to be done in a fixed practice methodology as per The Bureau of Indian Standard Specification.[23]

---

[21] Rule 4(2)(b-(i) The Manufacture Storage & Import of Hazardous Chemical Rules 1989; MoEF Notification S.O. 966(E). New Delhi.

[22] MoEF issued Batteries (Management & Handling) Rules, 2001.

[23] *Pramit Bhattacharya* – Waste Management Laws in India; Available at http://blog. ipleaders.in/waste-management; last seen on 02-05-2020.

Disaster Management Act, 2005

It defines a disaster or fiasco as "a disaster, setback, mishap, catastrophe, calamity or grave occurrence of event in any territory emerging from natural or artificial causes or coincidentally by accident or negligence, carelessness which brings about significant death toll or human torment or harm to and obliteration of property or harm to or debasement of condition and is of such a nature or extent as to be past the adapting limit of the network of the influenced region." Accessed.

The Water (Prevention and Control of Pollution) Act 1974

The specific law enacted for preventing & controlling of water pollution and to maintain/restore healthiness, the wholesomeness of water in the nation. It further lays down, the foundation of Boards for purpose of the prevention along with controlling of water pollution so as to complete the previously mentioned purposes. The Water Act, 1974 restricts and forbids the release of contaminants, impurities into water streams beyond the prescribed standards and the law states punishments of its non-compliance. At Central level, the Water Act 1974 has set up the Central Pollution Control Board which sets principles to prevent and regulating for abatement of water pollutant contamination. The SPCB work and function on the directions of the CPCB and the State Governments.

The Air (Prevention & Control of Pollution) Act 1981

A legislation enacted to prevent, avoid, regulate and abate air pollution by conferring powers to the same boards as of The Water Act 1974 at the Central and State levels towards achieving the objective of stated reasons.

The Indian Penal Code (IPC) 1860

The Indian Penal Code of 1860 has already listed the provision of solid left-over administration in *"Chapter XIV - offences influencing the public wellbeing, health, safety, comfort, suitability, courtesy and principled morals."* As this waste in solid form, ascends to different kinds of illness, infections and are hazardous to others wellbeing, now have to be treated as 'public nuisance' and shall be punishable. However in IPC, no direct specific section is listed which manages the issue of solid waste.

Code of Criminal Procedure, 1973

The provisions Sections 133–143 concerns for environment protection, being a procedural law deals with the procedure although does not states any definition of public nuisance.

Central Pollution Control Board Guidelines for Handling Wastes—As Advisory

The supreme, apex pollution monitoring body, Central Pollution Control Board established through-*"The Water (Prevention & Control of Pollution) Act, 1974 and The Air (Prevention & Control of Pollution) Act, 1981"* has issued explicit rules[24] for segregation wards, the quarantine/isolation facility centres, sample test collection centres, labs, ULBs along with shared biomedical waste treatment and disposal removal along with previous forms and practices of BMW Management Rules 2016. Highlighting the motto, the CPCB expressed that rules are primarily to consolidate explicit pre-requisites and obligations of people working for sewage treatment plants at healthcare centres besides segregating the wastes of quarantine homes and of non quarantine households.

According to the guidelines:[25]

1. For COVID-19 patients, the *"Confinement Wards"* of Healthcare Centres obligated to keep distinct shading oblique canisters/sacks/ compartments inwards, assorting legitimate isolation of squanders according to the BMWM Rules as amended and CPCB guiding principles on usage of the BMW Management Rules.

2. A safeguard, twofold coated sacks (exhausting 2 bag packs) utilizing in the assortment from Covid-19 segregation ward zones for guaranteeing satisfactory quality and no spills.

3. Collecting and putting away biomedical waste independently preceding giving over the equivalent to *"Common Bio-medical (Clinical) Waste Treatment & Disposal Facility (CBWTF)."*

---

[24] Covid-19 Managing Waste generated during patients treatment Guidelines; April 21, 2020; Online News website- Business standard; retrieved from https://www. businessstandard.com/covid-19-directives-for-handling-waste-on-patients-treatment; last accessed on 01-05-2020.

[25] CPCB, Ministry of Environment, Forest & Climate Change; retrieved from https:// www.tnpcb.gov.in/Guideline_COVID_19_waste.pdf; last accessed on 01-05-2020.

4. Separate, specifically labelled- collection container tagged as 'COVID-19' for storing the waste i.e. squanders, keeping in transitory extra space preceding giving to authorised CBWTF personnel. The biomedical left-over is to be lifted from isolation wards and is to be kept in CBWTF Collection van.

5. Again, from infected COVID 19 wards, the option to obligatory marking, sacks/holders utilized for collection of biomedical wastes, ought to be named as 'COVID-19 Waste. It is to be understood as *"adding that general waste not having contamination should be disposed of as solid waste as per Solid Waste Management Rules, 2016"*.

6. Maintaining distinct, different database w.r.t. COVID-19 wastes of detachment wards. Utilizing committed streetcars to carry assorted containers. A mark 'COVID-19 Waste' is to be made in all such things. The (internal and external) box of compartments/streetcars/trolleys which shall be used for Covid-19 waste, ought to be cleaned for storing with disinfectant of quantity 1 % sodium hypochlorite solution every day.

7. The "Report Opening" of activity of COVID-19 ward, to SPCBs[26] and respective *"Common Bio-medical Waste Treatment and Disposal Facility"* in specific area.

8. For timely collection and transfer of waste either as biomedical or general has to be sent to the provisional waste storage area, it has to be specific and for this task, special devoted sanitation labourers deputation is required.

9. All individuals need to follow steps as measures for ensuring safe handling, disposal of waste who is working in the quarantine camps/home-care for suspected Covid-19. The general waste solid in nature (family unit squander) produced from quarantine centres or camps ought to be given over to squander gatherers recognized by Urban Local Bodies or as according to the predominant nearby technique for discarding general waste.

10. The identification of biomedical waste, if any, produced from the quarantine centres/camps is gathered, the collection has to be in yellow-shaded sacks.

---

[26] State Pollution Control Board constituted under "The Water Act 1974 and The Air Act 1981" as authorities to function for prevention, control and abatement of water/air pollution.

11. Persons operating/working in quarantine camps or centres will call the *"Common Bio-medical Waste Treatment & Disposal Facility"* operators for gathering biomedical wastes, the moment it is generated.
12. The people who have been diagnosed with symptom of COVID-19 have to reside in their respective camps or homes as quarantining themselves for the 14 days as directed by hospitals or local authorities.
13. The disposal of biomedical leftover wastes generated in quarantine camps/isolation centres/homes shall be deemed as *'household hazardous waste'* as defined under The Solid Waste Management Rules 2016 & these guidelines.[27]

GLOBAL EFFORTS TO COMBAT COVID-19

The World Health Organization Concerns on Water, Sanitation, Hygiene and Waste Handling for COVID-19

For cleaning the utility gloves, reusable plastic covers with cleanser and afterwards water sterilization by using 0.5 percentage of sodium hypochlorite solution on every usage has been issued as mandate. Single usage hand-gloves (nitrile or latex) and gown outfits ought to be disposed off after each utilization and not to be reused/worn again. On expelling the PPE kits, the hands sanitation is required. If grey coloured water incorporates antiseptic in earlier scrubbing, it shouldn't be treated again or chlorinated. It's significant lies in for discarding in channels associated with a septic framework or in soak way pit only. The respective pit has to be fenced off on discarding its grey coloured water in a soakaway pit to prevent its tampering and to keep away from conceivable introduction on account of flood.[28]

UNEP Directions to Beat COVID-19

With the consistent aggravation and adverse impacts of COVID-19 upon human wellbeing, the concern has arisen where the economy is escalating step by step the governments are asked to treat all waste managements,

---

[27] Guidelines – Managing – the Treatment & Disposal of Waste during the treatment – COVID-19 https://www.tnpcb.gov.in/pdf_2020/Guideline_COVID_19_waste.pdf
[28] Special Brief - World Health Organization - "Water, Sanitation, Hygiene and Waste Management for COVID-19" available at http://www.who/publication/watersanitation-waste-management; last accessed on 02-05-2020.

such as medical, household and other hazardous waste so as to limit the conceivable auxiliary effects upon wellbeing and nature.[29]

The Basel Convention

The Convention characterizes "environmentally sound management of wastes" i.e. "squanders subject to its control as finding a way to guarantee that these squanders are overseen in a way which will ensure human wellbeing and the earth against the unfriendly effects which may result from such squanders." With specification, the Convention explicit that special rules favouring the earth administration shall be chosen by the Contracting Parties.

The States/Parties of the Basel Convention, have assented for framing essential provisions to guarantee – the dealing, handling of hazardous wastes, even on transboundary movement. For protecting human health and environment, the disposal place – right from its generation to treatment, from treatment to storage and to storage to recovery/final disposal shall be regulated.[30]

OECD[31] Principles for the Development of Waste Management Policies

1. *The Spring Mitigation Principle* – waste creation/generation of waste to be limited as far as its amount and it capability to cause contamination through fitting plant and procedure structures.
2. *The Integrated Life Cycle Principle* – during the generation, use, recovery and removal of waste, the substances and items have to be planned, designed and overseen to check the base ecological effect.
3. *An Anticipatory Preventive Measure Principle* – a precautionary measure is adopted in consideration of expenses, activity/inaction advantages, on a logical premise, regardless of whether constrained to accept that discharge of wastes in natural environment of substances, the wastes

---

[29] Waste Management a public service to combat COVID-19; Press Release – Chemicals & Waste on 24th March 2020 at UNEP. Available at https://www.unenvironment.org/waste-management-publicservice-fight-beat-covid-19; last retrieved on 01-05-2020.

[30] To control the transboundary movements of hazardous wastes and disposals – The Basel Convention; Retrieved from http://basel.int/Implementation/Technical/Guidelines; last accessed on 01-05-2020.

[31] The well-known Organization for Economic Co-operation & Development (OECD) – An international organization, to build better policies for better lives.

or vitality is presumably going to affect or harm to the wellbeing of humans or environment.

4. *The Integrated Pollution Governing Norm* – administration of hazardous waste necessitates the consideration for cross media and multi-media synergistic effects to be founded on a system;

5. *The Standardization Principle* – setting standards for environmentally, ecologically, sound management of hazardous wastes at every phase of its preparation, treatment, disposal, removal, recuperation and recovery;

6. *A Self-sustaining Rule* – nations which ought to guarantee that removal of waste produced inside their domain territory shall be undertaken, implying that being perfectly compatible with environmentally sound handling of wastes.

7. *The Proximity Principle* – The hazardous waste removal must occur as shut as conceivable to their point of generation with acknowledgment, recognition of financially, economically & environmentally sound management.

8. *The Transboundary Movement Principle*- controlling on the inter-state transit of waste for productive and environmentally comprehensive controlling of the left overs.

9. *The accountability through Polluter Pays Principle* – There shall be absolute liability for curing, remedying the consequences of the pollution, if actions could not prevent the contamination.

10. *The Rule of Dominance/Sovereign* – while framing the national waste management structure, every state party should keep the political, social and economic conditions. To accord with country's enactments, a nation may ban hazardous wastes importation.

11. *A Principle of Community Partaking* – Giving rights of accessibility to public for participation in information concerning management of hazardous wastes.

COVID-19 – A Pandemic Disease – Complicating the Sustainable Development Goals

The COVID-19 overall health pandemic rapidly changing the ways, we live and work. In the time of sustainable development and at a time, when the world is moving in the direction of accomplishing the SDGs, this ailment is complicating the SDG execution endeavor just as representing a genuine hazard to accomplishing focuses on communicable infections, training, life expectancy and decent work.[32]

The economic, financial stuns related to COVID-19, for example, the interruption of its modern creation, dropping commodity fares, financial budgetary market unpredictability along with rising uncertainty, derailing existing tepid economic growth and multifaceted intensified risks from its further actions. Thus, it incorporates a retreat from multilateralism, the discontent and distrust of globalization, increased debt risk misery, recurrent & severe climate shocks. Collectively it will make, sustainable finance more difficult and further undermine the ability to accomplish the Sustainable Development Goals (SDGs) by 2030.[33]

The Challenges to Overcome

1. Separate collection of increasing quantity of DHW (including Gloves, masks) is a challenge.
2. Waste collection staff lack "Personal Protective Equipment" PPEs/ regular supply of PPEs is a challenge because of getting contaminated.
3. Lack of training of sanitary staff to handle general waste discharged under COVI-19 pandemic especially asymptomatic citizens.
4. CPCB Guidelines says, "*Used masks and gloves generated from home quarantine or other households should be kept in paper bag for a minimum of 72 hours prior to disposal of the same as general waste*" – The possibilities exist of transmitting COVID via dry waste also.
5. Awareness among public to segregate dry and wet waste and domestic hazardous waste along with a system of segregated collection could not be established at instance.
6. Infrastructure mismatch or site conditions do require manual loading of waste, which indicates more possibilities of contamination.

---

[32] Sustainable Development Solutions Network organized virtual conference to examine the implications of COVID-19 for public health and SDGs on 27th April, 2020. Available at https://www.unsdsn.org/covid-19-webinar on 30.04.2020 at 2:55AM.

[33] United Nations Report on Financing for Sustainable Development 2020 -Inter-agency Task Force provides comprehensive assessment of progress; Retrieved from https://developmentfinance.un.org/developmentfinance.un.org; last accessed on 01-05-2020.

7. Waste processing and treatment plant operators suspects danger and may be are at risk. Regular training for plant staff on handling infectious waste is a challenge.

8. With lockdown and risks in waste collection, the informal recycling has almost stopped. There is a concern for PPEs for informal sector workers.

9. Door to door collection has been compromised to one-point collection in many localities, due to lack of staff/informal collectors in some of the areas. Vehicle collecting COVID waste is required to be disinfected, as they can also be the carriers of infection.

10. Monitoring, reviewing and verifying systems are required to avoid unknown leakages of contaminates to environment.

11. PPEs appropriate usage and removal among sanitary workers, their social distancing at collection centres and waste treatment plants.

Exit Strategies: Promoting Health Equity

For the development, recovery, treatment and removal of squanders i.e. wastes, a comprehensive controlling framework is required to limit its harm or causing damage to human health, wellbeing or harm to the environment. The mechanism to regulate the storage of wastes produced or generated, its transit from the generator to the site of its inevitable stockpiling, recuperation, reuse or removal is required. The obligation of care as a duty regarding the naturally sound management of all squanders i.e. wastes is to be set up with the responsibility. Prior to any waste to be moved, the level of characterization is to be marked in packaging for treatment. The idea of waste prevention, control, abatement and reduction incorporates several measures for a beneficial change in the waste management. The training is necessary for carrying out proper structured basis for control of waste treatment, the recycle the reuse and removal facility.

The Way Forward for Shared Responsibility and Solidarity

A positive approach for sustainable, just and resilient recovery, where the process will be translating the principles into practice. The world is battling the COVID-19 as global health emergency and its social and economic ramifications. It is also racing against the clock to avoid the environmental crisis around the corner. The pandemic situation has made a realization of preparedness when crisis hit and has shown the results for postponing the bold decisions which can led to have huge costs for climate change, biodiversity downfall, life-shortening air pollution and ocean acidification. Earth day being celebrated on 22nd April made to rethink on sustainability of environment, economic and social systems to have an integrated approach[34].

Still, far to go, as certain wastes are not yet classified to be treated/disposed in nature of recycle wastes, material recovery facility with piece vendors, recyclers along with corporates (keeping EPR suggestions) serving urban communities to earn incomes from waste. Certainly, it will help in closing the circular budget-economy loop, on expanding waste, reusing, recycling and recovery and lessening landfill area necessities. In addition, natural waste administration plants can assist cities accessibility for renewable energy sources or fuels such as biogas, substituting the fossil fuel demand also, in making urban areas greener. It is similarly significant for facilities to operate at full limit, with assured supply of raw materials as well as market demands for outputs. To reduce the burden on the city's sanitation frameworks and making recycling, treatment processes just like robust and reliable, an urgent necessity has arisen to set up impetus and showcase better mechanisms and systems. There is also a need to learn from COVID-19 crisis and articulate approaches to make waste management safer in case of such pandemic situations.[35] The Ministry of Environment Forest and Climate Change in 2016 year has notified a requirement for segregation, segregated waste treatments. Its implementation by the Ministry of Housing and Urban Affairs and respective State Urban Development Departments needs to be more efficaciously dealt. Generally, the most of cities lack appropriate linkages to collect segregated domestic hazardous waste and simply send it for handling & removal, despite SWM Rules 2016 year which already obligates linking domestic hazardous waste to hazardous waste disposal facilities.

---

[34] Tackling Coronavirus published on 22-04-2020 on http://www.oecd.org/coronavirus/ en/; last accessed on 01-05-2020.

[35] Dr. Suneel Pandey and Mr. Sourabh Manuja, Used Prickles- Masks & Plastic: Why India Need Smart Policies for Managing Squanders during Post-Covid19; Referred through https://www.news18.com/usedneedles-masks;plastic-india-need-strategies-manage-waste-post-covid19.html last accessed on 30.04.2020.

The disposal of Personal Protective Equipment[36] which includes all defensive kits, hand-gloves, covers, face-masks and other waste generated from emergency clinics, hospitals, medical facilities are equally significant. Such guidelines are being issued by Authority- Central Pollution Control Board (CPCB) for COVID-19 bio medical waste management issued an advisory to CBMWTFs for the diagnostics and quarantine, for functional/ operational of extra working hours and mandate for PPE kits for collection staff and vehicles. However, its a requirement of guaranteed limit building and direction, management to oversee municipal solid waste, especially particularly family unit, the risky waste.[37]

---

[36] Personal Protective Equipment's (PPEs) are *"protective, defensive gears intended to safeguard the health of workers by limiting the exposure to a biological agent (bacteria, viruses, fungi, other microorganisms and their associated toxins."*

[37] Sourabh Manuja; Waste Management Systems handle Pandemic disease as COVID-19 Retrieved From https://www.livemint.com/waste-management-system-handle-COVID-19-pandemic; last accessed on 30.04.2020.

Bio-Medical Waste Management: A Study on Assessment of Knowledge, Attitude and Practices in Health Care Centres during Pandemics like COVID-19

Dr. Rupinder Kaur*

ABSTRACT: Bio-medical waste has emerged as an issue of major concern not only to health care centres in particular and environment and public in general especially at present time when world is facing coronavirus. It can be infectious, toxic and causes risks to both people and the environment. Health care centres/Medical wastes produced from hospice care process are a hazard for both surrounding environment and the entities which depends on it. India generates about 600 tons of biomedical waste every day, of which only 90 per cent is treated. With Covid waste being generated at a faster pace and high volume, it is more challenging to see that it is disposed without causing additional health problems. On an average, about 2 tons of Covid waste is generated in each State from diagnoses, quarantine and treatment of the disease. It is a very complex process to properly manage such a huge health hazard waste by the management of the hospitals. "It is the duty of every occupier, (in the case of AIIMS, the Director, AIIMS) i.e. a person who has the control over the institution or its premises, to take all steps to ensure that waste generated is handled without any adverse effect to human health and environment" as per the Bio Medical Waste (Management and Handling) Rules in 2016. Reuse of such hazardous material is very harmful and can spread number of infectious diseases. Therefore the main aim of the study to have complete assessment of "knowledge, attitude and practices regarding the bio medical waste management in health care centers in a pandemic like COVID-19". The study is based on the primary survey conducted at Private hospital, Patiala, Punjab. The study reveals that medical staff at hospital is well aware of the regulations related to medical waste management but there is no in house treatment procedure of such waste in hospital. So study point out the need to provide awareness about,

* Assistant Professor, Amity University Noida, NOIDA, AUUP.

handling procedure and there must be proper equipment to handle and dispose of the medical waste.

Keywords: Bio-Medical Waste, Health Hazard Waste, Health Care, Medical Waste Management, Covid 19.

INTRODUCTION

Health care as an enterprise is an essential foundation for every civilized community. Pharmaceutical products, clinical equipment and instruments assists in aiding patients in hospitals, naturally, steers the creation of diverse medical and non-medical wastes. Medical waste means "any waste, which is generated during the diagnosis, treatment or immunization of human beings or animals or research activities pertaining thereto or in the production or testing of biological or in health camps." It is a continue issues as human progress. Bio-Medical waste generation can vary depending on number of factors such as hospital magnitude, category; patient ratio; degree of occupancy; geographic location; local waste management ordinances; waste disposal policies in hospitals. Environment and Public Health Organizations has reported that on an average about 1.7 kg per person per day healthcare waste is generated. Improper knowledge and inappropriate technique of handling biomedical waste can result in serious consequences on health and environment. Bio-medical waste processing facilities change the biological property or subdue the quality of clinical waste for causing disease. Dismantling facilities shatter clinical waste by mutilating it, or tearing it apart to render it less infection and unrecognizable as clinical waste. Once Bio medical waste is treated and destroyed completely, there is no need of further tracked of it. Their treatment and destruction facilities include incinerators, treatment operations, sterilize, or treat the waste with disinfectants, heat, or radiation. Therefore proper management of bio-medical waste is demand of today era. It is a challenge not only to health care centres but to entire human force. It is a worldwide Humanitarian issue. Medical waste management deals with handling and disposal procedure of waste generated during diagnosis and treatment of patients" in the hospitals and laboratory. As the generated waste is a potential source of transmission of diseases and handling such infected waste requires appropriate planning and strategies. If it is not disposed in an efficient manner then this dangerous waste may contain microorganisms that can badly affect the people who came in to contact of such waste directly or indirectly. Mismanagement of medical waste can adversely affect environment in number of ways like:

1. Contamination of Ground and Surface Water
2. Contamination of Quality of Air
3. Contamination of Municipal Solid Waste
4. Contamination of Soil etc.

Management of medical waste is an important part of infection control and hygiene programs in healthcare institutions. At present as the world is fighting to contain the spread of the coronavirus, the global pandemic is generating dangerous biomedical waste that requires special handling and treatment. India generates about 600 ton of biomedical waste every day, of which only 90 per cent is treated. With Covid waste being generated at a faster pace and high volume, it is more challenging to see that it is disposed without causing additional health problems. It is estimated that on an average, 2 ton of Covid waste is generated in each State from diagnoses, quarantine and treatment of the disease. "The health care intuitions are a major contributor to community-acquired infection, as they produce huge amounts of medical waste. Medical waste can be categorized based on the risk of causing injury and/or infection during handling and disposal. Wastes targeted for precautions during handling and disposal include sharps (needles or scalpel blades), pathological wastes (anatomical body parts, microbiology cultures and blood samples) and infectious wastes (items contaminated with body fluids and discharges such as dressing, catheters and I.V. lines). Other wastes generated in healthcare settings include radioactive wastes, mercury containing instruments and Polyvinyl Chloride (PVC) plastics. These are among the most environmentally sensitive by-products of healthcare." Inadequate or Improper waste management puts the people who come in to contact with such wastes at great risk. People who work in and out of such facilities should be protected by legal framework of the management system. This emphasizes that there is a need to evolve and implement better, safe methods and strategies for disposal of medical waste material generated by various health-care centres. In 2005, World Health Organization estimated that in general 85 percent of wastes in hospitals are not lethal, and 10 percent of wastes are contagious, and 5 percent of wastes are not contagious but lethal wastes. In United States of America, 15 percent of medical wastes is considered as toxic/infectious waste. In

India it ranges from 16 percent to 36 percent depends upon the total amount of waste generated. The proper management of health-care waste depends on "good administration and organization along with adequate legislation, financing, and active participation of trained and informed staff." The government of Indian, Ministry of environment, forest and climate has published manual called Bio-medical waste management, Rules, 2016 to efficiently handle/dispose of biomedical waste. Every health institute is bound to follow biomedical waste management regulations, 2016. The various modifications have been incorporated into the new regulations. There is need to ensure that all health institutions must follow new regulation and conduct the practice in more safely. Medical waste management is a long process, many step involved in this process that are collection, segregation, storage, transportation, treatment and disposal.

OBJECTIVES OF STUDY

The objectives of present study are:
1. To find the basic information about the way to dispose of medical waste by hospital.
2. To examine the knowledge, attitude and practices regarding waste management in hospital with special reference to Covid 19.
3. To analyze the waste management practices.

REVIEW OF LITERATURE

The various significant studies found in the literature which not only provides in depth knowledge and understanding but also reveals the problems being faced in implementation of biomedical waste management in the hospitals. Kishor J. *et al.* (2000) have conducted study at teaching hospital in New Delhi, on the awareness about BMW and infection control among dentists. The study by Peter *et al.* (2000), also emphasis on a need to create awareness among the health care centres staff and patients regarding the hazardous nature of waste. In similar study, Muduli K. *et al.* (2012) identified major health care waste management challenges like lack of Segregation Practices, lack of proper operational strategy, poor regulative measures, Lack of Green Procurement Policy, waste-picking and reusing. A study by Kumar R. *et al.* (2014) is mainly based on the 29 parameters related to various functions of HCW of north India. Bhardwaj M. *et al.* (2015) held a research study to find out the awareness and knowledge level of BMW among undergraduate medical students of Punjab. It was an observational descriptive study based on pre- designed and pre-tested questionnaire. The study was done on 110 second year professional medical students. It was concluded after research that 73.6% students were not known about the legislation of BMW. It was also revealed that majority of the students (71.8 %) had deficit knowledge about categories of BMW and its disposal in color bags. Almost 47.2% students didn't have the knowledge about the handling and disposal procedure of BMW. Hiremath R.N. (2016) presented study to assess "the level of Knowledge, Attitude, and Practices (KAP) about Biomedical Waste (BMW) management among 80 Health Care Workers (HCWs) at one of the Multispecialty Hospital in Eastern India." It was cross sectional descriptive study. It is cleared that there were various studies which emphasized the most common problems which are appeared due to the absence of waste management, lack of awareness about their health hazards, insufficient financial and human resources for proper management and uncontrolled disposal of biomedical waste. In light of findings, the present study is being conducted in Giani Lal Singh Hospital Patiala, Punjab.

MATERIAL AND METHODS

A cross sectional descriptive study was conducted in a multispecialty hospital having 200 beds, in Patiala district, Giani Lal Singh Medical College and Hospital, Patiala. There is a daily inflow of more than 100–200 patient in hospital out of which mainly are out-patients. Total medical staff of hospital is about 500 which consists of medical and paramedical staff. The Method used for the research is quantitative and in that the researcher adopted an instrument to collect the data with the consent of the healthcare facilities and personnel involved in the management and disposal of the wastes. The data was collected using different questionnaires, specifically developed for the research. "A total of 200 persons comprising doctors, nurses, laboratory technicians, ward boys, and sweepers of various departments who could be contacted during visits were interviewed. Temporary staffs are not included in the study. Site visits were conducted to support and supplement information gathered in the survey. The useful information about common practices in the management of the wastes was obtained from these visits." The forms contains data on the generation of waste and main aspects of segregation, collection, internal and external storage, transport, treatment, cost of the hospital waste administration and last dumping, along with this the knowledge, attitude and practices of handling the medical waste by the participants is also assessed.

RESULTS

A survey outcome exhibited that the regular normal waste adds to 79.77% of total hospital waste produced. The debris or wastes generated can be regular household or office normal waste which includes liquids, paper, and plastics and contains other materials which are not inherently contagious.

The main Classification of bio-medical waste are:

1. Pharmaceuticals
2. Contagious
3. Pathological
4. Sanitary effluents
5. Sharps

Consequently, clinical waste comprises of sharps, fluid, solid which are possibly deadly or toxic to the society and the nature. The phrase medical waste contain the following:

1. Type A Wastes – Biologically infectious wastes.
2. Type B Wastes – Blood and other bodily fluids.
3. Type C Wastes – Human body parts, tissues, organs.
4. Type D Wastes – Needles, Sharps, Syringes.
5. Type E Wastes – Dialysis wastes.
6. Type F Wastes – Other discarded material wastes.

The study revealed the portions for every type of wastes researched in hospital. Type D wastes contains the highest proportions (25–50%) of the total generated medical waste. The second highest portion is of type C wastes (10–40%). Generally, the hospital segregated the waste into following classifications:

1. The black bags/bins for normal waste.
2. The yellow bags/bins for contagious waste.

Frequently wastes were collected and transported to disposal facility. Such steps ensured to lessen the price of waste segregation and treatment in hospital. India already has the Biomedical Waste Management Rules, 2016; the CPCB issued specific guidelines to ensure segregation of Covid-19 waste to be disposed off in scientific manner. In addition to this, the waste should be properly secured in double-layered yellow leak proof bags, and labeled as waste generated from Covid-19 for clear identification. The storage bins, trolleys and vehicles transporting this waste should be disinfected regularly. The indiscriminate disposal of face masks, tissue papers and used sanitizer bottles can be potential sources of infection among municipal workers. They should be trained and provided with safety kit to handle the household waste during the pandemic to assist in halting the chain of transmission.

Knowledge, Attitude and Practice occupies an important role in bio medical waste management. This is an issue of "awareness, involvement and enlightenment of the staff of a medical institution to maintain it clean and by such an endeavor, to maintain the surrounding and the environment healthy. Once the doctor is aware of the issue that his institution and the genesis of bio medical waste that had great hazard for his neighborhood, he would react to the situation. The staff of the institution are most likely be influenced by his knowledge and interactions as regards the bio medical wastes and the invisible propensity of the wastes. That these wastes serve as the nidus of many iatrogenic diseases, the hospitals are great danger to the society in perpetuating infections and illnesses." The knowledge about bio medical waste will increase awareness and this will turn into practical aspect in the form of framing attitudes in the mindset of doctors and medical staff. The right attitude will help the medical staff to act in a way which is required to dispose the biomedical waste. Perfect knowledge and perfect attitude of medical staff is the best practice in this field. This practice will not help the old staff but it's a constant and long lasting concept to educate the patient and new staff. There is a need of continuing education of medical staff regarding dispose of the medical waste smoothly as new and better ways are developing day by day. Thus KAP i.e. (Knowledge, Attitude and Practice) is of utter importance in assessment of bio medical waste of healthcare institutions the present study finding has shown that, "almost all health care workers have general knowledge/understanding on health and environmental effect of medical waste if it is not handled properly. However there are still about 56% of waste handlers who are not knowledgeable on health and environmental effect of sharp waste as they lack training on how to take care and they do not know any injection safety policy, guideline and disposal policy. The survey also shows that, lack of knowledge among health workers and a lack of coordination among different ministries in handling care waste hinder safe handling of hospital waste. Furthermore high level of knowledge of hospital staff on sharps waste as ingredients of medical waste was, due to the familiarity of health workers with syringes and needles accidents that happen as a result of sharps injury. Knowledge of exposure to occupational hazard reported was lower for 75.0% in hospital. Hence it is the duty bound by the hospital management to make sure that it provides a sufficient knowledge on proper medical waste management. This will improve individual performance which will lead to the hospital performance and hence the maximization of quality healthcare provision." Furthermore, the study reveals that patients and attendants were not aware about the BMW and sometime contaminate the waste. Some of the respondents demand periodic seminars and proper equipment's. There is lack of sufficient equipment's in the hospitals at ground level. There is no in house treatment procedure of biomedical waste. The study also revealed that fourth class employee need to be well aware about the procedure of how this waste has to be disposed off.

CONCLUSION

Medical waste management has emerged as great challenge for the healthcare authorities especially at present when globally we are fighting with the deadly virus like coronavirus. It is not only threat to human but can also pollute environment. Education plays a strong role in bio medical waste management. Community awareness is the only way forward towards responsible waste management and containment of the virus. People should be made aware that the virus is active for three days or 72 hours. The waste generated should be kept separately in airtight containers and handed over to biomedical disposal staff for final treatment. Every member of community has to be informed about the bad/ill effects of such bio medical waste. Hence various methods like mass media should be used to educate the public in a comprehensive manner as it will minimize the impact of waste on human health. The responsibility rests not only with the hospitals and local bodies, but also the community, which needs to take keen interest in handling the waste so that it helps in breaking the chain of spreading the virus. There is a need to create awareness by special awareness programmers, organizing training in concerned local bodies, health departments, providing workers handling COVID-19 waste with adequate protective gear, adequate coordination with media and other concerned regulatory authorities. The health care centres should have transparent comprehensive approach in medical services to achieve better quality in disposal of medical waste Government has taken initiative in the form of Medical Waste Management rules book 2016 which has covered all most all the aspect related to handling and dispose of health hazard waste. The present study has explored about the BMW regulations and various health hazards in handling of biomedical waste with reference to pandemic like COVID-19. A pilot study also revealed that there is need to provide awareness about the handling procedure and there must be proper equipment's to handle and dispose of the waste.

REFERENCES

[1] Sharma, Anurag; Garg, Ravish; Srivastava, Anuj and Sharma, Neeraj, A Study about Knowledge, Attitude, Practices and Technologies of Biomedical Waste Management Techniques. *IOSR Journal of Environmental Science, Toxicology and Food Technology,* 9(12), 2015: 73–78.

[2] Bhardwaj, M. and Joshi, R., Awareness on Biomedical waste management (BMW) among undergraduate medical students of Punjab. European journal of pharmaceutical and medical research, 2016, 3(4), 263–265.

[3] Das, S.K. and Biswas, R., Awareness and practice of biomedical waste management among healthcare providers in a Tertiary Care Hospital of West Bengal, India. *International Journal of Medicine and Public Health,* 2016 Jan. 1;6(1):19-.

[4] Anamika, Gulati and Saini, Saini Vipin, Influence of Hospital Set-Up in Biomedical Waste Management: A Crosssectional Survey in Four Hospitals of West Delhi. *International Journal of Advancements in Research & Technology,* 5(6)2016; 321-44.

[5] Gupta, N.K., Shukla, M. and Tyagi, S. Knowledge, attitude and practices of biomedical waste management among health care

personnel in selected primary health care centres in Lucknow. *International Journal of Community Medicine-Public Health*, 2016; 3(1):309-13.

[6] Hiremath, R.N., Patil, S., Basundra, S., Ghodke, S., Edwards, T.S. and Malali, V.V. Knowledge, Attitude and Practices of Healthcare Workers (HCWs) Regarding Biomedical Waste (BMW) Management: A Multispecialty Hospital Based Cross-Sectional Study in Eastern India. *Journal of Krishna Institute of Medical Sciences (JKIMSU)*, 2016 Oct. 1; 5(4).

[7] Daljit, Kapoor; Nirola, A.; Kapoor, V. and Gambhir, R.S. Knowledge and awareness regarding biomedical waste management in dental teaching institutions in India—A systematic review. *Journal of clinical and experimental dentistry*, 2014 Oct.; 6(4): e419.

[8] Lakshmi, B.S. and Kumar, M.P. Awareness about Bio-medical Waste Management among Health Care Personnel of Some Important Medical Centers in Agra. *In International Journal of Engineering Research and Technology*, 2012; 1(7); 1–5.

[9] Muduli, K. and Barve, A. Challenges to Waste Management Practices in Indian Health Care Sector. *International Proceedings of Chemical, Biological & Environmental Engineering*, 2012; 32.

[10] Verma, L.K., Mani, S. and Sinha, N. Biomedical waste management in nursing homes and smaller hospitals in Delhi. *Waste Management*, 2008; 28: 2723–34.

[11] Kumar, S., Biomedical Waste Management Practices in Shimla City, 2011: A thesis.

[12] De Silva, C.E. and Hoppe, A.E. Hospital waste management in the South of Brazil. *Waste Manag*, 2005; 25: 600–5.

[13] Pandit, N.B., Mehta, H.K. and Kartha, G.P. Management of biomedical waste: Awareness and practices in a district of Gujarat. *Indian Journal of Public Health*, 2005; 49: 245–7.

[14] Abor, P.A. and Bouwer, A. Medical waste practices in a southern African hospital. *Int J Health Care Qual Assur*, 2008; 21: 356–64.

Biomedical Waste:
A Rising Global Concern

Mr. Abhinav Narayan* and Ms. Pratima Singh**

INTRODUCTION

The 21ˢᵗ century, a century of development and progress in each and every sector of the world has now proved to be an era of threat and danger too, as not all developments brought us good. Nuclear progression in nations was accompanied by threats of nuclear war, Bio-medical development lead to the emergence of bio-weapons and bio-medical wars, Industrial growth affected ozone and atmosphere and the list goes on.

One such sector is that of Biological equipment and waste that cannot be left behind. These bio hazardous substances have the capability of self-replication and can produce deadly effects upon biological organisms. These agents are not limited to virus and bacteria but now include human developed and cultured specimens consisting of plant viruses and experimental animal tissues. These biological stock releases a lot of waste and such used materials that are known as biological waste. These materials if not treated with care and safety, can lead to destruction and devastation of our environment.

Biological or Biomedical waste can also be defined as any waste produced during the research or medical activities like treatment, immunization or diagnosis of humans or animals. And therefore it's safe and ecological disposal becomes mandatory upon all of us, both socially and legally. Biological waste management needs a lot of concern and guidance in order to create a healthy and clean environment.

---

* Student, Amity Law School, NOIDA, AUUP.
** Law Graduate, Law College, Dehradun, Uttranchal University.

MEANING AND TYPES OF BIOLOGICAL WASTE

Biomedical waste can involve animal waste, stock, and cultures, blood, human wastes, and body parts, tissues, blood products, cell lines, and body fluids, etc. It also comprises recombinant DNA (rDNA), infection agent, human pathological waste and sharp instruments used by the health care sector like a medical syringe, glass, needles, scalpel or razors blades, etc.

Types of Biomedical Waste

Generated from clinics, laboratories, research centre, pathology labs, or hospitals, all kinds of biological waste can be broadly classified into certain distinct types of biological/Bio medical waste.

(a) *Radioactive Waste:* One of the most crucial and deadly kind of biological wastes is radioactive waste that generates from labs or research centers or industries and they generally are those unused radiotherapy liquid or lab research liquids. Any element that has come in contact f such liquid will also be taken as Radioactive Waste.

(b) *Sharps:* These are generated out of clinics, hospitals, labs and many such places where biological work is carried out. This includes wires, needles, glass, scalpels, razors, ampoules etc.

(c) *Chemical Waste:* Used in factories and labs, any solvent or liquids like mercury, uranium etc., Can be termed as a chemical waste.

(d) *Pathological Waste:* These are products from hospitals and labs and comprise of fluid tissues of human bodies, or blood, bodily fluids or infected animal remains and carve, etc.

(e) *Infectious Waste:* Anything that may cause infection is termed under this category like towel, swabs, excreta instruments, etc.

(f) *Genotoxic Waste:* One of the harmful type, these include medical waste that is either carcinogenic or mutagenic. Drugs used in cancer treatment also lies under this category.

(g) *General Non- Regulated Medical Waste:* Since they don't impose any threat of social or biological strata and therefore called as non-hazardous waste too.

BIOLOGICAL WASTE MANAGEMENT

One need to understand that though only 10%–25% of Bio Medical waste that is hazardous and rest 75%–90% is taken as non-hazardous yet, the safety and care that needs to be followed to dispose that 10%–25% should not be ignored. Biological waste management is very essential for the sake of safety and cleanliness of our environment. And therefore in the year 2007 in Geneva, World Health Organization issued certain guidelines for the disposal and management of Biological/Bio medical waste. It was advised that with right investment of resources and utmost dedication, the deadly effects of Biological waste to the people and surroundings can be reduced and therefore it was deduced that each shareholder connected to medical care activities or biologically concerned activities have to take it as their legal and moral obligation to safeguard the protection of others and must contribute in the act of appropriate supervision of Biological waste. It was also given by the WHO that government of States must design and create a body that would look after the maintenance and efficient management of biological waste disposal. WHO even advised the non-governmental organizations to take a call and contribute in their best capacity in the management and handling of biological waste disposal. World Health Organization released its very first version of handbook on safe management of waste in the year 1999 which is known as "The Blue Book'. And the second edition that got published in 2014, gave new methods and measures to control and manage the safe disposal of biological waste. Topics of concern like evolving pandemics, drug-resistant bacteria and climate changes etc. were very well enclosed in the second publication of "The Blue Book".[1]

BIOLOGICAL WASTE MANAGEMENT IN INDIA

A study[2] in 2018 done conjointly by an industry body revealed that by the year 2022 India is expected to produce 775.5 tons/day of medical waste as compared to 550.9 tons/day at that point of time. The study said that the growth rate of medical waste will increase by 7% annually at compounded annual growth rate (CAGR). The studies have always shown a clear concern regarding the biomedical waste disposal and management in India due to lack of resources, awareness, consciousness and cost price.

---

[1] Review of Health Impacts from Microbiological Hazards in Health-Care Wastes. Geneva: World Health Organization.

[2] Unearthing the Growth Curve and Necessities of Bio Medical Waste Management in India-2018.

But in recent years, there have been many changes observed regarding the handling of the biological waste disposal.

It was in the year 2019 that the Ministry of Environment, Forest & Climate Change initiated, amended and enforced the 'parent rules of 2016' for the concern of bio medicate waste management so that the situation of current biological waste disposal can be handled well. Some of the major clauses included were:

1. Any Healthcare amenities regardless of their capacity for beds need to frequently update the Biomedical waste management register and are supposed to display the monthly record on its website too. They need to follow the color coded scheme as given under Schedule 1 of the earlier rule book and must have to make available the annual report for the same on its website within the two years from the date of publication of Biomedical waste management (amendment) rules 2018.

2. Healthcare facilities that have beds less than 10 shall comply with the rule of output discharge standard measure for fluid waste produced by them as per the date 31st December 2019.

3. Duties of ministry of defense as per Schedule 3 : a report will be submitted to Central pollution control board after the complete scrutiny and intensive care of Healthcare Facilities that will include all Medical examination rooms, sick bays onboards, ships and submarines, station medical centres and field hospitals etc., functioned by Director General and Armed Forces of Medical Amenities.

Ground Reality of Bio-waste Management in India

As already discussed earlier, the rapid growth in generation of Biological waste in coming years demand a rapid and easily accessible solution yet the reality checks are quite different. Currently there are 199 common bio medical waste treatment facilities (CBWTFs) running[3] but to meet the demand of rapidly growing numbers, we still need a lot more than actually present. And due to high economic prices, setting up these facilities become one economically exhaustive task as there is a lack of funds.

Although the Bio Medical Waste Management legislation is active since 1998, which has also been revised and amended in past few years, yet

---

[3] According to CPCB 2017.

many areas of our country lack proper resources to eliminate the risk of bio hazardous waste. As per the source of CPCB, "compliance of rules is still an ongoing process in the country and law in many states is writ large. The legal obligation has been reduced to paper formality only and there is a lack of concern, motivation, awareness and cost factor in proper biomedical waste management." In an another observation by Centre for Science & Environment (CSE), in a study conducted in Jharkhand in 2017, it was found that many hospitals and nursing homes were violating the norms of Bio Medical Waste laws in regards to its segregation, collection, storage, treatment and disposal. Therefore an inference was drawn that most of the central and eastern sections of the nation, are also breaching the laws eventually.

New Biological Waste Management Rules

In the year 2016, a new set of guidelines were given for the better management of biological waste disposal. The new rules are distinct and detailed in nature as to bring positive change in Biological waste management in India. The new rules also includes health related facilities such as that of vaccination camps, blood donation camps etc. The rules also talk about the separation, wrapping, transportation and storage of these waste. To make segregation more prominent, it is being recommended and done in the first stage itself. Color coding has been suggested for different and particular type of waste so that its segregation and disposal treatment can be made efficient and easy both. For the elimination of emission of dioxins and furans from plastic and blood bags, pretreatment of laboratory waste is done as given by WHO guidelines. Bar code systems for bags/containers ensure tracking and identifying of bags for inspection and quality assurance. Authorized dealer are to be handled over with the recycling of polybags to ensure the control of various government agencies over such recyclers and their work. Recycling of waste has been given due importance in the new set of guidelines to conserve resources and to decrease pollution. Also the new rules have made emission standards for incinerators stricter to take a control over emission of dioxins and furans release. There has been an improvement in the intensive care sector Ministry of Environment, Forest & Climate Change is to evaluation HCF's once a year through State Health Secretaries & State Pollution Control Board, in addition to which, an advisory board on Biological/biomedical waste management is to meet every 6 months.

CONCLUSION

Amidst the century where the world is at a threat of Bio war will become the Third World War, it has becomes essential for each of us to show utmost consciousness in disposing and managing the biological/ biomedical waste as we know how deadly it can be if not contained, stored or handled with care. Biological development is a boon in disguise to the society as with all the possible developments and encouragements in this sector bring a possible threat of mishandled bio waste too that again causes great concern for the safety of our environment.

With establishments of more and more Biomedical Waste Management facilitators, we need to ensure better and much efficient disposal of biological waste. But the cost price and maintenance for the same are not supportive of the cause therefore the private companies with high economy must come forward to help the government in installing these units in both private and public sectors.

'Force Majeure' and where it Stands in the Present World Crisis

Ms. Richa Yadav* and Ms. Neelakshi Vats**

INTRODUCTION

The globe is on the standstill, the bustling streets, the blasting furnaces and chimneys, the tensed office hours the merry children hustling to and for all are restricted or rather quarantined into the comforts of their home. The World today is facing the gravest and unfortunate situation due to the outbreak of the SARS COVID-19. The COVID-19 has been officially declared a Global Pandemic by the World Health Organization through its press release dated March 11th, 2020. The only possible way advised to curb this pandemic was- LOCKDOWN. This led to serious punch to the economies world-wide. But, the knockout punch to the Indian economy has serious long-term consequences. Six weeks ago, the Nationwide lockdown announced be Prime Minister Modi placed the Indian Economy in the cold storage. The unprecedented economic freeze will take several quarters to revive. A Global recession as precedented may well be round the corner.

There has been an estimation made by the UN Department of Economic and Social Affairs (DESA) which hints towards the shrinkage of the Global Economy by at least 1% in the year 2020 due to COVID-19 Pandemic.[1] The estimated loss caused to the Global Economy is about $9 trillion as warned by Gita Gopinath of International Monetary Fund (IMF).[2] Amidst all the hardships the Governments across the World have been thriving to curb this unprecedented economic blow through various

*Assistant Professor, Amity Law School, NOIDA, AUUP.
** Student, Amity Law School, NOIDA, AUUP.
[1] Editorial, "Global economy could shrink by almost 1% in 2020 due to COVID-19 pandemic: United Nations", The Economic Times, Apr. 2, 2020.
[2] As per the statement made by Gita Gopinath (IMF), Coronavirus could lead to a loss of $9 trillion of global economy; Business Today; April 15, 2020; 23:37 IST.

measures. Looking at the current situation the regulatory bodies such as RBI and SEBI have relaxed the required deadlines until June 30th.

In the middle of this uncommon and bizarre footing one of the most deliberated and discussed argument is one that of *"FORCE MAJEURE."* Especially, in reference to the 'CONTRACTUAL OBLIGATIONS.' The current pandemic has rummaged almost all the industries functioning worldwide leading to a chaotic chain of events in the chapter of the world economy. The compelling number of people have been shut down into their homes, this thwarts the skillful functioning of businesses and industries and has majorly affected the contracts. The matters associated with the fulfilment of contracts and the contractual agreements have brought forth various aspects one of which can be termed as 'Force Majeure'. The 'Force Majeure' clause majorly impacted the formal contracts. With the ongoing disruption in the supply chains occurred due the coronavirus outbreak, creates a very strong possibility of postponement, interrupted or even suspended contracts.

'FORCE MAJEURE' AND VIS MAJOR

"Inevitable Accidents are defined as any mishaps that cannot been foreseen or prevented by due care or due diligence of any human being involved".[3] Another take on the concept of *'Inevitable Accidents'* could be termed as those incidents which are inevitable and unprecedented and cannot be avoided or prevented from happening by the exercise of ordinary care, caution and skill. These accidents are nowhere established to have a relationship with the parties involved in the accident further it doesn't even create a possibility for them where the action taken on their part can or could prevent an event.[4]

In the words of Sir Frederick Pollock:

> *"Not avoided by such precautions as a reasonable man, doing such an act then there, could be expected to take."*[5]

---

[3] Force majeure, *available at*: https://www.trans-lex.org/944000/_/force-majeure/ (Visited on 12 May, 2020).

[4] Anurag pandey, "Understanding the difference between act of god and force majeure" Academik, Feb. 3, 2015.

[5] Ibid.

Act of God (*VIS MAJOR*) is a much familiar and prevalent phrase in the legal fraternity a very sought-after defense to be used by the defendant side in order to save themselves from the conviction. The term holds to be the most referred defense provided in the *Inevitable Accident*. Act of God or *VIS MAJOR* are referred to the acts that are beyond the comprehensible precautions of the human beings involved.[6] The term was used for the first time in the legal fraternity by Lord Ellenborough, a very prominent jurist in the year1803. He stated,

> *"By Common Law, Carriers are insurers against every loss of property entrusted to their care, except losses arising from the Act of God, or the King's enemies."*[7]

The other defense available and the topic of interest is that of 'Force Majeure'. 'Force Majeure' in its French translation gives the meaning of *'A Superior or Irresistible Power'*. This indicates towards the occurrence of the event that can be said to be resulted from the course of nature and not so ordinary course of human behavior. They are majorly seemed to be used to pass off the liability for the mishaps occurring due to the natural and unavoidable chain of events that tend to intervene with the normal course of events and impede the parties involved. 'Force Majeure' clauses can be majorly found in the formal contracts especially in the supply and construction contracts, sometimes in the lease and the rental contracts too.

The United Nation Convention on the CISG[8] doesn't not specifically define term the word 'Force Majeure' but, Article 79, provides a very crisp definition of what the 'Force Majeure' clause provides and how it protects the non-contractual party in the event of such circumstances where the parties involved had no control of. Referring to the article it says:

> *"'Force Majeure' clauses excuse a party from performance if some unforeseen event beyond its control prevents performance of its contractual obligations."*[9]

---

[6] Krishnendra Joshi, "Act of God and Inevitable Accident" iPleaders, May 15, 2019.

[7] Edwin C. Goddard, "The Liability of the Common Carrier as Determined by Recent Decisions of the United States Supreme Court" 15 CLR 399–416 (1915).

[8] Contract of International Sales of Goods.

[9] Article 79, The United Nations Convention on the Contracts for International Sale of Goods (CISG).

In the natural and simple meaning both the terms referred i.e. the *vis major* and *force majeure* hold the same meaning but, in the usage especially in the legal terms both acquired a different connotation and are used very differently. On the one hand the term 'act of god' or '*vis major*' encompasses within it all the causes of the inevitable accident iterated by the elementary forces of the nature not remotely related to the man or any other either explicitly or impliedly.[10] Whereas, the definition of 'Force Majeure' is much more of a broader term which not only incorporates natural forces but, also tends to combine other causes which may not significantly be related to nature and can also seem to be connected to human actions either directly or indirectly, although the parties involved in such mishaps don't seem to have any control over the occurrence of such events.[11]

'FORCE MAJEURE' IN THE INDIAN CONTEXT

The Romans should be credited for recognizing the principle of the sanctity of contract, which can be hampered by one of the other principle '*clausula rebus sic stantibus*', which can be interpreted as "obligations under a contract are binding only as long as matters remain same as they were at the time of entering the contract".[12] This stands contrary to the principle of '*Pacta Sund Servanda*'[13] which can be interpreted as the 'the agreements should be kept', which is applicable in the civil as well as the international matters. The question that was brought in front of the judicial system was one where neither of the parties involved in the agreement were at fault. And, therefore, the impediment in fulfilling the contract was beyond their control. And thus, the contract stands frustrated and therefore, releasing both the parties from their obligations. Thus, it is established that the Doctrine of '*clausula rebus sic stantibus*' stands superior over the doctrine of '*Pacta Sund Servanda*'.

---

[10] Ratanlal and Dhirajlal, The Law of Torts, 92 (Lexis Nexis, Delhi, 25th edn., reprint 2009).

[11] Maulik Nanavati and Manvi Damle, "invoking-force-majeure-in-times-of-covid-19-and-its-impact-on-contracts" available at: https://www.livelaw.in/columns/invoking-force-majeure-in-times-of-covid-19-and-its-impact-on-contracts-156297 (Visited on 20 May, 2020).

[12] Lawrence Lieberman," The forgotten 'Force Majeure' clause and its relevance today under Indian and English law" Bar and Bench, Mar. 27, 2020.

[13] Art 26, Vienna Convention Law of the Treaties, 1969.

The Indian legal system was not introduced explicitly vide the legislative texts to the term of 'Force Majeure' until recently. The more prevalent alternative was the doctrine of Frustration of Contracts that had been fulfilling the void of the 'Force Majeure'. The Indian Contract act, 1872 does not specifically provide for any sort of definitions for the 'Force Majeure'. In the substitute, there have been sections that can be referred to whilst dealing with the circumstances which would otherwise be covered under the head of 'Force Majeure'.

In the recent developments the legislature has come across difficult circumstances and hardships. There have been time again cases in front of the Judiciary where the contracts had the categorical clause of 'Force Majeure' but, on the contrary there have even been contracts that remain frustrated due to the unforeseen events with no party being involved in happening of the said event.

Within the Indian legal system, the very first decision to establish the idea of 'Force Majeure' is the one given by the Madras High court in *'Edmund Bendit and Anr. v. Edgar Raphael Prudhome*[14] while pronouncing the judgement the judges cited a passage from the *Matsoukis v. Priestman*[15] and co., where the 'Force Majeure' has been defined as "causes you cannot prevent and for which you are not responsible".[16]

Both the English and the Indian law, doesn't provide 'Force Majeure' simply as something which is not within the ambit of control of the parties to the contract, on the contrary the meaning and the applicability changes and rests upon the wordings of that specific contract. It is the contractual language intended to anticipate unforeseen events and provided for what happens on their occurrence.[17] In the leading caselaw of *Dhanrajmal Govindram v. Shamji Kalidas*[18] decided by the 3 judges' bench where while interpreting the term 'Force Majeure' the words of Justice McCardie was referred from the case of *Le Beaupin v. Crispin*[19] where he gave a brief of what one can infer by 'Force Majeure' with an indication

---

[14] IRL (1925) 48 MAD 538 (MAD).
[15] [1915] 1 K.B. 161.
[16] Ibid.
[17] Ibid.
[18] (2002) 1 MAH Lj 774.
[19] (1920) 2 K.B. 714.

and relation drawing from its past. *The* term of 'Force Majeure' cannot be just tagged as a French adaptation of the Latin word *vis major*. It is unquestionably an expression that holds a broader importance. Problems emanated with a question as to what should be lawfully be enclosed or inserted within the head of *'Force Majeure'*. Jurists in their opinion have assented that though impediment of the dissent breakdown of machinery are some risks that cannot be seem to be associated with the term 'vis major' and therefore should be taken up within the ambit of 'Force Majeure'. The objective that can be inferred is to protect the obligated parties from the situations over which he exhibits no control. This can be the broadest connotation that can be provided to 'Force Majeure'.

'Force Majeure' Within the Frame of Indian Contrct Act, 1872

The Indian legal system highly relies on the concept of the Doctrine of Frustration. The general rule of the contracts speaks about the fulfilment of the contract and binds the parties to the contract towards a contractual obligation wherein any breach by the parties involved with the contract will result in the legal consequences over the defaulting party where the party at the receiving end will be compensated for the damages caused by the subsequent party involved in the similar contract. The Doctrine of Frustration poses to be an exception to the present rule.

The Doctrine of the Frustration of the contract on the other hand talks about basically, the impossibility of performance of the contract. The meaning that runs behind this doctrine is that the contract that was restricted or prohibited to be complied with was due an impediment caused beyond the control of the parties. Therefore, the performance of those contracts becomes what can be said as 'frustrated' in other words it can become complicated, or rather impossible to perform or sometimes even illegal.

The Indian Contract Act, 1872, does not provide specific definition 'frustration of contract'. However, one can find the term enshrined within the Article 56 of the said Act which reads as follows:

> *Section 56. Agreement to do impossible act-*
>
> *Which means, an agreement to an impossible act is in itself void.*

Contract to do act afterwards becoming impossible or unlawful-

Meaning, a contract to do an act, which after the contract is made, becomes impossible, or, by reason of some event which the promisor could not prevent, unlawful, becomes void when the act becomes impossible or unlawful.

Compensation for loss through non-performance of act to be impossible or unlawful:

Meaning, where one person has promised to do something which he knew, or, with reasonable diligence, might have known, and which the promise did not know, to be impossible or unlawful, such promisor must make compensation to such promise for any loss which such promise sustains through the non-performance of the promise."[20]

Article 56 of the contract act provides three instances where the parties can seek the defense of frustration of contract therefore it makes any agreement void where firstly, the act agreed to do is an impossible or secondly, due to the influence of some reason the act becomes unlawful for the promiser to comply with it or thirdly, the contract in the entirety becomes void when the act becomes impossible or unlawful.

A very landmark English case that draws the reference is the *Taylor v. Cadwell*[21] prior to this decision the laws related to contracts in the England were quite rigid. It was in this decision that the rigidity followed by the common law towards upholding the sanctity of the contract was loosened in a way. It was this case where it was upheld that if an unforeseen matter occurs during the performance of the contract that renders the act to be performed as impossible, thus, making the fundamental of the contract as impossible and thus, by insisting upon the performance would be unjust.

Another section within which the spirit of 'Force Majeure' and the doctrine of frustration can be found to be embedded is Section 32 of the Indian Contract Act, 1872. Section 32 reads as follows:

"Enforcement of contracts contingent on an event happening: contingent contracts to do or not to do anything if an uncertain future

---

[20] Section 56, Indian Contract Act, 1827.
[21] (1861–73) ALL ER Rep 24.

event happens cannot be enforced by law unless and until that event has happened. If the event becomes impossible, such contracts become void.[22]

The Court gave a very humble interpretation while pronouncing the decision in one of the recent judgements. The bench headed by Justice Arun Mishra in the case of *National Federation of Agriculture Cooperative v. Alimenta S.A.*[23] the question before the court was whether the National Federation of Agricultural cooperative (NAFED) was unable to comply with the contractual obligation to export the groundnut due to government's refusal? The second question involved is whether the NAFED could have been held liable in breach of contract to pay damages particularly in view of clause 14 of the agreement?

For the facts of the case NAFED is a canalizing agency of Government of India. NAFED entered into a contract with the ALIMENTA S.A. for the supply of 5000 metric ton of the groundnuts. Out of the required amount only 1900 metric ton could be shipped as the NAFED being the Government agency required the permission of the government before shipment. The said agreement and the transaction were governed by the "Force Majeure" and it included a prohibition clause whereby the contract would be deemed to cancelled in case of prohibition either by the executive orders or by the law in the face of Clause 14. The Supreme Court of India held that the frustration of contract in the present scenario is covered under the section 32 of the Indian Contract Act, 1872 as the NAFED being a canalizing agency was bound by the legislative orders and the law involved and this was known to both the parties and the clause 14 of the agreement renders the agreement to be a Contingent agreement thus, it remains frustrated and neither of the parties can be held liable for the same.

In another landmark judgement of *Energy Watchdog v. Central Electricity Regulatory Commission (CERC)*[24] where the fundamental basis of the contract remains unaltered the contract cannot be seemed to be said frustrated. Justice Rohinton S. Nariman whilst summarizing the entire "Force Majeure" held *"an unexpected price rise will not absolve the*

---

[22] Section 32, The Indian Contract Act, 1872.
[23] AIR (1989), SC 818.
[24] 2017 SCC OnLine SC 378.

generating companies from performing their part of the contract for the very good reason that when they submitted their bids, this was a risk they knowingly took. We are of the view that the mere fact that the bid may be non-escapable does not mean that the respondents are precluded from raising the plea of frustration, if otherwise it is available in law and can be pleaded by them....When a contract contains a 'Force Majeure' clause which on construction by the Court is held attracted to the facts of the case, Section 56 can have no application".

In the case of Satyabrata Ghosh v. Mungeeram Bangoree[25] the paragraph second of Section 56 has been referred to during the pronouncement of the judgement the judges explained the word "impossible". "The usage of the word in the Section does not indicate physical or literal impossibility. It can be inferred that the implementation of an act in actual sense may not be impossible, but it may be impracticable and useless from the point of view of the object and purpose of the parties. If an untoward event or change of circumstance totally upsets the very foundation upon which the parties entered their agreement, it can be said that the promisor finds it impossible to do the act which he had promised to do. It was further held that where the Court finds that the contract itself either impliedly or expressly contains a term, according to which performance would stand discharged under certain circumstances, the dissolution of the contract would take place under the terms of the contract itself and such cases would be dealt with under Section 32 of the Act. If, however, frustration is to take place de hors the contract, it will be governed by Section 56."[26]

In another similar instance, in Naihati Jute Mills Ltd. v. Hyaliram Jagannath,[27] the Court attracted the attention and mentioned the landmark and celebrated judgment of Satyabrata Ghose v. Mugneeram Bangur & Co.[28] Finally, the Court concluded that a contract cannot be rendered as frustrated merely on the pretext because the circumstances in which it was contracted have tend to altered. The Courts in general have no power to pardon a party from the obligations it was supposed to fulfill within the

---

[25] AIR 1954 SC 54.
[26] Prithviraj Senthil Nathan, "India: Legal Principles In Invoking 'Force Majeure' Clauses – Case Law Analysis" Mondaq, May 1, 2020.
[27] 968 (1), SCR 821.
[28] Supra 23 at 8.

contract merely because its performance has become erroneous owing an unanticipated turn of situations.[29]

In an English judgment namely, Tsakiroglou & Co. Ltd. v. Noblee Thorl GmbH,[30] in spite of the shutting down of the Suez channel, and in spite of the way that the standard course for transportation the products was distinctly by the way of the Suez canal, it was held that the agreement of offer of groundnuts in that case is not frustrated, despite the fact that it would need to be performed by an elective method of execution which was substantially more costly, to be specific, that the boat would now need to circumvent the Cape of Good Hope, which is multiple times the good ways from Hamburg to Port Sudan. The cargo for such excursion was additionally twofold. The House of Lords held that although the contract had become more harsh in the performance, it was not phenomenally altered. When the performance is possible, it is quite evident that a mere rise in freight price would not render either of the parties to claim that the contract was further made to discharge by impossibility of the act.

Further, there has been a test laid down seeking what cases can fall within the clamps of 'Force Majeure' it is:

- There are possibilities where the event that led to the party's non-performance as per the agreement or as under the contract falls in the ambit of 'Force Majeure' in the contract as it was decided in the case of *LeBeaupin v. Crispin*[31] that is to say that the said occurrence of event falls under the purview of 'Force Majeure' and the non-performance was caused due to the said event caused.[32]
- Another instance is where the event that led to the non-performance as well as the non-performance is not within the control of the party to the contract.[33] Thus, it can be concluded that economic hardships[34] like insufficient funds,[35] or the hike in product prices[36] do not fall

---

[29] Supra 25 at 9.
[30] 1961 (2) All ER 179.
[31] Supra 17 at 5.
[32] Supra 13 at 45.
[33] Supra 16 at 5.
[34] 1960 SC 588.
[35] The Condcadoro (1916) 2 AC 199.

under the ambit of 'Force Majeure' and therefore, defense under the same cannot be taken.

- The third instance can be derived where there was no reasonable care taken that could help in the avoidance or the mitigation of the event or for that matter even its consequences.[37]

Further, the parties to the contract claiming the defense of 'Force Majeure' should prove that there was no prior information about the happening of the said event resulting in non-performance available to the party. Or, he had any relation or acquaintance with the event. Because, any nexus drawn would render the defense to be baseless and just an act to save themselves from the obligations of the fulfillment of the contract.

'FORCE MAJEURE' AND THE CORONAVIRUS (SARS COVID 19)

The World Health Organization has officially declared coronavirus as a global pandemic in its official press release and media briefing on March 30, 2020. The present situations have affected the economies around the world. The times to follow post the pandemic is a situation of grave hardships especially for the economies a situation much graver than the 2008 recession. Amidst the present situation of SARS COVID-19 the Doctrine of 'Force Majeure' will now be brought under the purview of great scrutiny more specifically in relation to the matters related to the commercial contracts where the parties are unable to perform their obligations due to circumstances beyond their control.

The post pandemic situation would be a knockout punch over the economies and any amount of Sony Liston or Muhammad Ali punches cannot really save the day. The suppliers would be capable of fulfilling their obligations and in the evident cases this would result in the delay. They seek to render themselves free from their obligations. Similarly, the companies are not being able to meet the demands of their customers. On the other hand lessee whose property has been acquired during these time to cater the needs of the pandemic namely a school that has been taken up to be used as quarantine center, or a hospital that has been transformed as a COVID hospital in these cases the lessee seeks to abstain from the

---

[36] Supra 22 at 8.
[37] Supra 21 at 7.

payment of the rent to the lessor due to its inability to get a use out of the property, the real estate developers will be expecting a brief moratorium period due to these prolonged days of inactivity. Situation like these will attract the doctrine of 'Force Majeure' by the defending parties.

"On February 17, 2020, The China Council for the Promotion of International Trade (CCPIT), revealed that it had already issued over 166 "Force Majeure' Certificates' to firms in 30 sectors, covering contracts worth over $15 billion."

On the date of "February 19, 2020, the Department of Expenditure, Procurement Policy Division , Ministry of Finance" issued an "Office Memorandum" with respect to the 'Manual for Procurement of Goods, 2017', which provides for the matters related to procurement by the Government of India.

The Memorandum issued states Covid-19 clause as 'natural calamity' and therefore, it is liable to be effectively covered under the doctrine of "Force Majeure". It further states that "any *disruption in supply chain due to spread of corona virus in China or any other country*".

According to the previously mentioned memorandum, "the Ministry of New and Renewable Energy gave an Office Memorandum dated March 20, 2020" which coordinated all renewable energy executing organizations of the Ministry of New and Renewable Energy (MNRE) to treat delay because of disturbance of the gracefully ties because of spread of coronavirus in China or some other nation, as 'Force Majeure'.

In another appreciable and proactive move by the Supreme Court of India. The Hon'ble Supreme Court through a bench presided over by the Chief Justice S.A. Bobde, Justice L.N. Rao and Justice Surya Kant vide Order dated March 23, 2020 in the case for Cognizance for period of Limitation In re in Suo Motu Writ Petition No. 3 of 2020 ('the Order') "has taken 'suo-moto' cognizance of the dire situation arising out of the challenge faced by the country on account of Covid-19 Virus and resultant difficulties that may be faced by litigants across the country in filing their petitions/applications/suits/appeals/all other proceedings within the period of limitation prescribed under the general law of limitation or under Special Laws (both Central and/or State)."[38] The move made by the

---

[38] Extension of the period of limitation: a historical, proactive, commendable and timely order, available at: https://itatonline.org/articles_new/extension-of-period-of-limitation-

Supreme Court is under its power as referred in Article 141 and 142 of the constitution of India.

There have been several moves made by the finance ministry to deal with the economic crash. Since the parliament was not functioning the ordinances were passed vide notification dated 31.03.2020. The notification is called the 'The Taxation and other Laws (Relaxation of certain provisions) Ordinance 2020'. The amendment has been brought into the CGST Act, 2017 where 168A has been inserted giving the power to the central government extend the time limit in special circumstances.

In the present situation with extraordinary circumstances give out the results in the face of extraordinary consequences about the hardships faced around the world. Particularly in relation with the businesses, it can have effects beyond the imagination, as have already been predicted by the institutions. While at the rationale and factual side, it is quite evident that the organizations are already facing hard and tough times apart from the shortage of the funds and the minimization of the liquidity the ability to rum or carry out business activities freely are also being restricted and moreover delayed due to the impositions of lockdown across the nation and around the world as imposed by the state. Even with the greatest thinktanks available in the organization to lay out business plans or organize funds its highly unlikely to anticipate a crisis like these and chalk out the exit plans with minimization of the damages. Therefore, in the present times the organizations are busy analyzing and reviewing the existing contracts and agreements deliberating and trying to conceive out right plans and strategies to get over from the current phase of non-performance, delays etc.

CONCLUSION

The coronavirus crisis has given new relevance to the legal term "'Force Majeure'." It is a clause that can be found buried in many Contracts that lets a party off the hook in the event of some unforeseen contingencies. The Contractual Obligations have been regarded as the utmost important aspect and the sanctity of the contract is regarded to be held all times. The English as well as Indian Laws have been rigid in the matters related

---

a-historical-proactive-commendable-and-timely-order/ itaonline.org (Visited on 20 May, 2020).

to the contracts. *Taylor v. Cadwell*[39] has been the turning point where the judges gave flexibility in the fulfillment of the contract and eased out the air by rendering the party free from the obligation in the circumstances over which it can exercise no control this gives rise to the term of the 'Force Majeure' into the contracts.

'Force Majeure' has unanimously turned out to be the need of the hour. The entire world population webbed around and obligated with contract. The breakdown of supply chains has impacted most of the business and the manufacturing units. The economies are trying to establish the distorted order. Relaxations have been levied by the governments and various regulating authorities. The Supreme Court of India also took the suo-moto cognizance of the ongoing difficulties and eased the provisions regarding the filing of the suits.

One can infer that the 'Force Majeure' Clause is bound by its presence in the agreement and thus making the parties impliedly bound by it. The defaulting party cannot find its solace within the Doctrine of 'Force Majeure' in the event of commercial hardships or change and the fluctuation in the market prices of the good as these are the circumstances that are foreseeable and can be anticipated. Whereas the impediments which render the act and the fundamental basis of the contract impracticable and over which the parties had no control and was not anticipated.

One can take the examples of the present situation with the outbreak of the world pandemic. In the present situation the contracts that have been entered into prior to the outbreak of the COVID-19 can seek solace in the defense of 'Force Majeure' as this has been an unforeseen impediment and the situation has been declared as an pandemic by the World health Organization. On the contrary, the contracts that will be entered into post the implementation of the lockdown wouldn't be able to take the defense of 'Force Majeure' due to the pandemic as the situations prevalent around the world are known to both the parties and therefore the impediment not the unknown one.

The real estate industries would be also hit due the present lock down with stricter laws to safeguard the interest of the buyers into the RERA

---

[39] Supra 19 at 7.

ACT, 2016 there has also been a safeguard provided to the real estate developers in the form of SECTION 5 and 6 which provides a 'Force Majeure' clause. Whilst keeping in mind the hardships faced under the CGST ACT, 2017 the government has extended the dates for the compliance and the validity of the GST.

Moreover, even in the absence of the 'Force Majeure' clause one can always look towards the 'Doctrine of Frustration' that can always be invoked bide section 56 of the Indian Contract Act.

Corona is here to stay and the economies have to adapt to the new changes there needs to be new forms of business enterprises, new clauses to be look forward to in order to survive through the pandemic. This will change the lifestyles, the ease and way of doing businesses. Adaptability is the quality of man that has led it to be on the top of the food chain therefore, it is the adaptability that needs to be look forward to.

Debate on Centralization and Decentralization Amid Covid-19 Pandemic Outbreak

Dr. Rakhee Chauhan* and Dr. Meena Charanda**

On 11 March 2020 WHO announced that Covid-19, the viral corona virus that has shut down countries, halted travel, and forced the global society to engage in social distancing is an official pandemic. According to WHO "Coronavirus disease (Covid-19) is an infectious disease caused by a newly discovered coronavirus. Most people infected with the Covid-18 virus will experience mild to moderate respiratory illness and recover without requiring special treatment.... protect yourself and others from infection by washing your hands or using an alcohol-based rub frequently and not touching your face."[1]

The Coronavirus is a huge family of viruses that causes infections ranging from the usual cold to severe breathing patterns, but the existing virus is a different strain not seen before. Common signs of the novel Coronavirus strain include severe breathing symptoms for example fever, cough and problem in breathing.[2] The outbreak of corona started from China, Wuhan, ninth populous city of China. First case of anyone being infected by the Covid-19 virus dates back to November, 17, 2019 reported by the South China morning Post. By December 2019, these cases spread from one to another human being in Wuhan. Till now even the Chinese were unknown about the virus and most of the cases were labelled as 'pneumonia cases with unknown cause.' For the first time on December 21, 2019 that the suspected cases of pneumonia were quarantined. By the end of December, the rise up as anything in Wuhan, China. This was the time when the spread was reported in media not only in China but also outside the China. Dr. Li Wenliang was the first health worker who

* Department of Political Science, Kalindi College, University of Delhi, New Delhi,
** Department of Political Science, Kalindi College, University of Delhi, New Delhi,

warned about the SARS like illness urging medical community to use protection. By January the spread of the disease and cases of human transmission continued unabatedly. On January, 13, 2020 a Chinese woman visited Thailand from Wuhan with the infection of Corona virus. By this time many Corona infected Chinese citizens travelled from China to other parts of the world. On January, 15, Japan reported its first Coronavirus patient. Since first case in China in November 2018 Covid-19 Coronavirus infected millions of people and been declared a pandemic by the WHO in March. Dr. Li Wenliang, the whistle blower of the novel virus also died in China. All over the world almost 248,313 died due to the Coronavirus Pandemic till May 3, 2020 and more than 3,567,005 are Active Cases Globally.

The number of cases recorded in **USA** reached 1 million and above 60,000 deaths. Many of the Americans are taking benefits of unemployment given by the Government of United States of America, the number is climbed up to 26.5 million in the month of April, 2020. The present government, Trump Administration has predicted more in coming weeks, unemployment rate exceeding 16%. According to the Senior Economic Advisor in Trump Government, Kevin Hassett, USA is facing a major shock than the Great Depression of 1929. The main centre of the outbreak of Covid-19 is New York in USA, where almost 30% of cases occurred, other states effected are New Jersey, Illinois, Massachusetts, California, Pennsylvania and Michigan.[3] It is to be noted that earliest known case in U.S. was in February 2020. Primary elections due in U.S. in the month of March and April in states of Ohio, Georgia and New York have already postponed. American deaths from the novel virus passed Italy's tally which was the epicenter in Europe.

On January 31, 2020, the first confirmed case of coronavirus was reported in **Italy** caused by two Chinese tourists in Rome. The pandemic after that has taken a very harsh toll on Italy, where more than twenty-four thousand have died. More than 135,000 people in Italy are reported to have infected with the novel virus. From only three cases to having the highest death outside the China, the condition of Italy is really alarming during March-April. The hardest hit region in Italy is Lombardy, where almost 10 million people were hit by the impact of Covid -19. Italy is the one country which hit hardest by the pandemic. Italy is also a densely populated country in western nations. Italy is the nation of long-life expectancy and coronavirus poses serious threat to the older people. The spread of virus was undetected earlier so it spread like wildfire in some of the regions of Italy. The infection rate in Italy's is much higher than even China.

In **Spain,** Madrid and Catalonia are the two regions which have around 8,000 total confirmed deaths from coronavirus. The spread of virus was undetected in elderly in Spain. Experts accused the close ties of young and old people as the major reason behind the virus spread. It is said that more than eight million people around the age of 65 are living in Spain. The late response of the government results in rise of deaths that reach more than 20,000. The infection rate in Germany is lower in comparison of other countries. **Germany** recorded its first case of Covid-19 in January, 2020. Germany's vigorous and speedy testing program helped a lot and government also acted on data available to the health workers. German response is an example for the whole world to combat and the spread of virus. Total number of coronavirus cases in **United Kingdom** is 165,221, deaths reported are 26,097 by the end of April, 2020. There was a time when British Prime Minister Boris Johnson and Prince Charles both were infected with the deadly virus. Both recovered and the mitigation measures started all over the United Kingdom.

COVID-19 CASES IN ASIA

After emerging in China, Wuhan, in November, coronavirus spread to around 185 countries and regions. Four countries of **Southeast Asia** Malaysia, Indonesia, Thailand and Philippines witnessed a surge in cases. Governments of all four countries imposed comprehensive social restrictions in the cities suffering most from the infection. In Middle East, **Iran** has been hit very hard by coronavirus. More than 60,000 Iranians have contracted the virus and according to the sources in Iran about 4,000 have died however, some other sources estimates almost double the data. **Pakistan** government delayed nationwide lockdown till April, the result is the quick spread of virus 15,759 total cases and 346 deaths.

According to the World meter,[4] **China** has total 82,862 cases, 77,610 recovered and 4,633 deaths, further till April end currently infected patients' cases are 619. Raising concern all over the world is about the second wave in China, the origin points of the novel virus. Though

Wuhan is free of the infection but other cities like Beijing and Heilongjiang province, recorded some new imported cases and few local transmissions. Government is concerned about the second wave and sealed the borders so that travelers from other countries should not enter China.

In India infected cases climbed to 33,050 till 30 April, 2020 including 111 foreign nationals, 8324 cured/ discharged, 1 migrated and 1074 deaths. India documented its first coronavirus case on January 30, 2020 in the state of Kerala over the next four days two more cases in Kerala were reported. An affected person came to visit the state from Wuhan, China. And now confirmed cases of coronavirus are being reported from all over the country. States with the highest number of cases include Maharashtra on the top followed by Gujarat, Delhi, Uttar Pradesh, Andhra Pradesh, Karnataka, Rajasthan, Kerala and Tamil Nadu. First death due to the Covid-19 was reported from Karnataka on 12 March, 2020. Till March, 782,365 cases were reported all over the world after that WHO declared Covid-19 a pandemic and 37,582 deaths in 114 countries were confirmed till March globally.[5] Soon WHO declared the epidemic as a Global emergency. On March 10, 2020 Government of India has advised its citizens to evade the travels not necessary keeping in view the spread of the virus and strongly advised not to travel to certain countries such as China, Italy, Republic of Korea, Spain, France, Germany, Iran and Japan. e-visas were also suspended issued to the nationals of Spain, Germany and Japan. Patients of infected virus were isolated; many people were quarantined. Amid the scare of Covid-19 northeastern states sealed their borders with Myanmar. Restrictions were imposed on export of pharmaceutical ingredients. On March 22 first few policy decisions were taken and Prime Minister of India Narender Modi declared Indians to follow 'Janata curfew' voluntarily. And on March 24, 2020 at midnight, 1.3 billion people in India were facing an unprecedented situation when three-week lockdown was declared by the Government of India. To break the disease transmission chain the most important strategy is social distancing that means people should stay away from each other and the distance should be of six feet. However, WHO is clear that only lockdown or social distancing will not work. According to the Government of India polices, lockdown is just a measure to buy some time so that during and after the lockdown, the authorities will increase the number of testing so that more people with symptoms could be find, more people will be quarantine, treatment facilities will be enhanced and most important, would be to increase the number of health workers and frontline warriors.[6] Restaurants, malls, markets were also the part of complete shutdown. Colleges and schools were also the part of lockdown orders. Board exams of students of class X and XII were deferred till further notice by CBSE, personnel working in private or multinationals were requested to work from home. As the source of the spread is respiratory droplets it is necessary to distance. Only supportive care is available and vaccine or anti-viral treatment is yet to be discovered. Death toll related to virus is not only in thousands it's in lakhs and continues to rise with each day globally. India is under lockdown until May 3, 2020.

There are many reasons of spreading of infection in India:

- Social and religious gatherings
- Lack of proper protective equipment
- Low testing capacity in India
- Virus is beginning to spread in dense communities like Dharavi in Mumbai, Maharashtra
- Late response of the government
- Ignorance of majority of people about social distancing
- Illiteracy and poverty
- Non-reporting of the coronavirus infected patients at early stage
- High rate of migration
- Disregarding rules of lockdown
- Extended families living under one roof
- People don't follow general health and safety guidelines of government.

IMPACT OF THE LOCKDOWN ON STATES IN INDIA

UN High Commissioner for Human Rights Michelle Bachelet said; "The lockdown in India represents a massive logistical and implementation challenge given the population size and its density and we all hope the spread of the virus can be checked."[7]

India shut its $2-9 trillion economy with the declaration of lockdown on March 24, 2020. 250 districts have reported the infection. Almost 1/3 of the infected patients are from seven states, densely populated communities are facing the tough situation. Maharashtra is on the top of the chart of the recorded number of patients. Mumbai, the financial capital of India is the main hotspot.

Internal migration in India is very high. According to the census, 2011 around 450 million people migrate from one region to other and from one state to other. After the nationwide lockdown thousands of migrant workers stranded at the place where they live only for their bread and butter. Most of these moved towards far off places accessible only through trains. Prime Minister Modi announced the lockdown with barely four hours' notice. On March 28, 2020 thousands of migrants gathered at bus stations amid lockdown. Huge crowed thronged the Delhi-Uttar Pradesh border to go back to their native place. It created a massive problem not only for the governments of Delhi and UP but also for the migrant workers. Many of them started their journey on foot with small children and ladies, many on rickshaws or handcarts or cycles. Many of them stopped by the police on borders and sent back to Delhi. The governments didn't make arrangements for these people. Many of them died on the way to their homes. There was outrage against the governments indifferent attitude towards these migrants.

Unprecedent back to village migration, was seen from other regions too, such as Mumbai, Pune, Bangalore, Chennai, Kolkata. They could not stay in the city without any work and without food. Some of them even tried to flee in trucks and containers of milk. Clearly no policy maker has planned for these unorganized migrant workers. Social distancing is a luxury that a daily wager can't afford. Government is providing 500 rupees per month under the scheme but it is small fraction what they earned. On March 31, the Supreme Court of India instructed to ensure and provide sufficient food, beds, water, and other materials and also psychological counselling.

Broken supply chain lockdown was declared when the rabi crop wheat, mustard, jowar and soya etc. was ready to harvest. In some states the harvesting was allowed but non-availability of labour and machines are the major challenge. Further closure of markets and mandis would also be a problem. Not only this but transportation and storage will not be possible. Many of the perishable items like fruits and vegetables are dumped. Trucks are stranded on borders of state thus supply chains for the essential items have been disrupted.

Kharif crops are to be sown in many northern states, jute in West Bengal, sugarcane and rice in Uttar Pradesh, bajara in Rajasthan etc. Non availability of labour will be lost income for them and it will be difficult for the agriculturist to harvest this season. Allied sectors of agriculture will also suffer.

Fake news of unsafe non-vegetarian food during the Covid-19 infection have also became a challenge for the animal husbandry industry. Farmers who are farming for flowers are dumping their harvest. Forest dependent communities are also suffering due to restrictions.

No work means no food for those people who are daily wage workers in factories, construction workers, small shops, service providers like carpenters, electricians, plumbers, barbers etc. are sitting without work. With very little savings and without work for a long period means their survival is precarious.

Warriors of Covid-19 Attacked due to the growing infection, rising deaths, less knowledge, fake news, warriors of Coronavirus doctors, nurses and police are attacked. Healthcare workers are also demanding masks and protective gears. The unprecedented situation of Covid-19 has unsettled lives of all the citizens of India. No doubt that delay will result surge in cases but before the declaration a strong policy, keeping in mind all the classes of society, should be made. During lockdown police is also using force on law breakers and some of them are deploying innovative means to punish them.

Many of the **serious patients are facing problems** due to shutdown of nursing homes, hospitals and labs. As it is difficult to travel donors are also not available. With no transport, limited healthcare and restricted movements several patients are facing problems and taking self-medication. Many patients and their attendants are left stranded outside prestigious hospitals in Delhi.

For the **poor people** lockdown is a massive problem as many of them live in single room with limited money, no supply of water at some places, no space outside and without information. For them it is a humanitarian crisis for so long.

Students in Kota: Thousands of students, taking coaching for engineering and medical, were stuck in coaching hub Kota in Rajasthan amid lockdown. Madhya Pradesh, Assam, West Bengal, Uttar Pradesh, Gujarat, Punjab, Chhattisgarh in addition some other state governments made arrangements for the evacuation of a number of students. Students were going through mental agony and tension. Still in this situation students from Bihar are facing problems in Kota. A PIL was filed in Patna High Court also. Chief Minister of Bihar is strictly adhering to the guidelines on lockdown and opposed the move. Over 12,000 students from Bihar are still in Kota and trapped between the politics of lockdown and Bihar government.

On line Education there are several socio-economic factors that define Education System of India. Undoubtedly on line education will continue the pace of studies in schools and colleges but many of the problems around the whole discourse has hardly been in discussion. All India percentage of households having internet facilities stands at just 23.8%. with such a low percentage of net users it is almost incredible if net could be a mode of education for such a big country. Teachers and parents are two important pillars of the education system. For each lockdown is a reason of increased responsibilities. Progressive and innovative methods used by teachers need extra preparedness. Apart from responsibilities at home of cooking, cleaning and washing teachers are working round the clock. Extra responsibility means more working hours for educationist. Parents are also facing the same problem apart from their individual responsibility of 'work at home', they are taking care of their children and studies too. Closure of school means no mid-day meal for 12 crore students.

Domestic violence increased reports of domestic violence have increased all over the world. During lockdown women are confined with violent partners who have physically violent tendencies. According to statistics released by the UN, domestic violence increased 30% in France, 18% more calls in Spain 30% in Singapore and 35% in USA.[8] The National Commission of Women received 587 complaints in just 25 days between March, 23 April, 16. There are several personal and psychological problems people are suffering during lockdown. Apart from spending whole day with spouse many other problems are there such as job loss, salary cuts and uncertainty of future etc. Violence against women is a manifestation of the unequal power relations. UN Secretary General Antonio Guterres appealed to the governments to pay attention to the problem and prevent domestic violence.

Social and Psychological trauma it is said that man is a social animal it means that human beings can't live in isolation. They live with family or with interactive groups. Being isolated from family and friends it can be traumatic for most of the people and it can lead to long or short term psychological and physical health problems. During lockdown people who are with families even they are facing emotional void, anxiety and depression. It is traumatic and claustrophobic for low income families with many people in a small space.

POSITIVE EFFECTS

Low pollution levels lockdown for such a long period means close down of all the factories, shops, malls, markets, public transport, private vehicles, construction work is also stopped and the majority of people are also at homes. Data shows that many main cities are reporting lower levels of pollution all over the world. Nitrogen dioxide levels fell dramatically during lockdown. The skies are now clear, one can see the stars at night and

Cleaner rivers due to the lockdown, most of the industries are shut down, people's movement is also restricted, beauty of nature emerged again. Social media is full of such news and videos of cleaner Ganges in Varanasi and Haridwar. Polluted river Yamuna has also started appear clearer, toxic foam of chemicals from industrial waste, detergents and sewage is stopped. The improvement in the equality of water has been observed in other rivers also in India. But according to environmentalist this change is extra ordinary but short-lived.

Free wildlife as human beings are living inside wild animals are enjoying full freedom and exploring the area around outside their habitats. Due to quiet environment and less busy roads, elephants, spotted deer, sambhars are venturing out on main roads. In Delhi people can hear chirping of birds in place of horns and noise of factories and vehicles. Otherwise crowded streets and roads are now witness of some critically endangered species of wildlife.

View of Himalaya many of the cities situated around North India now can see Himalaya due to the drop in the pollution. Many enthusiasts shared beautiful pictures of Dhauladhars, a range of lesser Himalayas mountain from Jalandhar. Snow-capped mountains of Himalayas are also visible from the Saharanpur city of Uttar Pradesh for the first time in three decades.

Adoption of Healthy Behaviour basic hygiene practices to control Covid-19 spread, like washing hands, using sanitizer, distancing, staying home, eating home-cooked food are behavioral changes we need to continue even after the infection stopped.

Experiments in Education amid the lockdown all schools and colleges are also closed. But the alternative methods of education are working. NCERT has released an alternative academic calendar to facilitate 'stay at home' learning process for the students of the Primary Classes from 6-8 class students. It includes weekly academic plan to the teachers and interesting activities for the students.[9] By using on line methods students and teachers of schools and colleges will definitely learn the new methods and options of teaching and studying.

IMPOSITION OF LOCKDOWN

The lockdown that was imposed by the central government was under the Disaster Management Act-2005, Section 6(2)(i). According to it "The National Authority shall have the responsibility for laying down the policies, plans and guidelines for disaster management for ensuring timely and effective response to disaster."[10] before that a Janata curfew was imposed all over India on March 22, 2020. At many places Section 144 of the CrPC by District Magistrates was imposed. Already in comparison of some other federalism like USA and Canada, Indian federal system has a highly centralized arrangement. It also shows during the declaration of lockdown orders. A healthy working relationship between the centre and the state is must for the smooth sailing. If we define the federalism in India, it is a federal republic, with a parliamentary democracy under the broad framework of a written Constitution. Therefore, a national disaster or an emergency situation involve Centre, State and Municipalities/Panchayats along with other institutional actors. Not only chief ministers even Parliament was also not involved at any point of time.

Suspension of MPLADS Fund is Anti-Federal!!!

Under the Member of Parliament Local Area Development Scheme (MPLADS) each member of Parliament is allotted with ₹ five crores every year, in two instalments 2.5 crores each, for the development work of their respective constituencies. The scheme was launched in the tear of 1993 with ₹ one crore and raised to ₹ five crores in 2011–12. Central Government on April 6, 2020 declared suspension of scheme for two years. The circular from Ministry of Statistics and Programme Implementation, Govt. of India states that "Non- operation of Member of Parliament Local Area Development Scheme (MPLADS) for two years (2020–21 & 2021–22) for managing the health and adverse impact of Covid-19 on the society." [11] from the launching of the scheme this is the connection between the state and the people, between the MP and the voters of his constituency and between the government and the common people. The suspension of scheme would help government with ₹ 7,840 crore in two years. This money is to be transferred to the Consolidated Fund of India to augment resources for Covid-19 management.

Political experts have termed this move of the government as not in good taste and not according to the federal norms. This is alleged by many that it is also an effort to weak Members of Parliament and compact the whole problem. MPLADS fund is also used at the time of natural and man-made calamities. Many MPs have confidence in this fund as it could have complete the breaches in respite work left by the governments of centre and states. Many of the experts also believe that the fund could have played an important role for rapid responses. Congress MP Shashi Tharoor said in a tweet "MPLADS preserved the sense of direct responsibility for the well-being of constituents that is the hall mark of an Indian MP's work. Now the money will be allocated by the Centre will follow the priorities and preferences of New Delhi, rather than reflect 543 sets of local needs."[12]

Centralizing of Allocation of Funds

Shashi Tharoor in an article in Bloomberg Quint wrote "worse, by centralising the allocation of funds, the government has created significant delays in the devolution of funds to where they are most needed." He also pointed out that Kerala, the first and the most effected state in the initial stage received only ₹ 157 crore. This was the first instalment given by the centre to the state governments from the State Disaster Response Mitigation Fund. Though other states which are affected less but they received more of these funds from the centre. Gujarat, for instance, with just 122 Covid-19 patients, got ₹ 662 crore. Delhi's priorities are evidently not those of a distant southern state where the BJP has no presence worth the name.[13]

Lockdown Was Declared Without Consulting Any State

On March 24, 2020 Prime Minister declared lockdown all over India, in the process not a single state government was consulted. Acute problems faced by the state governments due to the unexpected announcement of the total lockdown. The problems faced by the state governments are discussed already-migrants stranded in states without work was the biggest problem. There was no solution effectively for the state governments as the borders were sealed and transportation stopped. Considering the uneven support structures that exist in different states, the process of framing rules and modalities of the lockdown demanded the participation of these states when the lockdown decision was announced on March 24.[14] Hemant Soren, Chief Minister of Jharkhand also said that all the chief ministers of the states are consulting with each other about the problems faced by them. But the prime Minister did not ask the states while imposing the lockdown. He also asked for the dedicated financial package to deal with the crisis.

No Consultation with any Opposition/Political Party

Normally any important policy decision specially that effects the whole country, all its people, most of the institutions, academic structures, political dimensions etc., are taken with the consultation of opposition and other important political parties too. The response to the Covid-19 pandemic has exposed major weaknesses in the cooperative federal structure of India. Rajya Sabha of Trinamool Congress leader, Derek O'Brien, in an interview alleged "if State Chief Ministers and Parliamentarians had been taken into confidence for the lockdown, we would have been at least one or two weeks ahead. This is not a decision which should have been taken by the centre. But more of all this later. There will be enough time for politics. No one must politicize this situation. We are extending all cooperation to the centre."[15]

Public Health and Sanitation are State Subjects

Public health and sanitation are subjects of the states. These two are matters falling exclusively within the legislative competence of the states

(Seventh Schedule of the Constitution of India, Entry 6, List II). The subject of constituting funds to tackle the challenge of the pandemic is not an issue of legislative competence. But the fact that states are vested with the exclusive authority to legislate on health-related issue is a good indicator of the crucial role that our Constitution-makers envisaged for states with respect to matters pertaining to public health.[16] so it's a question asked by the states and political experts that on what basis states capacity to raise money for the pandemic through their separate Covid-19 relief funds is weakened? In India the principle of cooperative federalism follows. It means that both centre and states must work together but within their domains and do not invade into each other spheres.

States Struggling for Revenue Amid Pandemic

With the lockdown many states are struggling for the revenue. States came to know about the lockdown through TV with just four-hour notice. Financial burden of migration, ramp up medical infrastructure, fell on unprepared states. The latest problem of banning alcohol is a bone of contention. States are spending a lot of revenue to ramp up health infrastructure and sale of liquor is a critical source of direct tax. With other banned items alcohol sale was also blocked by Prime Minister to contain the virus. States like Punjab reiterated to PM that for Punjab liquor sale is a major source of revenue estimated 7 billion rupees per day. Since only few vehicles are on road, petrol sales have also crashed. Though to make up this loss will not be possible for the state and Central government is not providing enough help. This fight over liquor is a series of problem in which the federal government has eroded the ability of states to raise the revenue.

Centralized Purchase

Leaders from Indian states are also criticizing centralize purchase of coronavirus medical and protective kits. On April 2, 2020 Ministry of Health and Family Welfare placed a centralized system of procurement for Covid-19 related medical supplies. By this the Central government had taken away the powers of state governments to procure ventilators and protective equipment for the health warriors.

State Dues

During the Covid-19 crisis, most of the states are complaining about the dues of states. GST introduced in 2017 is already a bone of contention between centre and states. Before the crisis states already demanded GST compensation the centre was holding. West Bengal, Punjab, Kerala, BJP led Gujarat has written to clear the GST compensation.

Central Teams for Violation of Lockdown

Central government decision to airdrop ministerial teams to check lockdown violations is deemed as interference in the internal affairs of the state. In the month of April four states Maharashtra, West Bengal, Rajasthan and Madhya Pradesh were identified by the centre to visit to check the violations, a team of officials also sent to Kerala in March 2019. States objected on this as intervention and unjustified on the part of the centre. It was stated that the centre should take states into confidence first and then coordinate and assist the states. Every type of federalism rests on mutual trust and coordination between the centre and states.

Financial Package for States

Manmohan Singh said "Success of lockdown is to be judged finally on our ability to tackle Covid-19. Cooperation between the centre and the states is key to success and the fight would very much depend upon the availability of resources."[17] Similar views were given by the Chief Minister of Rajasthan Ashok Gehlot, Chief Minister of Chhattisgarh Bhupesh Baghel and Chief Minister of Puducherry V Narayansamy during a meet of Congress-ruled states. On April 2, 2020 Centre released Rs. 17,287.08 crore to different states to deal with the challenges posed due to the Covid-19. But after that states are sending messages to centre to compensate for a slump in GST collections and also release of pending GST arrears. States are already suffering due to the lockdown additional spending on health infrastructure is severely straining the finances of states. Chief Ministers of almost all the states are demanding financial assistance to fight coronavirus. Except the agriculture sector, all other activities have been closed and the economy of the country is at standstill. Most of the chief ministers asked for the centre for sufficient funds during the video conferencing during lockdown.

LOCKDOWN/POST LOCKDOWN CHALLENGES

The lockdown was a surprise for all, the centre took the decision on its own and announce a nationwide lockdown without consulting anyone. This was the challenge for all the states. It causes serious problems but states worked on the solutions. The decision of partial lockdown was taken by the governments of Kerala, Karnataka and Odisha before the central government announced the full lockdown on March 24, 2020. The NDMA empowered both central and state governments to regulate the movement of people and goods nationwide but after the March 24 declaration centre is taking all the decisions and just impose decisions on states arbitrarily. Each and every state is taking decisions and making policies on their own and also developing models to fight against the novel virus. Kerala model is a well-known and most successful one, similarly Odisha and Rajasthan also prepared states accordingly. Some of the district administration such as Bhilwara in Rajasthan and Agra in Uttar Pradesh, are fighting against the Covid-19 within the broad framework of federalism.

As the lockdown is not the only part of the fight. To stop the spread is the biggest challenge before the states and that too with shrinking revenues, less help from the centre and with restrictions all over. Post lockdown will be a big challenge for whole country. States are working on modalities on their own but centre does not allow in such matters too. When Kerala, first state who flatten the curve, decided to open the restaurants based on its own risk assessment but centre pressurized the state government to cancel such a planning. Similarly, Government of Punjab was willing to open shops of liquor that was again denied by the centre. Here the role of centre should be of a mentor and not a master. States must be allowed to revive their revenue resources while working on the containment of the coronavirus.

Crisis in Jammu and Kashmir

The Union Territory of Kashmir is fighting on many fronts, one of them is Covid-19. Kashmir is under security lockdown since August 2019. There is a totally communication blackout since last August in Kashmir. 639 cases in total are reported in Jammu and Kashmir till the first week of May. Only in March 2020 that low speed internet facility was revived.

People living in the UT have no or little access to Facebook, WhatsApp and other social media platforms. People are unable to contact their friends and relatives. They hardly are getting connection for more than few minutes and that too for only white-listed sites. They are not getting vital information regarding the infection or disease or its treatment. Even on line education and work from home is the distant dream for the people living in Kashmir. Low speed communication system is also troubling the doctors and other health workers. As a part of India Union Territory of Jammu and Kashmir should get all the facilities like other states of the country.

Special Shramik Trains for Migrants, Tourists, Pilgrims, Students Without Consulting/Informing State Governments

Another extension of lockdown was declared on May 4, 2020, for another two weeks, the government permitted six special trains to transport migrant workers, tourists, pilgrims, students and other people who are stuck across India. The decision to run the trains shrouded in secrecy till the first train started at 5 a.m. on May, 1,2020 from Telangana, Limgampalli to Jharkhand, Hatiya carrying 12,00 migrants. For these six trains and subsequent trains it was decided by the policy makers that prices of the ticket will be compensated by the states from where the train will start or where it ends. Besides the sleeper-class ticket fare, Railways has charged ₹ 30 as superfast charge and an additional ₹ 20 per ticket.[18] Following a meeting between Railways and Home Secretary it was decided that migrant workers will be allowed to leave by trains. Again, state governments were neither informed nor consulted for the paying of tickets of passengers of these Shramik Specials. Various State Governments such as Bihar, Maharashtra and Rajasthan demanded that the Centre and the Railways bear the expenditure on humanitarian grounds. However, it was declared by Congress to pay the entire amount of special trains.

Things to Learn from Kerala

India detected its first case in January, 30, 2020 in Kerala, by March, the number increased. Situated in south-west of India has been recognized as having implemented best practices in the fight against coronavirus. Ever since the first case in Kerala has been on alert mode and trying to bring infection under control. Three months on and curve of Kerala has just flattened. Kerala spends the most on health sector in India and state has a very formidable primary health care system. In February Kerala was expecting a large number of foreign returnees from the Middle East and other countries. This is also to be noticed that 80% of the total number of cases are from people who travelled from the Gulf countries. Kerala has three international airports and a population of 3.5 crore people. Experiment in Kerala on first three cases can give a lesson on its coronavirus management to the whole country. Kerala already in 2018 has seen dangerous Nipah and Ebloa virus outbreak so state was prepared. Every facet of the WHO guidelines was strictly observed and obeyed, even the rumour mongers were identified from social media, every sector involved in the system cooperated. It was reported that patients who tested between March 9-March 20, Kerala and tested positive has a high rate of recovery at 84%, in comparison of Maharashtra of 5.5% and Delhi of 4.04%. Kerala community-based network, local bodies network and self-help groups of women are also helping the government. Kerala formed ward and division committees under local self-governing bodies. Continuous vigil also helped. The role of health minister K Shailja is working commendably in whole fight. She had won praise all over for her efforts to combat the coronavirus.

'Break the Chain' was the slogan given by the state government. The government took over vacant buildings, hotels, educational institutions, even train compartments were made quarantine care centres. Call centres for mental distress patients opened in the state, 241 counsellors were engaged to give relief to the infected people. The slogan given by the Chief Minister of the State Pinnarayi Vijayan was "Physical Distance, Social Unity" Relief packages were announced on time. the state also handled the problem of migrant workers very efficiently as they built shelters and distributed cooked meals wherever they were. Kerala government also opened the 'walk-in facility' so that people feel safe and can go for tests securely. Corona Safe Network has also been created with the Corona Care Centres and Corona Literacy Mission to create consciousness on the infection and tests of Covid-19. Everyone knows that battle is not won yet there is long way ahead but a robust health care system, a decentralized culture which give power to the grassroot workers, preparedness, community reach, mass screening with quarantine, timely tests and people to people contact have helped the state to tackle the biggest challenge of 2020.

The Way Forward.......

PM Modi held his fourth round of deliberations with the chief ministers of states on April, 27, 2020 to review the Covid-19 situation.40 days of lockdown are completed on May, 3, 2020. Some states urged to extend the lockdown and lockdown is extended till May 17, 2020. Is lockdown the only alternate left to fight with the coronavirus? Saving the lives of the citizens are important but the health of the economy is also vital and to be taken care of. No means of livelihoods and no excess to basic necessities available for a number of people. There will be widespread loss of employment and disruptions. Unlike the global financial crisis in 2007-08, it is a global health crisis. Medical infrastructure is working beyond their capacities. Mass testing is not possible in India, health system of most of the states is not robust, future of the vaccine in near future don't know. Economy even before the crisis was in shambles. Today people are at more risk of poverty and hunger than the coronavirus despite the help of government.

So, what is the need of the day? Restarting of economy, presentation of a sustainable plan and its implementation. The government will have to pay attention to the economic crisis. Our half of the population depends on agriculture, agriculturists are also affected by the lockdown. Migration back from villages to cities after the lockdown will not be so easy. Government also have to lend their industry a hand, a financial boost has to be given. Central government has to take care of demands of state governments also. Medium and small-scale industries will need help of the government. Start ups are the worst hit during the pandemic. Substantial measures have to be taken up to restart them. Most crucial part of the economy is the supply chain that is also hit during the lockdown. Lifting the lockdown will never be an easy process. It has to be done very cautiously and in a phased manner.

According to Indian Economist Raghuram Rajan, former RBI Chief and distinguished Professor of Finance at University of Chicago said "With the right resolve and priorities, and drawing on India's many sources of strength, it can beat this virus back, and even set the stage for a much hopeful tomorrow."

REFERENCES

[1] https://www.who.int/health-topics/coronavirus#tab=tab_1

[2] economictimes.indiatimes.com/news/international/world-news/

[3] https://www.livemint.com/news/world/us, accessed on April, 29, 2020.

[4] https://www.worldometers.info/coronavirus/country/china/

[5] https://economictimes.indiatimes.com/news/international/world-news/coronavirus-in-india, accessed on 30.4.2020

[6] indiatoday.in/india/story/coronavirus-pandemic-covid-19

[7] https://www.business-humanrights.org/en/india-un-chief

[8] https://theintercept.com/2020/04/13/coronavirus-lockdown-domestic-violence

[9] https://diigitallearning.eletsonline.com/2020/04/hrd-ministry, accessed on May 1, 2020

[10] https://www.ndmindia.nic.in/images/The%20Disaster%20Management%20Act,%202005.pdf

[11] https://www.mplads.gov.in/mplads/En/2008-english-circulars.aspx

[12] https://www.businesstoday.in/current/economy-politics/coronavirus-in-india-why-suspension-of-mplads-is-problematic/story/400771.html

[13] https://www.bloombergquint.com/coronavirus-outbreak/wrong-to-suspend-mplads-for-covid-19-shashi-tharoor

[14] https://www.epw.in/journal/2020/16/editorials/indian-federalism-and-covid-19.html, accessed on May 1, 2020.

[15] https://www.thehindu.com/opinion/interview/covid-19-we-are-witnessing-a-new-kind-of-federalism-says-trinamool-mp-derek-o-brien/article31312328.ece

[16] https://www.thehindu.com/opinion/interview/covid-19-we-are-witnessing-a-new-kind-of-federalism-says-trinamool-mp-derek-o-brien/article31312328.ece

[17] https://indianexpress.com/article/india

[18] The Indian Express, May 4, 2020.

COVID-19—Legal Challenges of Public Safety or Personal Liberty: A Checklist of New Laws Implemented

Dr. Geetanjali Chandra* and Ms. Devika Ramachandran**

ABSTRACT: The Covid-19 pandemic has reconstructed the entire globe in all aspects from public health to social terms, economic, legal, or constitutional terms. As a result, all countries have invoked emergency powers to support services and provide wide-ranging executive powers to counter the fast-spreading pandemic within their borders. Emergency powers often outlive the phenomenon that triggers the introduction of emergency powers, in the first instance when we look into the history. The world has witnessed several pandemics as well as epidemics throughout its history and some legal precedents were adopted regarding the power of government to prevent the spread of the highly deadly virus. Meanwhile, public health legislations give authority to governments, and also to regional health authorities, to undertake several activities to handle responses to public health events like Pandemics. Laws amending various legislative acts, including laws on emergency prevention and control and the Tax Code are implemented in most of the countries across the globe. It is seen that most of the Act tries to increase the availability of the health as well as social care professionals, release and ease the burden on the medical experts, and contain and slow the growth of the pandemic. In contrast, Emergency management legislation authorizes governments to facilitate and guide the coordination of responses to public health events as they change over time.

In this paper, the authors have focused on the new (temporary) Acts enacted by a few countries and also look into some countries that have amended the old Act in the current scenario. The paper throws light on the necessity of such new laws or acts for public safety. This research also aims to showcase how the Governments are aiding the society to prevent and respond to a variety of threats that comes from public health which has the potential to

---

* Head of Law Department, Amity Law School, Dubai.
**Visiting Faculty, Amity Law School, Dubai.

cross borders and endanger the health sector across the world. In this paper, authors have looked into the new temporary laws enacted and implemented by Australia, United Kingdom, United States, Singapore, United Arab Emirates, and India

Keywords: Pandemic Legislation, New Laws, Public Health Safety, Emergency Powers, Emergency Management Legislation.

INTRODUCTION

COVID-19, the pandemic of 2020, is a global health issue that has come with unique challenges to international law. From health to human rights to International trade to security, the global pandemic raises questions that will reshape the future. At this uncertain time, expertise is more important than ever in all fields of life. Almost all countries are well prepared for the challenges arising out of Covid-19, yet many experts suggests that clear thinking, sensitivity and diplomacy will be required as well. On January 30, 2020, the World Health Organization (WHO) declared Covid-19 a public health emergency, it developed certain tools, provided guidance as well as some training in order to support Nations so as to strengthen and maintain their capacities for a sudden detection of the virus. When there is an event that is preliminary determined to be an emergency situation in public health that has international concern, the Director General of WHO can seek the views of IHR established under Article 48. According to IHR, every country has to develop and prolong the ability to each country must develop and maintain the capacity to flare-up the risks in public health within its territory and to inform WHO of all events which may carry a public health emergency concern.

During the pandemic, WHO has given guidelines to help Nation's public health, the Director General of WHO has stressed that a strong health system will definitely act as a shield to protect any public health emergency and further came up with major operational planning guidelines to help countries navigate through these challenges. WHO has provided these guidelines so as to balance the demands of the response directly to Covid-19 and on the other hand it can maintain necessary health services and mitigate the risk of collapsing of the system. The guidelines include agglomeration of actions that can be taken immediately, and establish that Nations have to look into all the levels including national and regional levels to recognize, maintain and provide high quality health services to all.

Each Nations has its own responsibility and rights to identify essential services and prioritize them to maintain continuity of service delivery and make strategic shifts to ensure that escalation of limited resources provide maximum benefit for the society. Keeping the guidelines, every country has implemented and enacted their own laws to protect and safeguard the Public Health.

UNITED KINGDOM

In the wake of Covid-19, the UK government introduced emergency regulations to prevent further spread of the pandemic. On February 2020, UK parliament passed the Health Protection (Coronavirus Restrictions) (England) Regulations, 2020. This Act came into force immediately. The recent act passed was issued under the emergency procedure which is contained in Section 45R of the Public Health (Control of Disease) Act of 1984. This 1984 Act was amended by the Health and Social Care Act of 2008, a sunset clause of two years, which means the Act will get expired within a limited period, was also included in the Act.

According to the regulation, medical servants have the authority to hold back anyone with Covid-19 virus for the purpose of screening and to isolate for the specific period as required. According to the newly invoked regulations police constables or officers also have the power to detain people suspected to have Coronavirus.

Along with this, the Government has various other responsibilities or powers that come under Part 2 of the Civil Contingencies Act, 2004. The Part 2 provides and allows the authority to make regulations so as to deal with all emergency threats that may cause serious damages to the humans or their welfare. Here, emergency can mean any particular happenings that may cause or involve human sickness, deaths or even disruption to the medical services and even supply of food.

The UK government as a precaution has declared implementing further emergency legislation like Covid-19 emergency bill, if there is a chance of further spreading of Coronavirus.

UNITED STATES OF AMERICA

In the midst of Covid-19, United States of America declared a public health emergency in January. In US, the federal government has the authority to the national response of the pandemic and state or local health departments are standing on the front lines. Public Health Emergency declarations have been issued in each State and territory of the Country.

In United States of America, Covid-19 regulations are placed in three phases. All the three phases, the first phase, the "Coronavirus Preparedness and Response Supplemental Appropriations Act, the second phase, the "Families First, President Donald Trump signed and enacted the bill of Coronavirus Response Act", and the third phase the "Coronavirus Aid, Relief and Economic Security Act".

Both Phase 1 as well as Phase 2 focuses primarily on public health measures. Phase 2 along with health laws also provides labor, employment and tax provisions that will affect private sectors.

Some of the measures passed in US are:
1. Emergency Family and Medical Leave Expansion Act.
2. Emergency Paid Sick Leave Act.
3. Tax Credits for Paid Sick and Paid Family and Medical Leave.

SINGAPORE

Singapore's response to the Covid-19 has been held up by several countries around the world as a model. The country seemed to be successfully 'flattening the curve' up till late March. There was a sudden increase because of repatriation of Singaporeans as well as the students' who were stranded in other Nations. The last weeks of March and the first week of April clearly showed the need of stricter laws to be implemented. Singapore was relying on the powers of the provisions that were included in the old act of Infectious Disease Act, The Act was invoked during 2002 and 2003 when there was global severe acute respiratory outbreak.

On the 7th April 2020, the Singapore government passed the COVID (Temporary Measures) Act, 2020. CTMA included provisions which stated clearly under section 34(1) that the Minister can make regulations to prevent, protect or delay or otherwise control the spread of dreadful virus in Singapore. The Act includes in Part 2 restrictions on Individuals, Part 3 Restrictions in relation to premises and businesses and Part 4 miscellaneous which includes compoundable offences. Along with all these provisions

CTMA also grants the executive authority to issue control orders to prevent transmission of Coronavirus. Singaporean government never wanted to use the terms "emergency" or "lockdown", which were is used worldwide. They came up with a new term "Circuit Breaker". The new model drafted by the Government has powers to restrict many legal as well as constitutional rights of the country which will be lifted once the situation of COVID 19 comes under control.

UNITED ARAB EMIRATES

During the unexpected and unprecedented spread of the Covid-19, the UAE legislations provided for stricter preventive measures, obligations and penalties according to UAE Federal Law No14 of 2014 on communicable diseases (the 2014 Law), as amended and expanded by Cabinet Resolution 2016, now applies to Covid-19. The first legislative approach was taken by the UAE government and also issued in the year 1981 so as to prevent global pandemics and communicable diseases including Plague and Cholera during the 80's. In 1981 the law stated communicable diseases as transferable diseases. Transferable diseases here mean the one that is transferred to humans by the humans or animals or any other things. Penalties were also implemented in the 1981 Act for the violators.

After novel Coronavirus was declared as Pandemic, the Ministry of Health and Community Protection included it in the list of the Communicable diseases. The UAE ministry also confirmed that penalties will be applied as per Federal Law No. 14 of 2014. The violators, according to this act included all the medical professionals and staffs. It stated that if any one included in the Act intentionally fails to inform the authority the details of suspected person with virus or a non-report of the deaths due to the deadly virus are punishable under the law.

This law is applicable to everyone including friends, colleagues, family etc. UAE government, along with the 2014 law, has other rules and regulations circulated so as to prevent the spread of the Pandemic.

INDIA

As soon as World Health Organization declared Coronavirus as Public health emergency, India invoked provision of Epidemics Disease Act, 1897. This Act can be stated as a colonial-era on epidemics and legal experts suggested to repeal. The old Act has no provisions that give the power to the Center to interfere in any biological emergencies and the power as a whole remains with the State. This 123 year old Act has been used to contain various diseases in India including swine flu, cholera, malaria and dengue. In 2020 March, the Act was enforced across the country so as to stop the transmission of Coronavirus.

But, Section 2 contains provisions which state that if Center at any point of time thinks that spread of Epidemic diseases is becoming a threat and the provisions of the law are not enough then, they have the authority to take steps by publishing notice to the public or even prescribe temporary rules for the welfare of the society.

In April 2020, the Government of India declared the promulgation of an ordinance, The Epidemic Diseases (Amendment) Ordinance 2020, to amend the act, adding provisions to punish those attacking frontline health workers under section 3. Under this section, it states that if any person violates any regulation will be punishable according to section 188 of IPC.

CONCLUSION

The outbreak of COVID-19 currently is not under control, with high risk of spreading. Yet, governments across the globe have taken severe steps by implementing and enacting new legislations that help public health safety. Emergency measures within the ambit of laws are being imposed in most of the countries. The public along with authorities need to follow the Acts that have been implemented. This public health emergency teaches the government as well as the public to be alert and also to be prepared to prevent such pandemic situations.

REFERENCES

[1] "Clinical management of severe acute respiratory infection when novel coronavirus (2019-nCoV) infection is suspected". Published on 20 January 2020 by WHO.

[2] "Coronavirus is exposing all of the weaknesses in the US health system High health care costs and low medical capacity made the US uniquely vulnerable to the coronavirus". Published by Scott Dylan, on March 18th 2020.

[3] "WHO Director-General's opening remarks at the media briefing on COVID-19". Press Release by WHO on 11th March 2020.

[4] "Loss of sense of smell as marker of COVID-19 infection". Written by Hopkins, Claire on Ear, Nose and Throat surgery body of United Kingdom.

[5] China launches coronavirus 'close contact' app". Was be telecasted on BBC News on 11th February 2020.

[6] Ministry of Law and Justice (22 April 2020), The Epidemic Diseases (Amendment) Ordinance, 2020 (PDF), The Gazette of India, Government of India.

[7] Nair, Sangeeta (23 April 2020). "Epidemic Act amended: Penalty for any violence against health care workers increased to 7 years in Jail". Jagran Josh. Retrieved 25 April 2020.

[8] Awasthi, Prashasti. "Centre invokes 'Epidemic Act' and 'Disaster Management Act' to prevent spread of coronavirus". @businessline. Retrieved 2020-03-15.

[9] "A 123-yr-old Act to combat coronavirus in India; experts say nothing wrong". Livemint. IANS. 2020-03-14. Retrieved 2020-03-15.

[10] "To combat coronavirus, India invokes provisions of colonial-era Epidemic Diseases Act: A look at what this means". Firstpost. 12 March 2020. Retrieved 2020-03-12.

[11] https://en.wikipedia.org/wiki/Epidemic_Diseases_Act,_1897#Legal_provisions

[12] Website of UK government: www.gov.uk/coronavirus

[13] Article published in website twobirds... www.twobirds.com/en.news/articles/2020/uk/covid-19-uk-public-health-perspective.

[14] https://www.moh.gov.sg/policies-and-legislation/covid-19(temporary-measures)-control-order)-regulations

[15] https://sso.agc.gov.sg/SL/COVID19TMA2020-S254-2020?DocDate=20200407

[16] https://sso.agc.gov.sg/Act/COVID19TMA2020

[17] https://verfassungsblog.de/singapores-legislative-approach-to-the-covid-19-public-health-emergency/

[18] https://www.legal500.com/developments/thought-leadership/history-of-federal-law-no-14-for-the-year-2014-on-combating-the-communicable-diseases/

[19] https://gulfnews.com/uae/crime/uae-invokes-communicable-disease-law-to-tackle-covid-19-1.70588423

[20] https://u.ae/en/information-and-services/justice-safety-and-the-law/handling-the-covid-19-outbreak/2019-novel-coronavirus

[21] https://www.nortonrosefulbright.com/en/knowledge/publications/31a1e2d6/covid-19-now-within-the-uae-communicable-diseases-laws

[22] https://gulfnews.com/uae/covid-19-efforts-sheikh-mohammed-approves-draft-law-for-national-safety-1.1587468720344

[23] https://economictimes.indiatimes.com/news/politics-and-nation/how-india-is-fighting-coronavirus-with-a-colonial-era-law-on-epidemics/articleshow/74752473.cms?from=mdr

Malevolent Use of Biological Weapons: A Legal Ethical and Humanitarian Concern

Dr. Niteesh Kumar Upadhyay* and Ms. Bhumika Sharma**

INTRODUCTION

The entire humanity has always hoped for and also sought for a solution to avoid war of any sort. There is a movement from struggle to peace within the countries. The conventional desire for international war has faded with time. The history is replete with many examples of the efforts being made in the interest of peace at International level. The human civilization on its journey towards peace has been able to get varied degrees of achievements in almost all realms of life.

The science and technology have changed the human lives in both positive and negative contexts. Life-sciences and various other branches of science have successfully enhanced the quality of lives in general.[1] The advancements in information and communication technology have empowered the people, organizations and the States to a great extent. The progress in science and technology further benefits the life-sciences. The better access to communications technologies reinforces the extension of research at the Global level in various branches of the life-sciences. The advances in the other sciences too has been related to the reaction to the life-sciences. There is a tremendous chance of assemblage of knowledge from the diverse fields of sciences resulting into woes for the world. The weapons of mass destruction are one of the atrocious results of the same.[2] Nuclear,

* Assistant Professor of Law, Galgotias University.
** Ph.D. Research Scholar, Himachal Pradesh University, Shimla, India.
[1] David Weatherall, Brian Greenwood, Heng Leng Chee and PrawaseWasi, Science and Technology for Disease Control: Past, Present and Future (May 23, 2020, 09:10 PM), https://www.ncbi.nlm.nih.gov/books/NBK11740
[2] Gary Ackerman and Jeremy Tamsett, Jihadists and Weapons of Mass Destruction (May 20, 2020, 05:15 PM), https://fas.org/wp-content/uploads/2013/06/Jihadists__WMD1.pdf

biological and chemical weapons can be categorized as the main weapons of mass destruction. The cyber warfare is another looming front, having the potential to cause a Global catastrophe.[3] The sphere of weapons of biological constitution still remains unfamiliar to a certain point on account of two reasons i.e. eradication of the records and second reason being having the nature of classified information. There has been evident increase in its academic interest after the World War-I.

The biological threats may range from accidental, man-made (genetically modified) to naturally occurring. The timeline to counter the misuse of the life-sciences is relatively short due to their complex nature. Diverse schools of thoughts have prevailed with respect to the biological weapons. Their use of such weapons is alarming and horrid; thus, first school forbids the use of the biological weapons during the wars. The next school believes that they are hyped-up and are merely capable of temporary consequences. The last school holds that each weapon falling in this category may have extensive results. This further holds them feeble and inept. Since the World War-I, the International Scientific Community has been insisting for the reduction of the biological and chemical weapons. The Governments of various countries have been engaged to oversee; impede and counter them by expanding the scientific insight regarding them. The research in this area is still going on and is likely to gain momentum in the near future. The strides in the science and technology must go on while maintaining a watch over the risks and abuses. The wearing away of the ethical norms regarding the use of the biological weapons have made prevalence of the biological threats more common. Multifarious outlook to address the vulnerabilities of the former appears to be the solution. The paper starts with a brief review of the key legal factors in the following substantive parts.

HISTORY OF BIOLOGICAL WEAPONS

Biological weapons have been used in wars since ages and many historical texts and writings of jurists discuss regarding the instances when these biological weapons have created havoc. Even Kautilya's Arthashastra written way back in year 300 B.C. discussed about biological

---

[3] Supra Note 1.

weapons and their use for attaining military advantage over the enemy country[4].

One of the earliest examples of the use of biological weapons comes from Italy in year 1155 when King Barbarossa poisoned the water wells of Tortona with dead bodies of soldiers[5]. This technique of throwing dead bodies of humans and animals in water wells were very popular among Romans and Persians[6]. The year 1343, again saw a new version of weaponizing the dead bodies as biological weapons. In year 1343 Jani Beg ordered that their army men who died of plague should be catapulted to launch the dead bodies to the city. Thousands of dead plague bodies were thrown into the city walls of Caffa, Crimean Peninsula. The people attempted to dump as many bodies as they could in the sea but soon dead bodies poisoned the air and water supply which was carried by one infected person to other and created havoc at that time.

In year 1495, during Southern Italy battle, armed forces of Spain supplied the enemy forces of France with wine contaminated with the blood of leprosy patients.[7] This particular method of mixing wine with blood of infected people was an inefficient method of war because leprosy takes 15 to 20 years to develop and hence this method could have given a military advantage except mental satisfaction to the France army. Not just this, researchers have seen many failed attempts of biological weapons during war. For example, a confederate doctor tried to injure Union soldiers by giving them blankets infected with yellow fever and yellow fever is caused by mosquitoes. The same infected blanket techniques were useful for spread the disease small pox in year 1763 against British by Native Americans.

---

[4] Simon Whitby, Tatyana Novossiolova, Gerald Walther and Malcolm Dando, Preventing Biological Threats, (April 3, 2020, 11:15 AM), https://www.bureaubiose curity.nl/sites/default/files/2018-05/Bradford%20Textbook%202015.pdf

[5] Bruce E. Fleury, Biological Warfare: Using Germs as Weapons, (May 21, 2020, 06:30 PM), https://www.thegreatcoursesdaily.com/biological-warfare-using-germs-as-weapons

[6] C. Patrick Ryan, Zoonoses likely to be used in Bioterrorism, (May 18, 2020, 08:00 AM), https://www.ncbi.nlm.nih.gov/pmc/articles/PMC2289981

[7] Cassandra Willyard, Ancient Forms of Biological Warfare, (15 May, 2020, 04:45 PM), https://www.lastwordonnothing.com/2011/03/07/ancient-forms-of-biological-warfare

Throwing infected bodies, weapons containing rabies and other fatal diseases were very common in old days. Catapulting dead bodies was one of the methods which has been found to be used many times during wars. One more such example is of the Russian army throwing cadavers of plague victims in the city of Sweden[8]. Napoleon Bonaparte in year 1797 as war strategy tried to spread malaria in Mantua, Italy by flooding the plains. Napoleon wanted to weaken the resistance during armed conflict because if people get sick due of malaria, that will lead to weakening the army of enemy.

During world war one, Germany and French used anthrax and glanders as biological weapon against allies to dominate them in case of direct hostility. The race for acquiring biological weapon increased around the Globe after the First World War and by the time of Second World War, it was suspected that many states were developing biological weapons. The states which were being suspected were USA, Russia, Canada, France, Italy, Germany, Japan, Hungry and UK. UK developed cattle-cakes containing anthrax and produced millions of those but did not use it during or even after the war.[9]

After World War II, there were increase in allegations upon different states pertaining to use of biological weapons but most of such allegations could not be proved beyond reasonable doubt. For example, there was allegation on Great Britain that she had used biological weapon in Oman in year 1957. People's Republic of China also leveled allegations on United States of America that she caused Cholera epidemic in year 1961 in Hong Kong and apart from these, many other similar allegations against Iraq, Colombia etc. may be noticed.[10]

After the Second World War, many states started their attempt to research and further create biological weapons and in this the plan of Iraq during gulf war was the most controversial one. It is believed that around

---

[8] R. Roffey, A. Tegnell and F. Elgh, Biological Warfare in a Historical Perspective, (May 17, 2020, 10:30 AM), https://www.sciencedirect.com/science/article/pii/S1198743X 14626343

[9] Stefan Riedel, Biological Warfare and Bioterrorism: A Historical Review, (May 14, 2020, 08:55 PM), https://www.ncbi.nlm.nih.gov/pmc/articles/PMC1200679

[10] Franco Angeli, Weapons and the International Rule of Law, (May 23, 2020, 12:00 PM) http://iihl.org/wp-content/uploads/2019/03/Weapons-and-international-rule-of-law_Sanremo-Round-Table-2016-3.pdf

the year 1974, government of Iraq initiated her biological weapon project and started an institute called as AL Hazen Ibn Al Hautham. Though this institute attempted many trials but was shut down in the year 1978 without achieving much. This shut down of the institute was not the end of story of biological weapon development in Iraq and it is believed that during the year 1990, Iraq was trying to develop delivery means which can carry biological weapons through land and air. Apart from this, Iraq also had a visionary concept of creating a spray tank which could spray 2000 liters of anthrax over enemies. According to reports, a trial of these spray tanks was conducted but the attempt was not successful. Most of the weapons and prototypes developed were destroyed during the Gulf War. Hence, biological weapons and methods have formed an integral part of warfare in all times i.e. ancient, medieval, and modern. In future, a whole new range of these which will increase the injuries to human kind are possible.

DIFFERENCE BETWEEN BIOLOGICAL WARFARE AND CHEMICAL WARFARE

People often get confused between biological weapon and chemical weapons and the same has been mentioned many a times in research and news articles. Biological Warfare and Chemical Warfare have different characteristics. First and foremost, the differentiation is on the grounds of coverage like chemical weapons effect is limited to a few miles whereas on the other hand biological weapons can have effect up to thousands of miles including different countries and this is because biological agents multiply and mutilate very fast, hence are able to cover a very large area in short time and unlike natural epidemic it hits whole population resulting in collapsing of health, transport, economic and social system. Another point of differentiation is that detecting chemical weapons is possible in battle field whereas detecting biological weapons is not possible. Further defending against chemical weapons is possible whereas defending against biological weapons is really difficult.

Characteristics of Biological Weapons

Biological weapons have many characteristics which differ from conventional weapons. The one positive aspect of biological weapon is that use of these weapons does not destroy physical infrastructure including military installations, hospital, schools, temples and other cultural property. There is not a doubt that biological weapons will make them temporarily unusable due to the infectious biological agents but the use of the infrastructure can be restored after decontamination which will be comparatively much cheaper than building the whole structure again. Biological weapon though cannot destroy these physical infrastructures but this technique can be used to capture and conquer these buildings. For example, if country 'A' attacks on country 'B' with a biological weapon and know how to control the effects of these weapons than country 'A' can capture these physical infrastructures as soon as they are abandoned for some time by other country after administration of biological weapon.

Biological Weapons are Difficult to Detect

Biological weapons because of their unique nature and slow reaction in some cases may sometimes affect a person, plant or animal after weeks or maybe after years. The effects and usage of these weapons are really tough to detect unless responsibility of it is taken by some country. There are serious issues pertaining to biological weapons around the globe with regard to its Intelligence, Detection, Surveillance, and Diagnosis. Detection and surveillance of biological weapon is very tough as some biological weapon effects so slowly that it might take years to finally detect the effected person. There are many states which are still working on research and development of these biological weapons on pretext of measures for immunization and bio-safety, hence makes it really tough to control or keep a track of research and production[11]. These biological programs are tough to detect and it is difficult to prevent its effects during pre-clinical, clinical and trial stages. It cannot be said that any country developing biological weapon has full control over its property. There have been allegations by many newspapers around the globe thatCovid-19 is outcome of biological program of China but no doubt there is nothing substantial to prove it.

Biological Weapons Cover a Large Area

There is no doubt that there is substantial research which shows that biological weapons can be made in a way that their potency can be checked but due to factors like age, sex, climate, eating habits and immunity, the

---

[11] *Id.*

effect of biological weapon will be different on different communities. Furthermore, biological weapons may cover a very large area without any military distinction or military necessity and because of careers can reach to any part of the world and can seriously cover huge area which can prove to be dangerous for not just a particular community or state but also against the whole humanity itself.[12]

Small Amount is Needed

Many countries are alleged to be working upon tank and missile containing biological agents but one property of these biological weapons is that only a small amount of it is required to spread and act. Biological weapon work on either human, crops or animal and all the three transmit it very fast for one person, plant and animal to other. One person infects others and this chain keeps on going and that's why only a small amount of it is required because later it is transmitted by humans, animals and crops.

DIFFERENT BIOLOGICAL AGENTS HAVE DIFFERENT PROPERTIES AND HENCE GIVE FLEXIBILITY AND CHOICE

There are many biological weapons available with States and Armed Forces and they can choose which one they want to use according to the need or demand of time. There are a few biological weapons which can kill a large number of people, while few will only make them sick for some time, there are also weapons which will make a large area of population sick for particular time, and few will reduce the food and water supply by making it poisonous and hence military and states can use these weapons according to the military effect that they want to see .This property hence gives a great flexibility to the biological weapons.

Biological Weapons and Delayed Casualty

Most of the biological weapons take at least a week's time to show the effects which makes it a useless weapon for immediate retaliation or war. Since it takes few weeks to see the effects of these weapons on human,

---

[12] Supra note 10.

animals or plants, military as a result gets an interval time to plan for future course of action. So biological weapons can be used if a military wants to buy some extra time for planning of war strategies, development of weapons or building army as this will give them few weeks' time to prepare for the war and attack with the full Throttle.

Legality of Use of Biological Weapons

Disarmament and the control on the free use of the advancing weapons have been the concern of the International Community since the beginning of the Twentieth century. The incidents such as the disastrous wars or the wars within the confines of few countries have raised the attention for a stricter regime governing the array of dreadful weapons. The establishment of the League of the Nations and the United Nations during the different phases of the International history shows the significance of the need for the world peace. The chemical and the nuclear weapons have come under the purview of the international treaties quite early. Though with time, the need to bring revisions in the Treaties and the Protocols would always continue.

The Preamble of the Universal Declaration of Human Rights recognizes the need of furthering the development of friendly relations between the nations. It also clearly mentions that demining human rights in past has resulted in barbarous act which shocked the human conscience of mankind.

It is contended that even before 1925, the International Customary Law had restricted the use of biological weapons.[13] The definitive prohibition on the use of these weapons came in the form of the Protocol for the Prohibition of the Use in War of Asphyxiating, Poisonous or Other Gases and of Bacteriological Methods of Warfare in June 1925. The inclusion of bacteriological methods of warfare was at the instance of the Polish Government. The Geneva Protocol was applicable upon the signatory countries. The Protocol proved to be a failure in preventing the use of chemical and biological weapons.

---

[13] Jez Littlewood, Biological Weapons: Much Ado and Little Action, (May 22, 2020, 05:00 PM), https://www.jstor.org/stable/41821401?seq=1

The next major progress was made in 1972 with Biological and Toxin Weapons Convention (B.W.C.). The Convention became the maiden International Treaty for restricting the biological agents' use only for the peaceful purposes. The strength of the Convention lies in the possibility to include the latest means of biological warfare. The regular Review Conferences since 1980 have been able to keep the Convention quite effective. In 1991, V.E.R.E.X. was set up and in 1994. Protocol or the rolling text to the Convention was drafted. Again in 2002, a long draft Protocol was carved out. These steps show how the Convention has been moving to keep trends with the scientific developments[14].

The two hurdles in selecting the similar mechanism would be the existence of two differences between the biological and the chemical weapons and the agents. In case of the biological weapons, number and range of possible biological agents is wider as well as the reproduction of the biological weapons varies considerably from the chemical weapons.

The Biological Weapon Convention, 1972 also mentions in its preamble that state that party to this convention should work towards general and complete disarmament of weapons of mass destruction including chemical and biological weapons. This Convention also prohibits production, stockpiling and development of biological weapons for the sake of mankind and complete or partial destruction of human race. This Convention also prohibits development and production of weapons and equipment which can deliver or transfer the biological weapons. This Convention in Article 1 does allow development and research biological agents for the peaceful purposes but as the biological weapon research can serve dual purpose states have to take individual responsibility on ethical and legal grounds.

Apart from the primary Conventions and the Protocols, other relevant prohibitions also exist under the Draft Convention of the International Law Association for the Protection of Civilian Populations against New Engines of War, 1938.[15] Mendoza Declaration on Chemical and Biological Weapons, 1991 also emphasize on regulating the biological weapons. Brussels Treaty, 1948 read with its three Protocols prohibit the use of the biological weapons. The various countries in their respective Military

---

[14] Jenni Rissanen, The Biological Weapons Convention, (May 23, 2020, 06:15 PM), https://www.nti.org/analysis/articles/biological-weapons-convention
[15] Articles 6 and 9.

Manuals do mention restrictions on this aspect. Few states which mention prohibition of biological weapon in their military manuals are Australia, Burundi, Belgium, Bosnia and Herzegovina, Canada, France, Columbia, Chad, Germany, Italy, Kenya, Netherlands, USA etc. Almost half of the world prohibits use of biological weapon as part of their National Legal System under military manuals and at the same time many others prohibits use of biological weapons due to ratification to International Conventions, customary international law and customary international humanitarian law.

International Humanitarian Law and Biological Weapon

Any weapon can be used illegally and against the principle of just war. No one will deny a knife to a soldier but if the knife is used by him to kill civilians and I.C.R.C. Staff, then he is violating laws of war. All legal weapons can be used illegally for some purposes which are prohibited by different conventions and principles of just war. The understanding is a little different in case of a biological weapon as this is never treated as a legal weapon to be used during combat. The war brings with it two very important questions, first being that which all weapons can be used legally and second question is that if the first question is answered in the affirmative, whether the proposed use of this weapon is legal.

According to principle of just war, any combatant activity should take care of three important principles which are military necessity, proportionality and distinction. Biological weapons fail to justify and fulfill all the above three conditions of just war and all of these are discussed in detail below.

Biological Weapons and Military Necessity

This principle of just war puts obligation on all the combatants to do things which are a military necessity and gives certain military advantage. Biological weapons cannot be used for immediate retaliation as the after effects of biological weapons take at least a week's time or so and hence calling them military necessity will not be correct.

Biological Weapons and Principle of Distinction

The just war principle and principle of Geneva Conventions explain that during war, killing is allowed but one cannot kill everyone and also means and methods of such killing is also limited. Just war principle puts liability on combatant not to use any means and methods of warfare which have indiscriminate effect. If combatant uses indiscriminate use of any means and methods of warfare, he will be liable for individual criminal responsibility as per Rule 102 of Customary International Humanitarian Law.[16] If such indiscriminate attack was directed by commanders and military superiors these commanders will be held responsible for command responsibility defined under Rule 153 of Customary International Humanitarian Law[17]. Biological weapons by its nature do not discriminate between civilian, prisoners of war, old aged, women, medical staff, humanitarian assistance personals etc. and hence violate the principle of just war. Biological weapons can cause harm to a very wide area and may reach to one state from other state which might not even be participating in war and can also be dangerous for the country which is developing and using it in war. International Humanitarian Law does not allow weapons which cause indiscriminate harm and hence biological weapons fails to fulfill this criterion of just war and should not be used during war.

Biological Weapons and Principle of Proportionality

The Principle of Proportionality of attack is mentioned under Article 51(5)(b) of AP- I of Geneva Convention and also under Rule 16 of Customary International Humanitarian Law. This principle prohibits excessive use of force which is required to meet the military advantage anticipated. This principle says that if excessive force will be used it will definitely cause harm to civilian life, civilian property and objects and this is not the motive of any attack or war and gives no military advantage and hence not a military necessity. But, in case of biological weapons, the attack is indiscriminate and the affect is to a very large area and does not fulfill the requirement of principle of proportionality. The harm caused by biological weapon is always higher than the military advantage anticipated and hence these weapons should never be allowed during war because they breach the Customary International Humanitarian Law. This is the reason because

---

[16] ICRC, Rule 102 Individual Criminal Responsibility (May 23, 2020, 10:15 PM), https://ihl-databases.icrc.org/customary-ihl/eng/docs/v1_rul_rule102

[17] ICRC, Rule 153 Command Responsibility for Failure to Prevent, Repress or Report War Crimes (May 23, 2020, 10:25 PM), https://ihl-databases.icrc.org/customary-ihl/eng/docs/v1_rul_rule153

of which Rule 73 of Customary International Humanitarian Law prohibits use of biological weapon during armed conflict.[18]

Biological Weapons in Hands of Non-state Actors and Terrorists

One of the biggest concerns pertaining to biological weapons is that if these fall in hands of non-state actors and terrorists the world peace, security and life will be at danger. Also, there are suicide bombers and attackers who may plan these biological agents attack and can impact a large part of the society. Any country which is part of many treaties and convections cannot use biological weapons freely during war whereas non-state actors, if they do not have status of belligerents or insurgents cannot be bound by such laws of just war. The non-state actors can use these weapons for any purpose and one may never know what the reason behind it was. Terrorists also can make the peace and security worse by using biological weapon against any state and it can result in collapsing of the economy, health system and transport system of that country. The biological weapons hence not just create a fear among two hostile states but poses fear for humanity itself.

CONCLUSION

The life-sciences like any area of knowledge have benevolent and malevolent dimensions. The human history has impregnated how the knowledge of science and technology has been often used to destroy human lives and cause fatal incidents. With time, the society has shifted from the use of conventional means of warfare to chemical weapons to bio-weapons. The stage of up-gradation of the technological knowledge has resulted in more advanced weapons of destruction. During the historical times, examples of use of different kinds of weapons are found. The modern biological warfare emerged only after 1900s. The biological warfare possesses a peculiar character. They are arduous to detect; pounding effect over an extensive area; and elasticity in their use. Even a meager use of the biological agent may have a far-reaching impact. The International Humanitarian Law under the principle of Just War on the presence of military necessity, principle of necessity and principle of

---

[18] ICRC, Rule 73 The use of Biological Weapons is Prohibited, (May 23, 2020, 10:35 PM), https://ihl-databases.icrc.org/customary-ihl/eng/docs/v1_rul_rule73

distinction grants the use of weapons. Catena of provisions under international Conventions and Protocols continue to monitor the use of various kinds of weapons.

The modern life-sciences possess centripetal character, requiring the know-how of the experts from varied disciplines. The nature of these weapons makes it challenging to avert and thwart their occurrence. The impact of the biological weapons is shooting beyond anticipation. On the one hand, dialogues and reviews have allowed the regulation of the state of the art in the life-sciences. On the other, it is extremely onerous for the legal regulations to catch up with the rise of the life and other sciences.

SUGGESTIONS

- There is an eminent need to anticipate the development of new weapons from biological sources due to the interaction of various scientific fields. The integrated approach must encompass an all-embracing strategy against the contentious and abuse of the biological weapons.
- There is a need of few amendments in almost fifty years old B.W.C. for the on-going expansion of the biotechnology. The Verification Regime as existing under the Chemical Weapons Convention may be adopted under the B.W.C.[19]
- It is must to have strong decisions at both the International and National levels to regulate the exploitative and Anti-Humanitarian use of the biological weapons. The National Governments, scientists and the academicians must realise their responsibilities to ensure security against the biological threats.
- These roles have to be played by the biomedical science, national security along with the public health officials.
- In addition to the international regulation under the aegis of the U.N.; I.C.R.C. etc., self-governance prescribing the social and moral responsibilities of the life-scientists is utmost vital. The measures for conduct of the scientists with the regard to the life-sciences need to be laid down in a comprehensive form and accordingly be adhered to by everyone engaged in the research in life-sciences and allied fields.

---

[19] Christine Kirk, Bioterrorism and the Food Drug Administration, (May 24, 2020, 06:45 AM), https://dash.harvard.edu/bitstream/handle/1/8852149/kirk_bibliography.pdf?sequence=2

- Coordination and a chain of proper communication must come into play between the bio-scientists and the experts engaged in the security functions of the country.
- As the nature of the concern at hand is global, substantial cooperation is required evolve amongst all the countries of the world.
- There is a need of more active involvement of the international agencies involved in health and security in order to deal with aftermath of the biological disaster.
- There is a need to start a system of transparency and reporting pertaining to any on-going research in the life-sciences having the capacity to cause mass destruction. Such reporting must be made to the United Nations and its respective subsidiary organizations.
- Lastly, if any country is found guilty of initiating the biological weapons, the policy of boycott of such country for trade and other activities by the rest of the world needs to be implemented. Unless, such a fear is created, the countries would continue to in anti-humanity researches.

The Global scientific growth must continue while ensuring safety and security. The key to the same is the '5Rs' - Readiness (for prospective weapons), Restrain (against array of biological threats), Recognition (of proliferation of the progress in the life-sciences), Reduction (of the unethical use of the science and technological developments) and timely response (to any threats as a result of life-science). There are high hopes that the scientific community around the Globe would join hands to combat the uncertain and deceitful biological agents and weapons.

Implications of COVID-19 on the Corporate Realm with Reference to Mergers and Acquisitions

Ms. Swati Kaushal* and Ms. Shruti Gupta**

The outbreak of novel coronavirus in more than 100 countries is having a sway on the fiscal market, trade, operation of the business and most importantly social congregations everywhere in the world. One such market stimulated is merger and acquisition (hereinafter referred as M&A); in the beginning of this year it was predicted that this will be the paramount year of market of M&A[1] and ironically it turned out to be sloppier. M&A is one of the finest ways of expanding a business. The process of M&A can be said to be like the concept of marriage but here the difference is the two entities that come together are there for their individual definite purposes and are circumscribed by clauses of their agreement. In this façade of worldwide lockdown, the entities want to have an option to opt out from the deals and that's where Force Majeure clause comes into picture.

It is way too soon to predict the effect of COVID-19 on M&A in the period after COVID-19, but one thing which is very clear is that it is causing a breakthrough which is shaking up the deals which were in process before this period of lockdown. This research paper revolves around the sudden effect of the outbreak of COVID-19 in the market. The use of Force Majeure clause to get a way out of the deals which were pending or to get free from the contractual obligations. The process of Due diligence should be conducted with more precautions and read-

*Assistant Professor, Amity Law School, NOIDA, AUUP.
**Student, Amity Law School, NOIDA, AUUP.

[1] Russell Thomson, Susan Dettmar & Mark Garay, The state of the deal: M&A trends 2020, DELOITTE (June 5, 2020) https://www2.deloitte.com/us/en/pages/mergers-and-acquisitions/articles/m-a-trends-report.html.

through the analysis of financial position of the entity should be done very briefly. The Post-COVID-19 situation of the M&A market and the measures to be taken thereof.

RAMIFICATIONS OF COVID-19 PANDEMIC-A CORPORATE STORY

COVID-19 commonly known as Corona Virus is wide spread across the nations like USA, China, Japan, Australia, India and many more. The wide spread of this virus has caused a disruption in the working of economies in broad-spectrum. Now to circumvent dissemination of the virus, huge civic meetings/crowd are avoided and individuals are asked to lessen contact with others to the minimum. In China, to monitor COVID-19, citizens are asked to go out once in two days to do basic chores, all the production units or factories are shut down, students are given home education and all the public gathering are avoided.

"The outbreak is continuing to affect travel and events and in some instances, it's caused some Government offices to shut down".[2] The occurrence of the novel coronavirus has hindered the normal course of action in due diligence and it has also caused delay in closing of the deals which normally takes up maximum of 6 months' time. Because of the COVID-19 and unsolicited delay in due diligence it will eventually cause an impact on the value of the transaction.

Due to COVID-19, the operations of companies are shut down which means no or less production, this will impact the profitability of an organisation and moreover the turnover ratio. This will reduce the net value of the assets of the company, eventually reducing the valuation of the establishment or reducing the share value of the company in the concerned markets. On 11th March 2020, WHO has declared COVID-19 as pandemic which is not at all advantageous for the market.

---

[2] Mary Kathleen Flynn, Viral impact: How the coronavirus is affecting M&A and private equity, ARIZENT (June 11, 2020) https://www.themiddlemarket.com/news/viral-impact-how-covid-19-is-affecting-m-a-and-private-equity.

In an interview Coca-Cola Co. (NYSE: KO) CEO James Quincey said, "The outbreak of severe acute respiratory syndrome (SARS) in 2003 and 2004 was less of a concern than the current virus."[3]

The outbreak of the Coronavirus has impacted the demand and supply chain and caused huge losses to every other business of essential commodities during this pandemic. The instant change in demand and supply has made entities suffer a huge loss which has also rendered employees jobless. After the lockdown we can expect a 'U' shape recovery in demand and supply curve.

CAN COVID-19 BE CONSTRUED AS A *FORCE MAJEURE* EVENT?

Force majeure is a French word that in its literal sagacity means "greater force". 'The term force majeure was subsequently added in the common law realm in the 1900s and was borrowed from the Napoleonic Code[4], even though its origin can be outlined back to Roman law. The Black's Law Dictionary[5] defines *force-majeure* clause *"…as an event or effect that can be neither anticipated nor controlled. The term is commonly understood to encompass both acts of nature, such as floods and hurricanes, and acts of man, such as riots, strikes, and wars…"*[6] Further it defines force majeure clauses as "contractual provisions that address circumstances in which contractual performance becomes impossible or impracticable due to events that could not have been foreseen, and are not within a party's control". *"…It is important to note force majeure clauses do not generally provide for termination of an agreement; rather, they generally suspend a party's obligation to perform under the agreement for the duration of the force majeure event…"*[7] Ordinarily, this term in customarily used in English, with respect to its

---

[3] Amelia Lucas, Coca-Cola CEO says economic impact of coronavirus lockdowns is 'just starting to begin', CNBC (June 4, 2020) https://www.cnbc.com/2020/05/20/coca-cola-ceo-says-economic-impact-of-coronavirus-is-just-starting.html

[4] Refer, Lebeaupin v. Richard Crispin & Co [1920] 2KB 714.

[5] Bryan A. Garner, Black's Law Dictionary 657 (11th ed. Thomson Reuters 2019).

[6] Michael E. Kohagen, *The effects of COVID-19 on our interpersonal and business relationships grow each day*, Ward and Smith P.A. (May 28, 2020) https://www.wardandsmith.com/articles/covid-19-and-force-majeure-what-businesses-should-know.

[7] *Supra 6.*

roots from French understanding and it is also used in other aspects, including one that has roots in a principle of French law as "a contractual clause that is included in contracts to get away from the liability for natural and unavoidable catastrophes that interrupt the expected course of events and restrict participants of the contract from fulfilling obligations towards each other. This contractual clause confiscates liability for catastrophic events, such as natural disasters and warfare. Force Majeure also encompasses human actions, however, such as armed conflict. General discourse for events to constitute force majeure, they must be unforeseenable, external to the parties of the contract, and unavoidable". The requirements for an event to be considered as Force-Majeure are:

(a) It should proceed from a cause not caused by the defaulting party's default.[8]

(b) The cause should be inevitable and unpredictable.

(c) The cause should create execution of the contract completely not possible.

"…In the case of Halliburton Offshore Services Inc. v. Vedanta Limited and Ors. The High Court of Delhi allowed Force Majeure clause as, this pandemic is beyond the reasonable control of the Contractor and has a material adverse effect on the performance of Contractor's obligations under the Agreement. Hence, this event classifies as 'Force Majeure' and Contractor hereby serves the notice of Force Majeure pursuant to Section 15 of the Agreement and should be entitled for compensation and milestone adjustment under the provisions of the Agreement.…."[9]

Now, as we understand the essential conditions to constitute Force Majeure clause, usually it is interpreted very narrowly. There is very low probability that the contracts (of M&A) which were incorporated before this pandemic to have such clauses and to get out from the contract is more risky.

In Force Majeure clause, the substance is that due to incalculability of certain events like COVID-19, an element of uncertainty always exists and it can never be jettisoned under any given circumstances. Therefore, either party to the agreement can be held liable. It is considered more reasonable to extend or suspend the performance for a period of time.

---

[8] Refer, Dhanrajamal Gobindram v. Shamji Kalidas & Co MANU/SC/0362/1961.

[9] MANU/DE/0957/2020 para 22.

The Apex court in the judgment of *Energy Watchdog and Ors. v. Central Electricity Regulatory Commission and Ors.* (11.04.2017 – SC) categorically held that when alternatives modes of performance are available they cannot be force majeure[10].

Force Majeure & Vis Major

Vis Major simply means an act of god, in India vis. major is considered under law of contracts and law of torts. "…An act of God is a natural hazard outside human control, such as an earthquake or tsunami, for which no person can be held responsible. An Act of God may amount to an exception to liability in contracts or it may be an insured peril in an insurance policy…"[11]

"An event that directly associated solely from results of the incidence of natural causes that might not are prevented by the exercise of foresight or caution; a geological phenomenon.

Courts have recognized numerous events as acts of God—tornadoes, earthquakes, death, terribly high tides, violent winds, and floods, several insurance policies for property injury exclude from their protection injury caused by acts of God".

Acts of God provisions, conjointly known as "Force Majeure" clauses, relate to events outside human management, like flash floods, earthquakes, or alternative natural disasters. In general, these provisions eliminate or limit the liability for injuries or alternative losses ensuing from such events. The performance of a contract, the promise to perform is commonly discharged owing to the unforeseen circumstance and therefore the ensuing delay, expense, or alternative factors leading to what would otherwise quantity to a breach.

In the case of Dhanrajamal Gobindram v. Shamji Kalidas & Co[12] and Energy Watchdog and Ors. v. Central Electricity Regulatory Commission and Ors[13] the Supreme Court of India clearly differentiated between Force Majeure & vis major, it was held that "……. whilst also saving the non-

---

[10] MANU/SC/0408/2017.
[11] *Supra* 10.
[12] MANU/SC/0362/1961.
[13] MANU/SC/0408/2017 para 41.

performing party from the consequences of something over which it has no control".

The case of *The State Cooperative Election v. Ishwar Madhav Patange and Ors.*[14] has indirectly considered COVID-19 as a vis major (Act of God) event. In light of this judgment, it can be concluded that even the term "Act of God" in the Force Majeure clause can entitle the parties for relief.

The problem that arises here is that, in M&A agreements before COVID-19 struck such clauses were not incorporated but now after witnessing COVID-19 these clauses have been incorporated to deal with such situations in the future with a proper plan. Another point to be noted is that the contract is negotiated between the parties before signing and there are specified clauses which specify what all events will constitute an act of god and it also considered while determining the liability under any such clause. If any of party approaches the court, the court first looks into elucidation of phrases of the contract rather than focusing on law.

In broad-spectrum, force majeure and act of god is in strain with principle of *'Pacta Sunt Servanda'*. This is a well-established principle in international and contract law. It is believed that it should not be easy to escape the contractual liability because then there will be no accountability and fear of law. Now it is the duty of courts to determine what is foreseeable and what is unforeseeable so that liability can be determined.

Retaining the Pacta Sunt Servanda

Firstly, let's understand the concept of *Pacta Sunt Servanda*. "The pacta sunt servanda rule embodies an elementary and universally agreed principle fundamental to all legal systems (General Principles of Law). Although its good faith (bona fide) element runs through many aspects of International Law and the legal effect of certain unilateral statements rests on good faith—it is of prime importance for the stability of treaty relations (treaties)".[15] The often quoted Latin phrase means "no more than that agreement which are legally binding must be performed".[16] The 3rd line of

---

[14] Civil Application (St) No. 10472 of 2020 in Writ Petition No. 2924 of 2020.

[15] Anthony Aust, Pacta Sunt Servanda, Oxford Public International Law (May 12, 2020). https://opil.ouplaw.com/view/10.1093/law:epil/9780199231690/law-9780199231690-e1449

[16] *Supra* 11.

preamble to the Vienna Convention on the Law of Treaties clearly establishes the foundation of the abovementioned statement. This principle is believed to keep the sanity of the contracts. The concept of *rebus sic stantibus* stipulates that, *"...where there has been a fundamental change of circumstances, a party may withdraw from or terminate the treaty in question. An obvious case in point would be one in which a related island has become inundated. A fundamental change of circumstances, however, is not sufficient for termination or withdrawal unless the existence of the original circumstances was an essential basis of the consent of the parties to be bound by the treaty and the change radically transforms the extent of obligations still to be performed. In the present scenario, COVID-19 has changed the original statuses in few cases and therefore the principle if invoked can also be taken care of..."*[17]

From the above discussion, it can be understood that the parties in case of an international contact are accountable to the performance of the contract until and unless there is change of circumstances, which is a very rare case. Usually, in such agreement the parties to contract do have their own reservations, reservations here refer to certain circumstances, and if they occur the party is not bound to the performance of the contract. "The only limit we can say is to *pacta sunt servanda* is the peremptory norms of general international law known as jus cogens which means compelling law."

Juxtaposition of Material Adverse Effect Clause (MAE) and *Force Majeure* Clause

Material Adverse Effect is understood as an effect which is extremely high threshold. The definition of MAE is carved on the basis of type of arrangement, transaction and other aspects related to it. The exceptions to it are also dependent upon the interpretation of the definition of MAE as per the agreement. Normally, in a merger this clause is used to qualify the demonstrations and guarantees. The time between the finalization and signing of agreement of combination is very crucial and delegate. One can easily back out of the deal before signing of the agreement and without any repercussions.

---

[17] https://treaties.un.org/doc/Publication/UNTS/Volume%201155/volume-1155-I-18232-English.pdf

The clause of MAE comes into picture where, for example, a company A has promised to carry out an activity for company B, due to some reasons it is not able to do so, so this turns out to be MAE. Very often MAE and material adverse change are used interchangeably. *"…The important consideration while deciding about material adverse effect is that whether there is change in target's business that is consequential to the company's long-term earnings power over a commercially reasonable period, which one would expect to be measured in years rather than months…"*[18]

According to the data, the market witnessed a steep drop and many companies have paused their M&A deals. The Global M&A market has already witnessed its slowest first two months of a year. It has happened for the first time since 2005. To beat 2019 as the fourth strongest year for M&A on record, some dealmakers had been looking to 2020. It may take months or even years to recover from the effect of the virus, there's no certainty and the sway is swelling every single day.

If any claim arises on MAE, the very first consideration by court is to look into the interpretation of the terms of agreement and especially the MAE clause. The applicability of MAE will depend upon the inclusion of pandemic or any epidemic in the clause and the craving out of the terms of clause will be taken into consideration before anything. Also, if there is no such provision then it is next to impossible to incorporate material adverse effect clause. Also, if there is no such provision then it is next to impossible to incorporate material adverse effect clause. For example, "the February 20th 2020 Agreement and Plan of Merger between Morgan Stanley and E-trade Financial Corp. specifically carves out "epidemic, pandemic or disease outbreak (including the COVID-19 virus)" from events that could result in an MAE. Additionally, an impact that is this widespread across companies and industries will often be caught by a carve-out for changes in general market conditions". If there is no carve-out and it is a generic MAE clause, courts will then consider whether the buyer has shown the requisite substantial threat to the earnings potential of the target in a durational significant manner.

---

[18] Pavan Burugula & Maulik Vyas, M&A deals in India get delayed, called off, as virus spreads. Economics Times India (April 15, 2020) https://m.economictimes.com/markets/stocks/news/ma-deals-in-india-get-delayed-called-off-as-virus-spreads/articleshow/74546118.cms

The modification between Force Majeure clause and Material Adverse Effect clause, the major difference is that Force Majeure clause is incorporated when the event is unforeseeable or not predictable and the latter is incorporate on ability of non-performance of the Act. Also, it should be noted that force majeure is very narrowly interpreted in courts and is very rarely incorporated clause until now. Whereas, the Material Adverse Effect clause is interpreted on basis on craving out of the terms of agreement of the arrangement.

CONCLUSION

Due to COVID-19, it can be understood that there is an unprecedented effect on the market which was not anticipatable and naturally because of that there are many entities who have suffered massive losses. The confederation of clauses like MAE and viz. major should be incorporated in a contract so that both the parties are able to keep faith in each other and can commit for a long period of time.

The authors make following recommendations for the upcoming M&A:

1. The process of due diligence should be conducted with utmost care and surety.
2. The financial position of every entity is effected and it should be taken into consideration as well.
3. The M&A which were in process during the COVID-19 should undergo another round of due diligence to understand the COVID-19 effect on that organisation.

As stated above the contractual clauses which can be incorporated in the agreements while signing the M&A agreement, one should consider the interpretation of the clause before incorporation because the courts while deciding whether the clause can be invoked, look upon the interpretation of the clauses. The Courts in India usually give a very narrow interpretation for Force Majeure clause.

COVID-19 Pandemic: A Period of Global Crisis and Challenges

Ms. Ananya Kukreti*

ABSTRACT: *The outbreak of Novel Corona Virus or Covid-19 shook the entire world. It was first reported in Wuhan, a city in China but within few months it had spread all over the globe. Covid-19 has led to so many deaths and millions of people are infected. To control the spread of this virus Government has issued Nationwide lockdowns and advised their citizens to follow strict social distancing norms so that the spread of this virus can be controlled. According to World Health Organization (WHO), this virus is an animal based virus and declared this period as a Pandemic. Many countries have asked for an International level inquiry about the origin of this virus as they consider it as a laboratory made virus.*

This paper focuses on the origin of Covid-19, background, its effects that include deaths, economic crisis, etc. and the efforts taken by the world researchers, scientist and doctors all over the world to come up with a cure or a potential vaccine for it. The paper has stressed upon the crisis faced by the people because of Covid-19 and the various steps taken by the Governments, especially the Indian Government to tackle this situation. The Indian Government, to help its citizens, is issuing many new advisories and regulations and certain relaxation in payment of income tax payment and other payments are being issued. In order to follow the social distancing norms, courts are using virtual medium to discharge undisturbed, timely justice. Many offices are practicing work from home so that their tasks are performed and social distancing norms are followed. Covid-19 and the lockdown because of it has disturbed the livelihood of many people especially laborers and respective governments are coming up with norms to help them like, the Indian Government has ad vised all employers to pay their employees full wages without deduction for the period of lockdown according to the advisories issued.

The world wasn't prepared for such a devastating virus and hence faced the crisis. There is a need to come up with a global solution and certain strict

---

* Student, Amity Law School, Noida, AUUP.

regulations should be made to control the laboratory activities or trial taking place that deal with even more deadly virus, bacteria etc.

INTRODUCTION

The Covid-19 outbreak that was first reported in Wuhan, a city in China has now affected the entire world, resulting in lockdowns and social distancing to control the spread of this virus. World Health Organization (WHO), an International Organization has declared COVID-19 as a pandemic. This virus has brutally disturbed the normal life of the people all around the world. People have lost their jobs and economic condition of the entire world is affected. Thousands of individuals have lost their lives and millions are infected. People are following social distancing norms and there is lockdown throughout the world because of the severity of the virus and there is no medical cure or potential vaccine for it. Covid-19 brought a great disturbance in the life and business of people all around the world. Many well established firms are facing economic crisis. The Governments are shutting factories so that the people are maintaining proper social distancing because of these government norms many people especially laborers are facing major financial crisis, as the companies are not functional. Due to lockdowns people cannot travel to their respective homes due to flight, train, etc. services are shutdown.

This virus has infected millions of people and thousands are dead. Many assumptions are made regarding the origin of the virus, World Health Organization's (WHO) spokesperson stated that this Covid-19 virus is an animal based virus and it's not being constructed in laboratories but people are not satisfied and questions are being raised on the origin of the virus.[1]

US President Donald Trump has announced that his Government will investigate about the origin of the virus and has even stated that China will face serious consequences, if it found that it is intentionally responsible for Covid-19 pandemic. Countries are suspecting that this virus is made in the laboratory in China because of many reasons and have demanded an

[1] Article published in The Week https://www.theweek.in/news/india/2020/05/14/was-covid-19-made-in-a-lab-as-nitin-gadkari-sparks-fresh-debate-what-we-know-so-far.html

inquiry. Wuhan Institute of Virology National Biosafety Laboratory, which is four levels certified laboratory and is capable of conducting research activities' involving Ebola and other deadly viruses, is located only 32 km away from the considered epicenter of the virus.

In a research conducted scientist have identified relation of this virus with a previous bat virus SARS-CoV-2 and have considered that virus can most likely be the natural host. While other researchers consider it as a manmade virus. Some have proposed that insertion S1/S2 is unusual and have indicated it as a laboratory made virus.

STEPS TAKEN BY THE INDIAN GOVERNMENT

The devastating effect of this virus has even been seen in the developed countries like United States of America, Germany, Italy, etc. that have the best medical facilities in the world. The Indian Government, learning from the severity of the virus in Italy and Spain was bound to put entire lockdown in the country from 24.03.2020, to prevent the disease from spreading.[2] As a result of the lockdown, all public transports are shut and no public gatherings are allowed. The Nationwide lockdown was announced in pursuance of directions issued by the National Disaster Management Authority under the Disaster Management Act 2005.[3] The Home Ministry, Central and State Governments among other important authority had made sure that these regulations are properly followed throughout. According to Sections 2, 3 and 4 of the Epidemic Diseases Act, 1897, the government has the power to take certain measures, prescribe relief and pass regulations with respect to that epidemic disease so as to prevent its outbreak or limit the spread in the country.

The term "lockdown" basically means that the people have to stay inside their respective houses but, they can go out just to buy essentials commodities, and the people who are frontline workers during this pandemic like healthcare workers etc. are allowed to go out or one can avail such essential services. Incase if someone disobeys the regulations passed under Epidemic Disease Act, then that individual will be deemed

[2] Order dated March 24, 2020 vide No. 403/20202-DM-I(A) passed by the Ministry of Home Affairs, Government of India.

[3] Order date 24.03.2020 link : https://mha.gov.in/sites/default/files/ndma%20order%20copy.pdf

to have committed an offence under Section 188 of IPC and if someone does any negligent act that can lead to the spread of the virus or he/she willful does certain act to spread the disease are punishable under Section 268 and Section 270 of Indian Penal Code (IPC) respectively.

Due to the lockdown, the demand for the products has decreased drastically resulting in fall in the global market for crude oil, metals, fertilizers as well as trade. The lack of demand and foreign trade has reduced the investment by the foreign companies in India resulting in the fall in the economy of the country. United Nations has reported that the trade loss to India due to this outbreak is estimated to more than 350 million US Dollars. When the Government of India presented the Finance Bill for the year 2020–2021 it estimated India's GDP (Gross Domestic Product) growth rate as 10% but, according to the economist this rate is far from the reality. According to the statement by Chief Economist at Goldman Sachs as on 9th April 2020, the estimated economic growth of India is as less as 1.6%.[4]

Covid-19 has greatly affected all the industries, markets are closed, flights are shut down, hotels are vacant, factories are closed resulting in no production and hence these sectors have no choice except to cut the wages of the workers. This lockdown has stressed a lot on supply of essential products, looking into the present scenario, the production of other items are put to a halt and the production of essential commodities has been increased but due to stopping production of other items and decreasing the manpower it has resulted in bringing down the overall production graph. Due to this lockdown restriction, the commercial activities have slowed down which has impacted the domestic growth, it is the hardest time for the world economy. As per the report of International Labor Organization, 40 crore workers just from the unorganized firms have lost their jobs. In India, according to Centre for Monitoring Indian Economy (CMIE) estimation on 7th April 2020, the unemployment rate has increased to 23% of which 31% is the urban unemployment.[5]

---

[4] Article published in Economic Times https://economictimes.indiatimes.com/markets/ expert-view/goldman-sachs-revised-global-growth-forecast-for-2020-to-2-and-that-of-us-to-6-prachi-mishra/articleshow/75065449.cms

[5] Article published in Mondaq link: https://www.mondaq.com/india/operational-impacts-and-strategy/936014/coronavirus-covid-19-and-indian-economy

In order to cope up with and minimize the effect of Corona Virus The Union Finance and Corporate Affairs Minister, announced certain relief measures on 24th March 2020. It stated much needed, important and crucial relief measures in areas of Taxes, Corporate Affairs, Banking sector and Commerce, Insolvency and Bankruptcy Code, etc. to boost the economy. Even Reserve Bank of India (RBI) on 9.04.2020 came up with its Monetary Policy Report where it published different aspects of economy, especially the effect of Covid-19 on Global Growth.

Many foreign officials that are working in India have left for their native countries looking at this pandemic situation. All the visas for India stand suspended till 15th April 2020 expect the visas of diplomats, UN or International Organizations, employment and other visas. In case where a foreign national is already there in the country then in that case his visa can be extended for which they have to contact to the Foreign Regional Registration Office.

Work from home process is being adopted by most of the countries all around the world. Ministry of Home Affairs came up with the guidelines on 24.03.2020 that all the establishments where possible should allow their employees to work from their respective homes and pay them full remuneration for their work and establishments that are being closed because Covid-19, the employees of such establishments will be deemed to be on their duty. Even the employers of the commercial units or shops during the lockdown period have to pay full wages to their workers, on due date. The Ministry of Labor and Employment issued an advisory on 30.03.2020 that the employer has to pay full salary without deduction to the employees this includes the contract and casual workers as well.[6] The owners are advised not to deduct the salary of the worker, if he avails the quarantine leave and the employees cannot be forced to utilize their annual leaves if employee is in self-isolation.[7] In this time of hardship and economic crisis all around the world, employers are advised to pay full wages to the laborers during the period of lockdown. Even the State Governments have issued orders were employers are asked not to deduct the wages of their employees. In Kanpur, a circular was issued on 25.03.2020 that directed all the Trade Unions of Uttar Pradesh to pay their workers and further report about it accordingly, if someone is not able

---

[6] https://labour.gov.in/sites/default/files/file%201.pdf
[7] https://pib.gov.in/PressReleasePage.aspx?PRID=1607911

to pay the wages he should go through the advisories issued by the Government.

The Government has granted multiple relaxations on account of Covid-19. The Employees Provident Fund Organization issued a notice on 1st April 2020, that stated for introduction of a package under Pradhan Mantri Garib Yojna, according to which the Government will be paying 24 percent wages in the worker's Employees Provident Fund (EPF) account if the establishment has less than 100 employs and 90% of whom have wages less than Rupees 15,000 per month, there are certain conditions that are implied to it.

Employees Provident Fund Scheme, 1952 has also been amended by the Ministry of Labor and Employment. According to the amended scheme, the commissioner may on a written request or application from any member of an establishment that is located in affected zone of the outbreak (here Covid-19 pandemic) can permit non-refundable advance from Employment Provident Fund that cannot be more than 3 month's basic wage or maximum seventy five percent of the total amount standing to his credit in the fund.

The Ministry is issuing advisories for the unorganized construction workers and has advised the State Governments to transfer the fund in the account of the construction workers from funds collected by Labor Welfare Boards. Skill development and Entrepreneurship Ministry, on 30th March 2020, made it mandatory for the establishments to give full stipend amount to the apprentices during this period of lock down.[8]

The last date of filing of Unified Online Annual Returns of last year (2019) has been extended up to 30th April 2020. This has been extended under the eight Labor Acts. The Jurisdictional Authority is advised not take any legal action in this regard. The Acts that are mentioned under the unified annual return filing include:

1. Payment of Wages Act, 1936
2. Minimum Wages Act, 1948
3. Contract Labor (Regulation and Abolition) Act, 1970
4. Maternity Benefit Act, 1961
5. Building and Other Construction Workers Act, 1996

---

[8] Press release link: https://pib.gov.in/PressReleasePage.aspx?PRID=1607911

6. Payment of Bonus Act, 1965
7. Inter-State Migrant Workmen Act, 1979
8. Industrial Dispute Act, 1947

Considering the demands of public for opening some important activities and for improving the economic condition of the Government, both the Central and State Governments are announcing relaxations from time to time so that more economic activities can be started during this difficult period. It is predicted that the Gross Domestic Product may further fall down, especially in India which is not immune to global recession. Hon' Prime Minister Shri Narendra Modi has already asked the Economic Task Force to make policy measures to handle and cope up effectively with this economic issue and come up certain recovery measures to support the Indian Economy.

VIRTUAL COURTS

In order deliver uninterrupted justice even during the times of a pandemic where lockdown is imposed everywhere and norms of social distancing are being followed, Supreme Court of India decided to deliver justice through online medium. The Supreme Court bench consisting of Chief Justice of India S.A. Bobde, Justices D.Y. Chandrachud and L. Nageswara Rao issued guidelines for the court functionings through video conferencing so as to maintain social distancing.[9] The Supreme Court has asked the District Courts and High Courts to follow online medium through virtual courts and e-filling method to disperse justice.

JUDICIAL PRECEDENTS OF VIRTUAL COURTS

CASE: Krishna Veni Nagam v. Harish Nagam[10]

This was the case of transfer petition under Section 13 of the Hindu Marriage Act, 1955. Here, the parties were not located in the jurisdiction of a same court. Taking in view the difficulty faced by the litigant, they were referred to participate in their matrimonial dispute case through video conferencing.

---

[9] Suo Moto Writ Petition (Civil) No. 5/2020.
[10] Transfer petition (CIVIL) No. 1912 of 2014.

The Apex Court held that it is appropriate for the court to use new and advanced video conferencing technology where both the parties are facing the same jurisdiction issue with the condition being that the parties who have requested for virtual hearing of their case have to appear in person in the video conferencing. Though the Supreme Court overruled it in the case Santhini v. Vijaya Venketesh[11] by 2:1 majority. Ex-Chief Justice of India Dipak Mishra and Justice A.K. Khanwilkar held that the courts couldn't direct video conferencing in cases of transfer petition. Though the third judge Justice Chandrachud was in favor of the previous judgment and wrote that, the Family Courts Act, 1984 was enacted when there was no such advancement in technology but now the distance can be covered by use of technology and virtual methods.

The pros and cons of virtual courts are still a matter of debate, the cons include lack of knowledge and accessibility to use online medium, cyber security threat, the quality of justice may be affected, etc. whereas the pros include speedy delivery of justice, use of less paper, etc. During the lockdown period where social distancing has to be followed, the courts have adopted online method for delivering justice.

The Chairman of Bar Council of India (BCI) wrote a letter to Chief Justice of India[12] SA Bobde addressing the issues in virtual hearing and opposing it. Though the medium of online is a positive step taken by the courts especially the Supreme Court and High Courts where most of the matters are of urgency, many advocated are not able to adapt to this method. Few lawyers belong to such areas and background that for them video-conferencing and e-filing process is quiet new and tough.

Many lawyers raised concern that in the online proceedings of the case only the judges, counsels and the party concerned can be a part of it. It was held in the case Naresh Shridhar Mirajkar & Ors vs. State of Maharashtra & others that due to virtual courts the right of Public hearing is being violated, as others cannot be a part of the video conferencing proceeding. The Supreme Court of India issued a press note stating that at this difficult period virtual court is the medium of delivering Justice and the aim of both Open court and online court is the same that is discharging justice. It further stated that "Open Court hearings cannot be claimed as a matter of

---

[11] Transfer Petition (Civil) No. 1278 of 2016.
[12] Letter BCI: D: 1372/2020 (Council) dated 28.04.2020.

absolute right and process of adjudication itself does not demand an Open Court".[13]

FORCE MAJEURE

Covid-19 has brought great destruction to life and business and has resulted to the major question of whether the parties who are in contractual relation but are not able to perform the contract have to face any contractual liability or is there any defense of "Force Majeure"[14] available? Force Majeure is an event that is not under the control of the parties or 'a supervening event over which none of the performers have any control'. This Pandemic has led to lockdowns all over the world and due to lockdowns there has been failure in performance of the contract by the parties.

The Government, in the memorandums that are issued by the Ministry of Finance and other departments has declared this Covid-19 period as a 'Force Majeure' event and has directed the departments to invoke the 'Force Majeure' clauses. Even though the government has declared this period as natural calamity and 'Force Majeure' laws have been invoked, it is valid only if a party proves that failure in performance of the contract is related to this issue or contract involved travelling etc. Though the court or the Arbitral Tribunal decides the complexity of the situation in a particular case.

CONCLUSION

Debates are being conducted all over the world about the origin of the virus, is it a natural virus, a laboratory made that is intentionally used as a bioweapon or it has accidentally escaped from the laboratory. Governments of various countries demand for an international inquiry about the origin of virus, US has even threatened China of facing serious consequences if they are knowingly responsible.[15] The world wasn't prepared for Covid-19

---

[13] Supreme Court of India, Note on open court hearings, 2 May 2020, retrieved fromhttps://images.assettype.com/barandbench/2020-05/06c7b93c-c27a-4702-9b16-5a47841aa88f/Note_on_Open_Court_Hearing.pdf

[14] Derived from a French phrase meaning 'superior force'.

[15] Article in The Week Week https://www.theweek.in/news/india/2020/05/14/was-covid-19-made-in-a-lab-as-nitin-gadkari-sparks-fresh-debate-what-we-know-so-far.html

that lead to the death of thousands of people, economic crisis etc. Till now there is no cure or a vaccine for this virus. Doctors, researchers and pharmaceutical companies are working 24 hours to find a solution for it. The Governments of various countries and United Nations have invested billions to come up with the cure or vaccine.

In order to control the spread of the virus Governments across the world have issued lockdowns in their respective countries and have asked to maintain social distancing. Even in this situation, the work has not stopped (except the few like manufacturing, travel etc.) as they have opted to turn to the digital medium. Employees are working from their respective homes and are following social distancing norms, work from home is a new trend that is being practiced everywhere. The courts are using the virtual medium to discharge justice through e-filling and video conferencing.

In India, the Government has come up with various regulations to help their citizens in all possible way, though due to lockdown people are facing a lot of economic crisis. The Government has advised the employers to pay full wages to their employees for this period of lockdown and have come up with certain norms to help the workers and laborers.

In order to prevent any such incident in future, certain strict regulations and precautions need to be introduced relating to the laboratory research or clinical trials all over the world as everyone will face the consequences of such researches and trials. The entire world has come to a halt and is facing crisis because of a virus. This issue need to be taken seriously and should be worked upon together in peace and harmony.

Biological Weapons and Biological Warfare

Ms. Vaani Vishal*

ABSTRACT: The on-going outbreak of the COVID-19 Virus, popularly known as the—Corona Virus, has led to various suspicions arising that this Virus which is said to have been originated after the consumption of an under-cooked bat. It is in reality a Biological Weapon that has been leaked from laboratories in China. Due to this increasing threat of terrorism, the need to evaluate the risk posed by various microorganisms as biological weapons along with their development through the course of time and the usage of such biological agents needs to be understood better as well. Biological warfare agents risk being more formidable than conventional. During the span of the past century, the progress that has been made in the biotechnology and biochemistry industries has simplified the development and production of such weapons. In addition to this the most dangerous potential is held by genetic engineering. Ease of capability to produce biological agents and the broad availability of such biological agents and the technical know-hows relating to them has further lead to a spread of biological weapons and an increase in desire to have them among developing countries. This paper aims to examine the concepts of biological warfare, biological terrorism and its evolution and development through time, it's utilization, the attempts made to control its proliferation throughout history, it's effect of humans and the ecosystem at large, the Conventions and Laws governing Biological Weapons and Warfare among other topics of concern relating to Biological Warfare and Bio-terrorism, along with a focus questions that may arise in one's mind while reading about the topic at first glance; Are biological Weapons and Chemical Weapons the same?; Do Biological Weapons only affect the biodiversity?; and Whether there has been any non-compliance to the Convention that overlooks Biological Weapons and Biological Warfare. The threat of bio-terrorism is very much real and significant in today's times; it is neither in the realm of science fiction nor is it confined to a particular nation.

---

* Student, Amity Law School, Noida AUUP.

INTRODUCTION

To understand Biological Warfare and Bio-terrorism we firstly need to understand what a Biological Weapon is. A biological weapon (bio-weapon) may be defined as a biological organism, and a substance that is directly derived from living organisms, and can be used to cause death or injury to humans, animals, or plants.[1] Diseases and biological toxins have been used as weapons of war throughout recorded history, from at least as early as Biblical times to the present day. Historically, bioweapons were used primarily, although not exclusively, for direct attacks against human populations. Biological warfare has historically involved the use of plant and fungal toxins (hellebore, ergot), animal carcasses, human cadavers, disease-contaminated clothing or blankets, and fecal matter.[2,3]

We can also say that apart from the catastrophic effects of biological warfare on the biodiversity and the environment, the danger of biological weapons lies in their low cost and rapid spread, as well as the easy preparation, transport, and use of such weapons.

Biological weapons are considered the most dangerous of all known Weapons of Mass Destruction. They are used to deliberately cause epidemics among humans; destroy the environmental components including water, air, and soil; and target crops and livestock. Some examples of diseases used in biological warfare are anthrax, smallpox, plague, cholera, avian flu, etc.

Unlike nuclear and chemical bombs, biological weapons do not have any odor or colour and therefore cannot be detected. Additionally, biological weapons are dangerous because of their effects on untargeted organisms in a military attack, and the clinical symptoms they create may be difficult to distinguish from normal diseases. Pathogens of biological weapons remain in nature for several years and are able to survive in harsh environmental conditions.[4]

[1] Christopher G.W. Cieslak T.J. Palvin J.A. Eitzen EM Jr. (1997). Biological Warfare: A historical perpective. *Journal of the American Association,* 278: 412–417.
[2] Kortepeter M. Christopher G. Cieslak T. Culpepper R. Darling R. Rowe J. McKee K. Jr. Eitzen E. Jr. (2001). *Medical Management of Biological Casualties Handbook.* 4th ed. Fort Detrick (MD): US Army Medical Research Institute of Infectious Diseases.
[3] Bioscience.oxfordjounals.org
[4] http://www.ecomena.org

When micro-organisms or toxins derived from living organisms are used intentionally to cause death or diseases in humans, animals, or plants on which we depend is known as Bio-terrorism.[5]

Bioterrorism is a growing threat and meticulous strategies and programs are being formulated globally to increase the awareness, preparedness and mitigation of these threats for tackling the problem responsibly since the use of biological weapons can inflict great trauma upon civilian population.

With the threat of bio-terrorism higher than ever, it is a well-established fact that the capability of a biological weapon to create immense panic and unimaginable fear has drawn the terrorists to despicably use biological agents for causing terror attacks. Moreover to add to the grievance, this era of biotechnology and nanotechnology has created an easy accessibility to more sophisticated biologic agents apart from the conventional bacteria, viruses and toxins. These biological weapons have the capability to cause large-scale mortality and morbidity in large population and create civil disruption in the shortest possible time.

If such weapons are used by a Nation against another Nation and by subversive groups within a nation as a maneuverer by hostility is generally referred to as Biological Warfare, and the use of these biological weapons for terrorist activities is generally referred to as Bio-terrorism.[6] Biological warfare and bio-terrorism can be used interchangeably, but usually bio-terrorism refers to acts committed by a sub-national entity, rather than a country.

The draft of Model State Emergency Health Powers Act of 2001, (MSEHPA) drafted by the which is a document designed to guide legislative bodies in the United States of America as they draft laws regarding public health emergencies, defines bioterrorism as:

The Intentional use of any microorganism, virus, infectious substance, or biological product that may be engineered as a result of biotechnology, or any naturally occurring or bioengineered component of any such microorganism, virus, infectious substance, or biological product, to cause death, disease, or other biological malfunction in a human, an animal, a

---

[5] *Ashford, D.A., Kaiser, R.M., Bales, M.E., Shutt, K., Patrawalla, A., McShan, A., Tappero, J.W., Perkins, B.A., Dannenberg, A.L. Emerg Infect Dis. 2003 May; 9(5):515-9.*
[6] https://link.springer.com

plant, or another living organism in order to influence the conduct of government or to intimidate or coerce a civilian population.

Biological Defense against Biological Warfare or Bio-terrorism can be described as the use of medical measures to protect people against such Biological Weapons. Biological Defense includes coming up with proper antidotes such as medicines and vaccinations. Biological Defense also includes the medical research, preparations and precautions taken in order to defend the people from attacks of Biological Weapons.

HISTORY AND EVOLUTION OF BIOLOGICAL WARFARE AND BIO-TERRORISM

Infectious diseases can be recognized for their potential impact on people and armies as early as 600 BC.[7] The crude use of filth and cadavers, animal carcasses, and contagion had devastating effects and weakened the enemy.[8] Polluting of wells and other sources of water of the opposing army was considered a common strategy that continued to be used through various European wars, during the American Civil War, and even into the 20th Century.

Military leaders of the middle ages recognized that victims of infectious diseases could end up becoming weapons themselves.[9] During the siege of Caffa, a well-fortified Genoese-controlled seaport (now Feodosia, Ukraine), in 1346, the attacking Tartar force experienced an epidemic of plague.[10] The Tartars, however, converted their misfortune into an opportunity by hurling the cadavers of their deceased into the city, thus initiating a plague epidemic in the city. The Outbreak of Plague that followed forced the retreat of the Genoese forces. The plague pandemic, famously known as the Black Death, swept through Europe and North Africa in the 14th century

---

[7] Eitzen E.M., Jr, Takafuji E.T. Historical overview of biological warfare. In: Sidell F.R., Takafuji E.T., Franz D.R., editors. Medical Aspects of Chemical and Biological Warfare. Washington, DC: Office of the Surgeon General, Borden Institute, Walter Reed Army Medical Center; 1997.

[8] Eitzen E.M., Jr, Takafuji E.T. Historical overview of biological warfare. In: Sidell F.R., Takafuji E.T., Franz D.R., editors. Medical Aspects of Chemical and Biological Warfare. Washington, DC: Office of the Surgeon General, Borden Institute, Walter Reed Army Medical Center; 1997.

[9] Ibid.

[10] *Wheelis M. Emerg Infect Dis. 2002.*

and was probably the most devastating public health disaster in recorded history. Though, the ultimate origin of the plague remains uncertain: several countries in the Far East, China, Mongolia, India, and central Asia have been suggested.[11]

The Caffa incident was said to have taken place in 1348 or 1349 by Gabriel de Mussis. Gabriel de Mussis was a notary born in Piacenza north of Genoa.[12] Two important claims were made by Gabriel de Mussis firstly that, the plague was transmitted to the citizens of Caffa by the hurling of diseased cadavers into the besieged city, and second that the Italians fleeing from Caffa brought the plague into the Mediterranean seaports.[13] In fact, ships carrying plague-infected refugees (and possibly rats) sailed to Constantinople, Genoa, Venice, and other Mediterranean seaports and are thought to have contributed to the second plague pandemic. However, taking into consideration the complexity of the ecology and epidemiology of plague, it may be an oversimplification to assume that a single biological attack was the sole cause of the plague epidemic in Caffa and even during the 14th-century plague pandemic in Europe.[14] Nonetheless, we can say that the account of a biological warfare attack in Caffa is plausible and consistent with the technology of that time, and despite its historical of the diseases caused being as weapons.

During the same 14th-century plague pandemic, which killed more than 25 million Europeans in the 14th and 15th centuries, many other incidents indicate the various uses of disease and poisons during war. For example, bodies of dead soldiers were catapulted into the ranks of the enemy in Karolstein in 1422. A similar strategy using cadavers of plague victims was utilized in 1710 during the battle between Russian troops and Swedish forces in Reval.[15]

The use of biological weapons include those practiced during the middle ages when diseased carcasses and bodies were catapulted over enemy walls

---

[11] Henschel AW. Dokument für Geschichte des schwarzen Todes. Archives fur die gesammte Median, 1842.

[12] De Mussis and the great plague of 1348. A forgotten episode of bacteriological warfare. *Derbes V.J. JAMA, 196(1).*

[13] East or west? The geographic origin of the Black Death. *Norris J. Bull Hist Med. 1977 Spring.*

[14] *Ibid., 6.*

[15] *Ibid., 3.*

in attempts to induce sickness in humans or animals in Europe; during the French Wars, the British supplied Native Americans with smallpox-infected blankets.

During World War II, Japanese Unit 731 experimented with biological weapons on prisoners of war in Manchuria, resulting in more than 1000 deaths.[16]

During the Indo-Pakistan war of 1965, a scrub typhus outbreak that took place in north-eastern India came under suspicion.

In 1984, the salad bars at two restaurants in the Dalles, Oregon, were contaminated with Salmonella by followers of Shree Rajneesh. The perpetrators of this bioterrorist action were attempting to sicken citizens and prevent them from voting in an upcoming election.[17]

In 1995, after the gulf war, Iraq was found to have produced bombs, rockets, and aircraft spray tanks containing Bacillus anthracis and botulinum toxin.[18]

In the incident usually known as Japan Subway Sarin Incident, nerve gas sarin was released by perpetrators of a Religious Movement Aum Shinrikyo in the Tokyo subway system in 1995 killing 13 people, severely injuring 50 and causing temporary vision problems for nearly 1000 others.[19]

In India mysterious outbreaks of plague were observed in Surat (Gujarat) and Beed (Maharashtra) in 1994[20] and in district Shimla (Himachal Pradesh) in 2002.[21]

After the terrorist attacks on 11 September 2001, the biological attacks with powders containing B. Anthracis sent through the mail during

---

[16] Biological warfare. A historical perspective. Christopher G.W., Cieslak T.J., Pavlin J.A., Eitzen E.M. Jr. JAMA, 1997.

[17] A large community outbreak of salmonellosis caused by intentional contamination of restaurant salad bars. Török T.J., Tauxe R.V., Wise R.P., Livengood J.R., Sokolow R., Mauvais S., Birkness K.A., Skeels M.R., Horan J.M., Foster LR. JAMA, 1997.

[18] Iraq's biological weapons. The past as future? *Zilinskas RA. JAMA. 1997.*

[19] Aum Shinrikyo: once and future threat? *Olson KB. Emerg Infect Dis. 1999.*

[20] India wakes up to threat of bioterrorism. *Sharma R. BMJ. 2001.*

[21] Pneumonic plague, northern India, 2002. *Gupta ML, Sharma A. Emerg Infect Dis. 2007 Apr.*

September and October 2001 reignited biological warfare research and preparedness in U.S.[22]

In October 2001 anthrax scare reached Mumbai, when offices of both chief minister and deputy chief minister received a mail with white powder.[23,24]

On numerous occasions during the past 2000 years, the use of biological agents in the form of disease, filth, and animal and human cadavers has been mentioned in historical recordings. The following table (Table 1) mentions a few of the most known instances apart from the above mentioned that where biological and chemical warfare took place in the past 2000 years.

Table 1: Few Instances of Biological and
Chemical Warfare in the past 2000 years[25]

Time	Event
600 BC	Solon uses the purgative herb hellebore during the siege of Krissa.
1155	Emperor Barbarossa poisons water wells with human bodies in Tortona, Italy.
1346	Tartar forces catapult bodies of plague victims over the city walls of Caffa, Crimean Peninsula (now Feodosia, Ukraine).
1495	Spanish mix wine with blood of leprosy patients to sell to their French foes in Naples, Italy.
1695	German and French forces agree to not use—poisonous bullets.
1710	Russian troops catapult human bodies of plague victims into Swedish cities.
1763	The British distribute blankets from smallpox patients to Native Americans.
1797	Napoleon floods the plains around Mantua, Italy, to enhance the spread of malaria.

---

[22] Collaboration between public health and law enforcement: new paradigms and partnerships for bioterrorism planning and response. *Butler JC, Cohen ML, Friedman CR, Scripp RM, Watz CG. Emerg Infect Dis. 2002.*

[23] Times of India. Anthrax scare reaches Mantralaya via mail. October 25, 2001. http://timesofindia.indiatimes.com/city/mumbai/Anthrax-scare-reaches-Mantralaya-via-mail/articleshow/904876048.cms.

[24] *Ibid. 6.*

[25] http://www.ncbi.nlm.nih.gov

Time	Event
1863	Confederates sell clothing from yellow fever and small pox patients to Union Troops during the US Civil War.
World War I	German and French agents use glanders and anthrax.
World War II	Japan uses plague, anthrax and other diseases; several other countries experiment with and develop biological weapons programmes.
1980–1988	Iraq uses mustard gas, sarin and tabun against Iran and ethnic groups within Iraq during the Persian Gulf War.
1995	Aum Shinrikyo uses sarin gas in Tokyo subway system.

What is a Chemical Weapon? Is it different from a Biological Weapon?

Chemical and Biological Weapons are weapons of mass destruction. An effective attack where a chemical or biological agent was used could easily kill thousands of people.[26]

A chemical weapon can be described as any weapon in which a manufactured chemical is used in order to kill people. The first chemical weapon known to have been used effectively in battle was chlorine gas; it burns and destroys the lung tissues. Chlorine is not a rare chemical; it is used by most municipal water systems today in order to kill bacteria. It is easy to produce chlorine from common table salt. In World War I, the German army is said to have released tons of the gas in order to create a cloud that the wind carried toward the enemy in order to kill the enemies.[27]

Chemical weapons in today's modern times tend to focus on agents with much greater killing power, meaning that it takes a lot lesser amount of the chemical to kill the same number of people as it may have taken in the past. For example, when one sprays their lawn or garden with a chemical to control aphids, they are, in essence, waging a chemical war on aphids.

Humans tend to think of a chemical weapon as a bomb or missile that releases highly toxic chemicals over a city. But in 1995, a group Aum Shinrikyo released sarin gas, which is a nerve gas, in the Tokyo subway. Thousands were wounded due to this incident and 13 people were killed.[28]

---

[26] http://www.ikhsan-plato.blogspot.com

[27] www.nmun.org

[28] www.swts.com

There were no giant bombs or missiles that were involved—the terrorists used small exploding canisters in order to release the gas in the subway.[29]

On the other hand, a bacteria or virus, or in some cases toxins that come directly from bacteria[30] is used in a biological weapon in order to kill people. For Example, if one were to dump a load of manure or human waste into a town's water well, it would be classified a simple form of biological warfare since the human and animal manure contains bacteria that are deadly in a variety of ways if they are consumed by humans.

Thus, we can say that the main difference between Biological Weapons and Chemical Weapons is that in biological weapons[31] pathogens or diseases are used in order to cause destruction, while in chemical weapons any of the variety of ways are used to inflict death by chemical exposure.

Risk Categories of Biological Weapons

Based on the priority of the agents to pose a risk to the National Security and the ease with which they can be disseminated, these biologic agents are classified and labelled as Categories A through C.[32]

Category A agents are the highest priority agents and include organisms that can be disseminated easily or transmitted person-to-person. They have the potential for major public health impact as they can cause high mortality and create public panic and social disruption and require special action for public health preparedness.

Category B agents are the second highest priority agents and include organisms that are moderately easy to disseminate; these agents cause moderate morbidity and low mortality and require specific and enhanced disease surveillance.

Category C agents are the least highest priority agents out of the three[33] and include emerging pathogens that could be engineered for mass dissemination in the future because of availability, ease of production and

---

[29] *Ibid., 6.*

[30] www.mialnmun.it

[31] www.gambassa.com

[32] Biological and chemical terrorism: strategic plan for preparedness and response. Recommendations of the CDC Strategic Planning Workgroup. *MMWR Recomm Rep. 2000.*

[33] www.scribd.com

dissemination and have the potential for high morbidity and mortality and can cause major health impact.[34]

The following is a table (Table 2) which mentions a few biological agents that come under the above mentioned categories and the diseases cause by a few of the agents.

Table 2: Critical Biologic Agent List

Biological Agents	Disease
Category A	
Variola Major	Smallpox
B Anthracis	Anthrax
Y Pestis	Plague
Clostridium Botulinum (Botilinum Toxins)	Botulism
Francisella Tularensis	Tularemia
Filovirus (Marburg and Ebola)	Viral Haemorrhagic Fevers
Arenavirus (Lassa, Argentine/Junin)	Viral Haemorrhagic Fevers
Category B	
Coxeilla Burnetti	Q Fever
Brucella Spp.	Brucellosis
Burkholderia Mallei	Glanders
B. Pseodomallei	Melioidosis
Alphaviruses Venezuela Equine Encephalitis Eastern Equine Encephalitis Western Equine Encephalitis	Encephalitis
Rickettsia Prowaekki	Typhus Fever
Toxins	Toxic Syndromes
Chlamydia Psittaci	Psittacosis
Category C	
Emerging Pathogens (Nipah Virus, Hantavirus, tick-borne encephalitics virus, tick-borne haemorrhagic fever virus, yellow fever, multi drug resistant tuberculosis, etc.)	

---

[34] http://link.springer.com

The Effects of Biological Weapons

After defining the biological weapons and mention some of its example. Knowing the damage that occurs because of biological weapons and their impact on the environment and living organisms around us and to humans is very important. There are many negative effects of Biological Weapons on our life.

It can change the disease that meant only to kill and injure humans as genetic strands of DNA can mutate it might changes into another thing that could effect and kill other living species like animals and plants. This means that Biological Weapons have a longer and lasting effect on us, much longer than the length of the conflict, effects so grave that some Biological Weapons pose a threat to the future generations. The genetic mutation can manifest itself in many different forms. New born babies will go through prematurity because of the genetic mutation; also the number new born babies with birth defects will increase. It is also known that a person will become susceptible to many different forms of diseases which will weaken their immune system.

In addition to this another disadvantage is that some of the biological agents last for really long time, studies show that anthrax can live up to 50 years in soil.

A biological weapon does not have any one specific target but it has the power to affect people, animals and plants within its impact radius making it hard to control the damage caused.[35]

The Economic Effects of Biological Weapons

The outbreak of Foot - Mouth Disease (FMD) in Britain demonstrates that even countries with a well-organized and technologically sophisticated veterinary services infrastructure are susceptible to introduction of highly infectious pathogenic agents into their livestock populations. The economic consequences of a disease epidemic affecting livestock are severe for any country, whether industrialized or developing. For example, the total costs of containment and eradication of the 1997 FMD outbreak in Taiwan approached $15 billion. Direct and indirect losses to the British economy associated with the 2001 FMD outbreak are expected to be $12 billion to

---

[35] http://www.ukessays.com

$14 billion.[36] Losses in meat and livestock export revenue amounted to approximately $14 million per week. Estimated losses to the tourism industry because of restrictions on travel in affected areas were estimated at around $350 million per week in March 2001, or 25 times (2,500%) higher than concurrent direct losses in the agricultural export sector. Total economic losses to the national tourism industry during the peak of the FMD epidemic in March 2001 were estimated at more than $4 billion and are still rising.[37] The potential for catastrophic social and economic consequences from biological weapon disease epidemics is proportionally higher in developing countries, where doctors, veterinarians, antibiotics, and medical or veterinarian treatment and quarantine facilities are in short supply.

Technical and logistical capabilities for countering the impacts of disease threats from bioweapons and emerging infectious diseases may be handicapped by the on-going proliferation of drug-resistant disease strains of important diseases such as tuberculosis (*Mycobacterium tuberculosis*) and malaria (*Plasmodium* spp.). Improper use and inappropriate uses of antibiotics to suppress diseases and infections in both humans and animals are contributing to the emergence of drug-resistant strains of many important human and animal pathogens. The current widespread use of antibiotics in livestock feeds, now banned only in the European Union, may have serious epidemiological consequences.[38] Nearly half of all antibiotics used in the United States are dispensed in animal feeds, despite growing scientific concern over.

Incomplete treatment regimens, inappropriate clinical applications, adulterated medicines, and both inadvertent and deliberate sub-therapeutic uses of antibiotics are resulting in the evolution—through human selection—of highly resistant and highly virulent strains of disease organisms. In effect, the current situation represents an ongoing, essentially

---

[36] Office International des Epizooties. 2001. Biological agents as potential weapons against animals. *Biological Warfare Technical Brief, November 2001 draft*. Geneva: World Health Organization Office.

[37] Dudley J.P. and Woodford M.H. (2002). Bioweapons, bioterrorism, and biodiversity: The potential impacts of biological weapons attacks on agricultural and biological diversity. *Science and Technical Review.*

[38] McDonald L.C. (2001). Quinupristin-dalfopristin-resistant *Enterococcus faecium* on chicken and in human stool specimens. *New England Journal of Medicine.*

uncontrolled field experiment in the cultivation and proliferation of antibiotic-resistant microbe populations. This problem may well be aggravated by fear of exposure to bioterrorist attacks—witness the panic-inspired purchases and consumption of antibiotics by American citizens after the anthrax attacks during September and November 2001. Subsequent events proved that such concerns were not entirely unwarranted—5 of the 21 people known to have contracted anthrax as the result of exposure to contaminated mail subsequently died as the result of undiagnosed or tardily diagnosed pulmonary anthrax infection.[39]

Global Legislative Preparedness against Biologic Disasters

The Geneva Protocol signed in 1925 is a customary International Law that prohibits the use of asphyxiating, poisonous or other gases and of bacteriological methods of warfare. Biological and toxin weapons convention of 1972 was the first multilateral disarmament treaty signed by about 170 countries that forbids Nations from developing, producing, stockpiling or otherwise acquiring biological agents or toxins that have no justification for peaceful or defensive purposes. In 2001, Model

State Emergency Health Powers Act (MSEHPA or Model Act) was drafted to help America's State Legislatures in revising their public health laws to control epidemics and respond to bioterrorism.[40] USA PATRIOT Act was also signed into law in 2001. The title of the act USA PATRIOT stands for Uniting and Strengthening America by providing appropriate tools required to Intercept and Obstruct Terrorism Act of 2001.[41] A new federal law—Public Health Security and Bioterrorism Preparedness and response Act was passed in US in 2002.[42] This Act deals with Nation's preparedness for bioterrorism and other public health emergencies, by enhancing controls on dangerous biological agents and toxins, protecting safety and security of food and water supply, the prompt approval of safe and effective

---

[39] http://bioscience.oxfordjournals.org

[40] The Model State Emergency Health Powers Act: planning for and response to bioterrorism and naturally occurring infectious diseases. *JAMA. 2002 Aug 7; 288(5):622–8.*

[41] Effects of the USA PATRIOT Act and the 2002 Bioterrorism Preparedness Act on select agent research in the United States. *Proc Natl Acad Sci U S A. 2010 May 25; 107(21): 9556-61.*

[42] U.S. Food and Drug Administration. Bioterrorism Act of 2002.

new drugs that are critical to the improvement of the public health and the review of human drug applications and the assurance of drug safety. In 2004, US Congress passed the Project Bio shield Act, which funds the government to purchase and stockpile new vaccines and drugs to fight anthrax, smallpox and other potential agents of bioterrorism.[43] The Indian National Crisis Management Committee approved a model of standard operating procedures for preventing and responding to a bioterrorism attack in March 2007. According to this model, the Ministry of Home Affairs (MHA) is in charge of coordinating command, control and preparedness measures as well as post-attack response mechanisms, but primary responsibility for responding to attacks lies with the State Governments.

Strict legal and regulatory laws dealing with quarantine and jurisdictional concerns must be framed and implemented at an International Level to restrain catastrophic bioterrorist attacks and penalize the Nations and terrorist groups with illicit intentions.[44]

Biological Weapons Convention

During the late 1960s, public and expert concerns were raised Internationally regarding the indiscriminate nature of, unpredictability of, epidemiologic risks of, and the lack of epidemiologic control measures for biological weapons.[45] In addition, more information on various nations' biological weapons programs became evident, and it was obvious that the 1925 Geneva Protocol was ineffective in controlling the proliferation of biological[46] weapons.[47]

---

[43] Project BioShield: what it is, why it is needed, and its accomplishments so far. *Russell PK. Clin Infect Dis. 2007.*

[44] *Ibid.,* 6.

[45] Stockholm International Peace Research Institute (SIPRI) The Problem of Chemical and Biological Warfare, Vol. 1. The Rise of CB Weapons. New York.

[46] http://www.baylorhealth.edu

[47] US Arms Control and Disarmament Agency. Arms Control and Disarmament Agreements: Texts and Histories of the Negotiations. Washington, DC: US Arms Control and Disarmament Agency; 1996.

In July 1969, Great Britain submitted a proposal to the UN Committee on Disarmament outlining the need to prohibit the development, production, and stockpiling of biological weapons.[48]

Furthermore, the proposal provided for measures for control and inspections, as well as procedures to be followed in case of violation. Shortly after submission of the British proposal, in September 1969, the Warsaw Pact nations under the lead of the Soviet Union submitted a similar proposal to the United Nations (UN).

However, this proposal lacked provisions for inspections. Two months later, in November 1969, a report regarding the possible consequences of the use of biological warfare agents was issued by the World Health Organization.[49]

Following the above mentioned report in 1972 the "Convention on the Prohibition of the Development, Production, and Stockpiling of Bacteriological (Biological) and Toxin Weapons and on Their Destruction," was developed and is now popularly known as the BWC.

This Biological Weapons Convention (BWC) was introduced as a legally binding treaty that outlaws biological arms. After being discussed and negotiated in the United Nations' disarmament forum starting in 1969, the BWC opened was for signature on April 10, 1972, and was enforced on March 26, 1975. The BWC currently has including Palestine, and four signatories (Egypt, Haiti, Somalia, Syria, and Tanzania). Ten states have neither signed nor ratified the BWC, these states being Chad, Comoros, Djibouti, Eritrea, Israel, Kiribati, Micronesia, Namibia, South Sudan and Tuvalu.[50]

The BWC is a multilateral treaty which is of indefinite duration and is open to any country.[51]

This treaty regime mandates that all states-parties need to consult with one another and cooperate, bilaterally or multilaterally, to solve compliance

---

[48] Stockholm International Peace Research Institute (SIPRI) The Problem of Chemical and Biological Warfare, Vol. 4: CB Disarmament Negotiations, 1920–1970. New York: Humanities Press; 1971.

[49] http://www.pubmedcentral.nih.gov

[50] https://www.armscontrol.org

[51] armscontrol.org

concerns. The regime also allows states-parties to lodge a complaint with the United Nations Security Council (UNSC) if they believe other member states are violating this convention. The UNSC has the power to investigate the complaints, but this power has never been invoked till now.[52] The UNSC voting rules give China, France, Russia, the United Kingdom, and the United States veto power over the decisions of the UNSC, including the ones relating to the conduct investigations under BWC.

Under the BWC the following are the bans that are implemented on the member states that have ratified the Convention; the Convention firstly bans the development, stockpiling, acquisition, retention, and production of biological agents and toxins that come under the type and under the quantities that have no justification[53] for prophylactic, protective or other peaceful purposes and weapons, equipment, and delivery vehicles that are designed with the intention to use such agents or toxins for hostile purposes or during armed conflict. Secondly, it bans the transfer of or offering assistance in acquiring the agents, toxins, weapons, equipment, and delivery vehicles.

Under this Convention it is further required that the states-parties destroy or divert to peaceful purposes the "agents, toxins, weapons, equipment, and means of delivery" described above within nine months of the convention's entry into force if the state parties had possession of any such agents. The BWC did not ban the use of biological and toxin weapons but after reaffirmation in the 1925 Geneva Protocol, such uses were prohibits. This Convention does not ban bio-defense programs that may be undertaken by the member states.

The States-parties/ member states had convened a review conference was to take place every five years in order to review upon and improve the implementation of this treaty. The following are the finding and improved implementations that took place after every review conference that has taken place since the Convention came into being:

---

[52] https://www.reachingcriticalwill.org

[53] www.howardnema.com

Second Review Conference

The second BWC review conference took place in 1986, in this review conference the member states agreed to implement a set of confidence-building measures as an effort to enhance the confidence of the member states as well as promote cooperation among the member states.

After the review conference took place it was observed that the member states should undertake these politically binding measure:

- Exchange data relating to high-containment research centers and laboratories or on centers and laboratories that specialize in permitted biological activities that are relating to the convention.
- Exchange information in-case an abnormal outbreaks of infectious diseases takes place.
- Encourage the publication of biological research results related to the BWC and promote the use of knowledge gained from this research in order to spread more information regarding it.
- Promote scientific contact on biological research that relate to the convention.

Third Review Conference

The third BWC review conference took place in 1991. In this review conference the scope of the first measure of the Convention was expanded to include national biological defense programs and the second and fourth measures were slightly modified as well. In addition to this, the following three measures were also added to this list:

- The member states shall declare legislation, regulations, and introduce "other measures" pertaining to the BWC.
- The member states shall declare any offensive or defensive biological research and development programs in existence in their states since January 1, 1946.
- The member states shall introduce vaccine production facilities.

These endeavors had been largely unsuccessful since a vast majority of member states had consistently failed to submit declarations on their activities and facilities relating to biological offence and biological defense in their possession.

The 1991 review conference appointed a group of "governmental experts" to evaluate the potential verification measures for use in a future compliance protocol to the BWC. This group subsequently considered 21 such measures and submitted a report to a special conference of states-parties which was held in 1994. Building off of this report, the conference tasked a second body, known as the Ad Hoc Group, with the power of a legally binding protocol to the BWC in order to strengthen the convention.

Ad Hoc Group

The meetings of the Ad Hoc Group took place between January 1995 and July 2001. The aim of this Ad Hoc Group was to finish its work before the fifth review conference, which was to begin in November 2001. During the course of the negotiations, the Ad Hoc Group developed a protocol that envisioned states submitting to an international regulatory body declaration of treaty-relevant facilities and activities. This regulatory body would have the power and authority to conduct routine on-site visits in to facilities declared by the member states and also has the power to conduct inspections of suspected facilities and activities as well.

However, in regards to the above mentioned suggestions a number of fundamental issues proves difficult to resolve, the scope of on-site visits and the role these regulatory body shall in the regime was on such issue. In March 2001, a draft of the protocol was submitted by the Ad Hoc Group's chairman. This draft contained language which attempted to strike a compromise on disputed issues. However, in July 2001, during the Ad Hoc Group's last scheduled meeting, the United States rejected the draft and any further protocol negotiations, claiming that such a protocol could not help strengthen compliance with the BWC and could hamper the interests of the U.S. national security and commercial.[54]

Fifth Review Conference

The fifth BWC review conference was the one that many experts thought could resolve the fate of the Ad Hoc Group. The fifth review conference was suspended on its last day, December 7, 2001, after the United States tabled a controversial proposal to terminate the Ad Hoc Group's mandate and replace it with annual meetings of the member states to the BWC. The

---

[54] asipss.com

United States was the only country that favored the revocation of the group's mandate. The fifth review conference was resumed by the member states in November 2002, but the member states failed to agree on any verification measures, including the proposed protocol by the Ad Hoc Group.

Sixth Review Conference

The meetings for the sixth BWC review conference took place between November 20, 2006 and December 8, 2006. The sixth review conference was the first successful review conference to have been conducted since 1996, an agreement on a final document was reached on.

This conference produced a list of four work programs to be held each successive year until the next review conference in 2011.

Like every other agreement ever made some issues were brought up. Some of these issues that enjoyed broad-based support did not make it into the work program. The proposals to reform confidence-building measures on the basis of the participation of the member stated where the existing mechanisms are poor, was strongly opposed by the United States and Russia. The primary factor behind bio-terrorism being dropped from the list of agenda items during the conference was Russia.

The member states agreed to address the BWC's institutional deficit through the creation of the Implementation Support Unit (ISU), which is staffed by three permanent employees based in Geneva making it a permanent body. The permanent staff members were to be paid by the BWC and were housed in the UN Department of Disarmament Affairs in Geneva. Prior to this, the BWC review conference was only supported on a part-time basis.

The ISU's mandate was introduced with the aim of providing administrative support for the BWC as well as facilitating confidence-building measures between the member states to the Convention. The ISU, among other things, served the responsibility to ease communication between the member states, as well as compile and disseminate confidence-building measures submitted from member states.

After the sixth review conference was concluded in 2006 the ISU has strengthened in terms of budget and staff. Despite the initial opposition from U.S.A., a proposal made by the European Union (EU) to allow states parties to make additional, voluntary contributions to the ISU was accepted during the 2007 annual meeting. The United States originally objected to the proposal on the grounds that it would increase the responsibility of the ISU. This problem was resolved through a statement stressing that the ISU has only three staff members, and any contributions are only designed to assist the ISU in completing its mandate. During the 2008 annual meeting of the member states, a $2 million dollar donation was made to the ISU by the European Union in order to pay for two additional staff members for the following two years.

Seventh Review Conference

The seventh BWC review conference took place in December 2011. The Final Declaration of the seventh review conference document concluded that —under all circumstances the use of bacteriological (biological) and toxin weapons is effectively prohibited by the Convention and affirms the determination of States parties to condemn any use of biological agents or toxins other than for peaceful purposes, by anyone at any time."[55]

Eighth Review Conference

The eighth BWC review conference took place in November 2016. At the end of the conference, delegates agreed to a future one-week meeting of states-parties at the end of the year and a five-year extension of the BWC Implementation Support Unit.[56]

Has Non-Compliance to BWC Taken Place?

Due to difficulty in verifying the compliance, many concerns about the violation of BWC prohibitions have persisted throughout the Convention's history. At several review conference Member States have openly accused other Nations of non-compliance to the convention. During the Third

---

[55] Seventh Review Conference of the States Parties to the Convention on the Prohibition of the Development, Production and Stockpiling of Bacteriological (Biological) and Toxin Weapons and on Their Destruction; https://www.unog.ch/80256EDD006 B8954/(httpAssets)/E7D8D6E2C5258849C1257B6E0033A1D3/$file/BWC_CON F.VII_07.pdf

[56] https://www.armscontrol.org

Review Conference which happened in 1991, Australia, the United Kingdom, and the United States brought forth accusations that the Soviet Union had developed biological weapons. Similarly, during the first session of the Fifth Review Conference which took place in 2001, the United States made allegations against four States Parties, i.e. Iraq, Iran, North Korea, and Libya. The allegations were a few high-profile cases where the abovementioned four states had developed biological weapons even though ratification of the BWC had been done by all four states.

THE SOVIET UNION

The Soviet Union can be taken as the most striking example of noncompliance to the BWC; it is known to have had operated a massive biological weapons program, despite its status as a BWC State Party, since 1972. The Soviet Union is said to have begun its biological weapons program in 1928 under the Red Army. In the early 1970s, around the time when the BWC was concluded and signed by the Soviet Union and other Member States, the leaders of the Soviet decided to expand its program substantially by exploiting advances in science and technology, conducting further research, and creating infrastructure to produce biological weapons. These activities were organized under an institution which was established in 1973 and was called *Biopreparat*, This Institution served as a civilian cover for military research. This program involved hundreds of facilities employing as many as 60,000 people, and had a large budget of hundreds of billions of rubles. The Soviet program succeeded in weaponizing a number of dangerous pathogens, including those which cause smallpox, plague, tularemia, glanders, Venezuelan equine encephalitis, anthrax, Q fever, and Marburg fever. Furthermore, it did research on other highly dangerous viruses such as the Ebola and yellow fever viruses.

Although, the West suspected that the Soviet Union was not in compliance with the BWC, they were not aware of the details of *Biopreparat* and its work. The suspicions of many other nations were heightened after a strange outbreak of disease took place in 1979 in the Soviet Union's city of Sverdlovsk, where approximately 70 people were infected with anthrax, many of who were fatally affected. The Soviets claimed the incident was due to tainted meat. The reality had however had been that there had been an accident at a nearby military microbiology facility which resulted in the escape of anthrax spores that drifted downwind through the town.

The allegations of Soviet non-compliance persisted throughout the Cold War, with the Soviets repeatedly denying that they were violating their commitments under the BWC. Shortly after the dissolution of the Soviet Union, the Russian President Boris Yeltsin admitted in a speech telecasted on the televisions that the allegations against the Soviet Union of non-compliance to the BWC were true. In April, 1992, Yeltsin issued a presidential decree which outlawed any activities within the Russian Federation that were not in accordance with the Convention.

Although, after the issuance of the Presidential Decree by Yeltsin under which a promise to end the funding for any biological weapons research, the concerns relating to Russia's compliance to the BWC still remained. Therefore, the United States, the United Kingdom, and Russia agreed to begin a trilateral process that would help to alleviate suspicions and build confidence. One aspect of the trilateral process was a series of visits to non-military facilities in each of the three countries. Site visits were conducted in all three countries, but failed to alleviate concerns. There were plans to extend the visits to military facilities, but these never materialized due to the differences. The trilateral process came to a halt in 1994 and no visits have taken place since. The concerns relating to Russia's activities in its military biological laboratories continue and its compliance to the BWC still remains in question.

IRAQ

Iraq's non-compliance to the BWC is well documented due to an international process that was established following the Persian Gulf War in 1991. UN Security Council Resolution 687 signified the conclusion of the war and initiated an important disarmament process. According to this resolution Iraq was required to declare all of its weapons of mass destruction and ordered that they be destructed. The United Nations Security Council (UNSC) established a special body called the UNSCOM, the main roll of the UNSCOM was to carry out inspections of Iraq's chemical, biological, and missile capabilities and to provide for their destruction. UNSCOM worked on this from 1991 to 1998, uncovering Iraq's BW program, some of which dated back to the early 1970s.

It is now known that Iraq's biological weapons program produced botulinum toxin, anthrax bacteria, aflatoxin, ricin, and wheat cover smut fungus, and initiated a program on several viral agents. To deliver the weaponized agents, Iraq produced bombs, missile warheads, aerosol generators, and spray systems. It also came to knowledge that Iraq imported Western technology and many of its researchers acquired their knowledge in Western countries. Iraq is said to have spent an estimated $200 million on its programs.

Iraq ratified the BWC in 1991 as a condition of the cease-fire agreement ending the Persian Gulf War. Although, Iraq claims to have ended its biological weapons program in 1991, it is still widely believed that Iraq maintained the program throughout the 1990s. These beliefs are supported by Iraqi efforts to try to conceal its program from UNSCOM inspectors while the inspection was underway. In 1998, Iraq suspended cooperation with UNSCOM that left many issues unresolved. The UNSCOM was disbanded and replaced with the UN Monitoring, Verification and Inspection Commission (UNMOVIC). In 2002, the United States and United Kingdom released detailed reports about Iraqi non-compliance, charging that Iraq is using dual-use facilities and mobile laboratories to continue its work on biological weapons. On November 8, 2002 the UN Security Council adopted resolution 1441 required that Iraq grant unrestricted access to UNMOVIC inspectors. The inspections resumed again from November 27.

OTHER STATES

In contrast to the biological weapons programs of the Soviet Union and Iraq, only limited information is available on other BWC States Parties that have been suspected of being in non-compliance to it, including South Africa. It is believed that South Africa has had a smaller scale program. Although no allegations of non-compliance have ever made against South Africa, recent research suggested that some government officials had been involved in illegal activities. Much of what is now known has been learned from the work of the South African Truth and Reconciliation Commission (TRC) as part of their effort to reconcile with South Africa's apartheid past.

South Africa began its program in 1981 under the apartheid regime, under the auspices of the South African Defence Force. South Africa had signed the BWC in 1972. Documentary and testimonial evidence have shown that the program was both defensive and offensive in nature and was carried out both for external (regional security) and internal purposes (domestic opposition). Although the program is thought to have involved anthrax and cholera, it is also believed that the program also included work with other agents, including plague, salmonella, and botulinum toxin. The program also included also a fertility project, aimed at producing contraceptives that could be administered to women without their knowledge. The program ended in 1993 under considerable pressure from the U.S., UK, and others, around the time of a regime change.

Several other States Parties to the BWC have been accused by other states or have been under suspicion of conducting research, developing, and/or producing biological weapons. These allegations have been made in a variety of settings, including formal meetings of States Parties (review conferences), public speeches, and reports published by the accusing country or non-governmental entities. Because of the lack of publicly available evidence, it is difficult to determine the true extent of activities and whether they cross the line from being legitimate defensive programs to violations of the Convention. However, it is certain that the history of non-compliance and the real possibility that prohibited activities are continuing are perhaps the most significant threats to the BWC.[57]

CONCLUSION

Biological weapons are unique because of their invisibility and their delayed effects. These factors allow those who use them to inculcate fear and cause confusion among their victims and help them to escape undetected. A Biological Warfare attack does not only cause sickness and death in a large numbers but it also aims to create fear, panic, and paralyzing uncertainty in the society. The main goal of using Biological Weapons is to cause disruption of social and economic activities, the breakdown of government authority, and the impairment of military responses. As demonstrated by the—anthrax letters in the aftermath of the World Trade Centre attack in September 2001, the occurrence of only a small number of infections created an enormous psychological impact and everyone felt threatened and nobody knew what would happen next.

---

[57] www.nti.org

The choice of the Biological Warfare agent depends on the economic, technical, and financial capabilities of the state or organization that produces the Weapon. Viruses such as Smallpox, Ebola, and Marburg virus may be chosen because they have a reputation for causing a more horrifying illness. Images on the nightly news of doctors, nurses, and law enforcement personnel in full protective gear have the power to cause widespread public distraction and anxiety.

Biological Warfare attacks are now a common possibility seeing the progress nations are making across the World. The medical community as well as the public needs to become familiar with epidemiology and control measures in order to increase the likelihood of a calm and reasoned response if an outbreak should occur. In fact, the principles that help clinicians develop strategies against diseases are relevant as the medical community considers the problem of biological weapons proliferation. For the medical community, further timely education focusing on recognition of this threat is necessary as they are a few of the people who fight the outbreaks in the frontlines.

To combat a bioterrorism attack focus should be laid on developing full international cooperation amongst nations for dealing with this problem since formal international scientific collaborations will need to be created and international laws against use of biological weapons will have to be framed. Response against any bioterrorist event will necessitate co-ordinated efforts of public health departments (surveillance, laboratory response network, alertness of medical and paramedical faculties) and administrative systems including intelligence agencies, army, law enforcement machinery and civil administration for protecting the public and promoting its welfare. From the perspective of medical and public health communities the challenges to be faced include comprehensive detection and assessment, mass casualty management and implementation of preventive, curative and specific control measures for containing the further spread of the disease. Oral and maxillofacial surgeons can contribute to terrorism response plans and complement the medical fraternity in overcoming the overt catastrophic incident. They should be trained mandatorily in a core set of competencies that will enable them to respond to a significant bioterrorism attack by helping to contain the spread of the attack and participating in surveillance activities as appropriate upon direction of proper authorities.

REFERENCES

[1] Eitzen E.M., Jr and Takafuji, E.T. Historical overview of biological warfare. In: Sidell FR, Takafuji E.T., Franz D.R., editors. Medical Aspects of Chemical and Biological Warfare. Washington, DC: Office of the Surgeon General, Borden Institute, Walter Reed Army Medical Center; 1997. pp. 415–423. Available at http://www.bordeninstitute.army.mil/cwbw/default_index.htm; accessed July 6, 2004. [Google Scholar]

[2] Robertson, A.G. and Robertson, L.J. From asps to allegations: biological warfare in history. Mil Med. 1995; 160:369–373. [PubMed] [Google Scholar]

[3] Wheelis, M., Biological warfare at the 1346 siege of Caffa. Emerg Infect Dis. 2002; 8:971–975. [PMC free article] [PubMed] [Google Scholar]

[4] Norris J. East or west? The geographic origin of the Black Death. Bull Hist Med. 1977; 51:1–24. [PubMed] [Google Scholar]

[5] Henschel, A.W. Dokument für Geschichte des schwarzen Todes. Archives fur die gesammte Median, 1842; 2:26–59. [Google Scholar]

[6] Derbes, V.J., De Mussis and the great plague of 1348. A forgotten episode of bacteriological warfare. JAMA. 1966; 196: 59–62. [PubMed] [Google Scholar]

[7] Christopher, G.W., Cieslak, T.J., Pavlin, J.A. and Eitzen, E.M., Biological warfare. A historical perspective. JAMA. 1997; 278: 412–417. [PubMed] [Google Scholar]

[8] Henderson, D.A., Inglesby, T.V., Bartlett, J.G., Ascher, M.S., Eitzen, E., Jahrling, P.B., Hauer, J., Layton, M., McDade, J., Osterholm, M.T., O'Toole, T., Parker, G., Perl, T., Russell, P.K., Tonat, K. Smallpox as a biological weapon: medical and public health management. Working Group on Civilian Biodefense. JAMA. 1999; 281: 2127–2137. [PubMed] [Google Scholar]

[9] Sipe, C.H., The Indian Wars of Pennsylvania. Harrisburg, PA: Telegraph Press; 1929. [Google Scholar]

[10] Hugh-Jones, M. Wickham Steed and German biological warfare research. Intelligence and National Security. 1992; 7:379–402. [Google Scholar]

[11] Stockholm International Peace Research Institute (SIPRI) The Problem of Chemical and Biological Warfare, Vol. I: The Rise of CB Weapons. New York: Humanities Press; 1971. [Google Scholar]

[12] Kadlec, R.P., Zelicoff, A.P. and Vrtis, A.M. Biological weapons control. Prospects and implications for the future. JAMA. 1997; 278: 351–356. [PubMed] [Google Scholar]

[13] US Arms Control and Disarmament Agency. Arms Control and Disarmament Agreements: Texts and Histories of the Negotiations. Washington, DC: US Arms Control and Disarmament Agency; 1996. [Google Scholar]

[14] Harris, S.H., Factories of Death. New York: Routledge; 1994. [Google Scholar]

[15] Mitscherlich, A., Mielke, F. Medizin ohne Menschlichkeit: Dokumente des Nürnberger ärzteprozesses. Frankfurt am Main, Germany: Fischer Taschen-buchverlag; 1983. [Google Scholar]

[16] Harris, S., Japanese biological warfare research on humans: A case study of microbiology and ethics. Ann, NY Acad Sci. 1992; 666:21–52. [PubMed] [Google Scholar]

[17] Manchee, R.J. and Stewart, R., The decontamination of Gruinard Island. *Chem Br.,* 1988; 24:690–691. [Google Scholar]

[18] Poupard, J.A. and Miller, L.A. History of biological warfare: Catapults to capsomeres. *Ann NY Acad Sci.,* 1992; 666:9–20. [PubMed] [Google Scholar]

[19] US Department of the Army. US Army Activity in the US Biological Warfare Programs. Washington, DC: US Department of the Army; 1977. Publication DTIC B193427 L. [Google Scholar]

[20] Yu, V.L. Serratia marcescens: historical perspective and clinical review. N Engl J Med. 979; 300:887–893. [PubMed] [Google Scholar]

[21] Carter, G.B. Biological warfare and biological defence in the United Kingdom 1940–1979. Royal United Service Institute Journal. 1992; 137:67–74. [Google Scholar]

[22] Stockholm International Peace Research Institute (SIPRI). The Problem of Chemical and Biological Warfare, Vol. 4: CB Disarmament Negotiations, 1920–1970. New York: Humanities Press; 1971. [Google Scholar]

[23] WHO Group of Consultants. Health Aspects of Chemical and Biological Weapons. Geneva, Switzerland: World Health Organization; 1970. [Google Scholar]

[24] Stockholm International Peace Research Institute (SIPRI). The Problem of Chemical and Biological Warfare, Vol. 3: CBW and the Law of War. New York: Humanities Press; 1973. [Google Scholar]

[25] Stockholm International Peace Research Institute (SIPRI). The Problem of Chemical and Biological Warfare, Vol. 5: Technical Aspects of Early Warning and Verification. New York: Humanities Press; 1971. [Google Scholar]

[26] US Army Medical Research Institute for Infectious Diseases. Medical Management of Biological Casualties Handbook. 4th ed. Frederick, MD: Fort Detrick; 2001. [Google Scholar]

[27] Meselson, M., Guillemin, J, Hugh-Jones, M., Langmuir, A., Popova, I., Shelokov, A., Yampolskaya, O. The Sverdlovsk anthrax outbreak of 1979. Science. 1994; 266:1202–1208. [PubMed] [Google Scholar]

[28] Caudle, L.C., III. The biological warfare threat. In: Sidell FR, Takafuji ET, Franz DR, editors. Medical Aspects of Chemical and Biological Warfare. Washington, DC: Office of the Surgeon General, Borden Institute, Walter Reed Army Medical Center; 1997. pp. 451–466. Available at http://www.bordeninstitute.army.mil/cwbw/default_index.htm; accessed July 6, 2004. [Google Scholar]

[29] Abramova, F.A., Grinberg, L.M., Yampolskaya, O.V. and Walker, D.H., Pathology of inhalational anthrax in 42 cases from the Sverdlovsk outbreak of 1979. *Proc. Natl Acad Sci.,* USA. 1993; 90:2291–2314. [PMC free article] [PubMed] [Google Scholar]

[30] Zilinskas, R.A. Iraq's biological weapons. The past as future? JAMA. 1997; 278:418–424. [PubMed] [Google Scholar]

[31] Ashford, D.A., Kaiser, R.M., Bales, M.E., Shutt, K., Patrawalla, A., McShan, A., *et al.* Planning against biological terrorism: lessons from outbreak investigations. Emerg Infect Dis. 2003; 9(5):515–519. doi: 10.3201/eid0905.020388. [PMC free article] [PubMed] [CrossRef] [Google Scholar]

[32] Chaudhry R. Botulism: A diagnostic challenge. *Indian J. Med Res.*, 2011; 134(1):10–12. [PMC free article] [PubMed] [Google Scholar]

[33] Anderson, P.D., Bioterrorism: toxins as weapons. J. Pharm Pract., 2012; 25(2):121–129, doi: 10.1177/0897190012442351. [PubMed] [CrossRef] [Google Scholar]

[34] Nair, P. QnAs with Vern L. Schramm. Proc Natl Acad Sci USA. 2011; 108(10):3829. doi: 10.1073/pnas.1101040108. [PMC free article] [PubMed] [CrossRef] [Google Scholar]

[35] Roxas-Duncan, VI and Smith, L.A. (2012). Of beans and beads: ricin and abrin in bioterrorism and biocrime. J Bioterr Biodef S2:002. http://www.omicsonline. org/of-beans-and-beads-ricin-and-abrin-in-bioterrorism-and-biocrime-2157-2526.S2-002.php?aid=4686%3faid=4686. Accessed, 23 Nov. 2014.

[36] Christopher, G.N., Cieslak, T.J., Pavlin, J.A., Eitzen, E.M., Jr Biological warfare: a historical perspective. JAMA. 1997; 278:412–417. doi: 10.1001/jama.1997.03550050074036. [PubMed] [CrossRef] [Google Scholar]

[37] Torok, T.J., Tauxe, R.V., Wise, R.P., Livengood, J.R., Sokolow, R., Mauvais, S., Birkness, K.A., Skeels, M.R., Horan, J.M. and Foster, L.R. A large community outbreak of salmonellosis caused by intentional contamination of restaurant salad bars. JAMA. 1997; 278:389–doi: 10.1001/jama.1997. 03550050051033. [PubMed] [CrossRef] [Google Scholar]

[38] Zalinskas, R.A. Iraq's biological weapons: the past as future? JAMA. 1997; 278:418–424. doi: 10.1001/jama.1997.03550050080037. [PubMed] [Cross Ref] [Google Scholar]

[39] Olson, K.B., Aum Shinrikyo: Once and future threat? Emerg Infect Dis. 1999; 5(4):513–516. doi: 10.3201/eid0504.990409. [PMC free article] [PubMed] [CrossRef] [Google Scholar]

[40] Sharma, R. India wakes up to threat of bioterrorism. BMJ. 2001; 323:714. doi: 10.1136/bmj.323.7315.714a. [PMC free article] [PubMed] [CrossRef] [Google Scholar]

[41] Gupta, M.L. and Sharma, A. Pneumonic plague, Northern India. Emerg Infect Dis. 2002; 13(4):664–666. doi: 10.3201/eid1304.051105. [PMC free article] [PubMed] [CrossRef] [Google Scholar]

[43] Butler, J.C., Cohen, M.L., Friedman, C.R., Scripp, R.M. and Watz, C.G. Collaboration between public health and law enforcement: new paradigms and partnerships for bioterrorism planning and response. Emerg Infect Dis. 2002; 8(10):1152–1156. doi: 10.3201/eid0810.020400. [PMC free article] [PubMed] [CrossRef] [Google Scholar]

[44] es.scribd.com

[45] Times of India. Anthrax scare reaches Mantralaya via mail. October 25, 2001. http://timesofindia.indiatimes.com/city/mumbai/Anthrax-scare-reaches-Mantralaya-via-mail/articleshow/904876048.cms. Accessed 23 Nov 2014

[46] Centers for disease control and prevention. Biological and chemical terrorism: strategic plan for preparedness and response. MMWR Recomm Rep 2000; 49 (No. RR-4):1–14 [PubMed]

[47] www.ncbi.nlm.nih.gov

[48] link.springer.com

Author Index